GET EX ☑ W9-BRW-718

You are on the threshold of discovering
that living healthfully is not
an art that we must learn, but simply
an instinctive way of life
to which we can return.

FOOD—Enjoy irresistible menus that keep
you young and help you get in shape.
WATER—Find out what is in your tap water
and what is the best water for your body.
AIR—Learn how to breathe so you will feel
less stress in your life.
SLEEP—Discover how to sleep deeply and
restfully *every night* and why naps keep you
young and healthy.
SUNSHINE—Get the most nutrients you can
from the sun without harming your skin.
EXERCISE—Feel more fit with an easy,
stress-free program for all ages that gives you
a workout *every day*.
LOVING RELATIONSHIPS—Let age-old
strategies increase the love in your life, make
sex more fulfilling, and enhance your spiritual
growth.

THE DIAMONDS HAVE ALREADY TRANSFORMED THE
LIVES OF MILLIONS OF READERS THROUGH *FIT FOR
LIFE*, THE #1 DIET BOOK OF ALL TIME, AND *FIT FOR
LIFE II: LIVING HEALTH*. PLEASE TURN THIS PAGE TO
FIND OUT WHAT JUST A FEW OF THEM HAVE TO SAY
ABOUT THE PROGRAM IN THIS BOOK.

NORTH AND SOUTH, PEOPLE HAVE FOUND TO FEELING **FIT FOR LIFE II:**

"I finished reading *Living Health*, and I didn't think it was possible, yet you topped *Fit for Life*. . . . Never in my life have I felt this alive, happy, and healthy."

—**R.N.W.**
Markham, Ont., Canada

*   *   *

"I can never thank you enough for all that you have done for me as well as thousands of others. You have opened a bright new door to my future. . . . I love being outdoors and sleeping with the window open—and I don't get sick or have the allergies like I used to."

—**A.W.**
Fort Wayne, Ind.

*   *   *

"I am a vocational nurse who works in a traditional medical setting. I am, however, a true believer in Natural Hygiene. . . . Thank you for the book *Living Health*! It has been invaluable to myself and my family."

—**A.D.W.**
Austin, Tex.

EAST AND WEST—
THE RIGHT ROAD
GREAT IN
LIVING HEALTH

"The program has worked wonders for my diabetes. . . . Bought a whole new wardrobe of dresses yesterday. My daughter was amazed."

—F.J.
Blakes, Va.

*   *   *

"I have yo-yoed all my life on diets and since being on your program, I have lost and maintained [my weight] and have enjoyed every mouthful of food. This has been something I've been looking for for years! Bless you!!"

—S.L.P.
Seattle, Wash.

*   *   *

"I had cervix cancer four years ago and have been doing a lot of reading on eating right. Your books have been a real help for me. I especially enjoy your recipes. . . . My daughter and I are both feeling a lot better. I can't believe the difference in our skin. . . . It's great to be able to stop using the prescription drugs."

—C.R.
Rockland, Maine

*   *   *

"My husband and I . . . adhere to a life-style of Natural Hygiene. I am presently in my 7th month of pregnancy with our first child and have enjoyed outstanding health and energy throughout my pregnancy. I am still jogging 2 miles per day, 6 days per week."

—N.L.
Midland, Mich.

*   *   *

"Thank you, thank you so much for . . . *Living Health* . . . I feel great, and am so enthusiastic about all that I have learned that I can't help but talk about it to all my friends. . . . And last, but not least, thank you for telling us in a manner in which we could understand things . . . just as if you were here talking to us."

—P.N. & J.M.
Wooster, Ohio

*   *   *

"I have read both your books and love them. I have also tried your diet and have lost 17 lbs. in 3 weeks and I feel like a new man."

—R.S.
Fallbrook, Calif.

*   *   *

"I have lost 25 lbs. in 7 weeks! . . . Thanks Gang, one more happy person in the world."

—J.B.
Cocoa, Fla.

* * *

"We are a family of 5. . . . I never dreamed that the preventative nutritional approach to lifelong health could really be put in our own hands. And another beautiful aspect is that we don't have to spend our life savings to have health and vitality."

—E.J.
Winston-Salem, N.C.

* * *

"I have just completed reading *Living Health* and in my opinion it is the most important book on health and food that I ever read. I am 80 years of age and intend to follow the natural way to eat for the balance of my days."

—A.W.
Santa Monica, Calif.

* * *

"I have been following your book *Living Health* for the past 6 weeks and have noticed a dramatic change in the way I feel. . . . I have my children eating right now and am slowly convincing my husband to change over."

—E.M.
O'Fallon, Mo.

* * *

"I've learned more workable information from your book than a whole year of nutrition classes I've been attending. The results when tested upon oneself are immediate. I really feel better. . . . My energy is there!"

—D.H.
Chicago, Ill.

*   *   *

"I am 15 years old and a competitive gymnast . . . I've lost 8 pounds and am stronger than ever. Before starting your program I used to go to a workout and about half way through I'd totally run out of energy. Well, that hasn't happened once. I always have so much energy. . . . My mother went on the program with me. She says she's never felt better, and has lost 15 pounds."

—J.W.
Reno, Nev.

*   *   *

"We are in our 70s, retired. . . . Thanking you for making our life easier and better."

—Mr. and Mrs. J.H.W.
Ocala, Fla.

*   *   *

"In case there is anyone who doubts that this way of eating and living will result in a state of improved health and well-being, I can give myself as an example that it most definitely will. . . . I have become more healthy than I have ever been in my life, have more energy than anyone I know. . . . I am going to buy *Living Health* for every member of my family."

—A.G.
Seattle, Wash.

*   *   *

Copies of these and other signed testimonials are on file and may be examined at Warner Books, 666 Fifth Avenue, New York, N.Y. 10103.

Also by Harvey and Marilyn Diamond

FIT FOR LIFE
A NEW WAY OF EATING

Published by
WARNER BOOKS

FIT
FOR LIFE II:
LIVING HEALTH
HARVEY & MARILYN
DIAMOND

WARNER BOOKS

A Warner Communications Company

For God and for all God's children

WARNER BOOKS EDITION

Warner Books, Inc.
666 Fifth Avenue
New York, N.Y. 10103

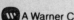 A Warner Communications Company

Printed in the United States of America

This book was originally published in hardcover by Warner Books.
First Printed in Paperback: August, 1988

10 9 8 7 6 5 4 3 2 1

ACKNOWLEDGMENTS

We wish to express our heartfelt gratitude to Warner Books for its consistent effort to bring democracy to the field of health, for the professionalism of its dedicated staff, with special recognition to Larry Kirshbaum and Nansey Neiman for their strength and understanding.

Many thanks to Norman Brokaw, Mel Berger, and Irene Webb of the William Morris Agency for their continued advice and support.

Special mention must also be made of the great health reformers, our mentors and predecessors, who under extreme pressure and persecution fought the battle for freedom of choice in health care: Isaac Jennings, Russell Trall, John H. Tilden, Sylvester Graham, Florence Nightingale, Herbert M. Shelton, and all those others far too numerous to mention.

To all those present day health reformers without whose work ours could not be done, we are eternally grateful.

To our parents, Irving Diamond, who lost his life in his prime because he had no recourse other than a system of treatment that ignored his biological needs. To Sophie Diamond, whose love for us always came through. And, to Fran and Bernie Horecker, whose fifty year love affair and commitment to excellence gave us the understanding that love is the glue that holds everything together.

Additionally, our unbounding love to Beau, Lisa, and Greg, who once again tiptoed through their summer vacations out of respect for the work being done in their home.

Thank you all and God bless all of you . . .

And God bless Ita, who is always there to help.

CONTENTS

PREFACE

HARVEY AND MARILYN:

This is a book about your body and what you can do to take care of it. It's a manual that leads you, step-by-step, to a practical and sensible health lifestyle. Embracing and distilling for you much of the most current information from many health-related fields, it gives you an understanding of the impact of exercise, nutrition, breathing, sunshine, sleep, water, love, sex and much more on your health. It clears out the confusion you may be feeling and guides you, with a new competence and confidence, in knowing exactly what *you can do* to look and feel your best. And it doesn't leave anyone out. From toddlers to teens, from parents to grand-parents, this book offers the commonsense, SAFE solutions you have been searching to find.

This book is bursting with new information that will change your relationship to your body. Having just completed a 17-city tour nearly two years after the publication of **Fit for Life**, we have had ample opportunity to witness the incredible results being reaped by hundreds of thousands of people on the **Fit for Life** program. From weight loss to vast improvements in health, the evidence is in. This is something that is working for people over the long term, freeing them from a dependence on drugs and treatments and allowing them to eliminate, on their own, many of their health problems. Looking and feeling better than ever before in recent history, they are asking for much more information to give them an even greater control over their bodies.

This is an era of great advances in "self-care." There is so much you can learn to do to live more healthfully. It is more and more obvious that all the treatments and "cures" in the world cannot bring *lasting* health if you are not willing first to live a healthier existence. Years of physical abuse—smoking, drinking, overeating the wrong foods, lack of rest or exercise—can only interfere with good health. Emotional instability is also incompatible with good health. And when the result is overt ill health, drugs and surgery serve only as Band-Aids. To repair the damage of disease you must live more healthfully. But more to the point, to *prevent* disease you must live more healthfully. In all likelihood you know this already. This book tells you how to build on that instinctive knowledge.

There is plenty of information coming to light now about what a healthier existence involves. And as you come into contact with this information, what becomes obvious is that there are also plenty of well-trained, knowledgeable people schooled in many different philosophies who can assist you in your "self-care" quest. All of these specialists—doctors of hygiene, chiropractic, osteopathy, medicine, psychology, acupuncture, as well as physical therapists, midwives, homeopaths, massage therapists and exercise and posture specialists—can assist you when their particular expertise is relevant to your needs. None of them, however, can do the job *for* you, and none of them should be relied upon to do so. The challenge is for you to weigh what they have to say, use what seems to apply to your situation, and reject what doesn't. No practitioner should be treated as the ultimate and only authority on the subject of health care. Each can offer you the benefit of what he or she has learned, but it is up to you—using your common sense, instincts, past experience, present needs, and future goals —to decide whether what a practitioner concludes is true and helpful to you. That is how *you* remain in charge.

We have written this book as a suggested blueprint for a health-producing life-style. After a combined twenty-nine years of study on the needs of the human body, we are presenting to you in lay terms what we have found is necessary in order to lead a healthy life. Here as well are explanations of how you can fulfill your health needs easily and routinely as part of your *normal way of life*. Not that some change won't be required—it will. In order for this program to work for you, you have to be willing to apply at least some part of it. And as you make those first modest changes, you will get positive results that spur you to do more.

Changing is fun. And if you can visualize your new health-style as involving not the breaking of old habits but the making of *new* ones, you will feel very positive and excited about what the future holds for you.

Although change sometimes hurts, it is an important phenomenon. The only thing constant in this world is change. As Benjamin Franklin once said, "When you're finished changing, you're finished." Can you imagine how horrendously monotonous your life would be without it?

There is only one thing that can bring about fresh change, and that is new information. We don't claim to have the only answer or the best answer. What we have is a philosophy of health care, an approach to living that has been working for a great number of people.

There was a time when we were in pain and searching for relief, and we were fortunate enough to come into contact with a field of study that, although totally new and foreign to us, brought us the healing and well-being that we so desperately needed. As we began to share our work in this field with others, we saw them achieve their health goals as well. We personally have witnessed thousands of people improve their health using only a small part of this information. With the publication of our first book, millions have begun to improve their health!

What we are presenting here is a health life-style that, put into practice, can vastly improve your well-being. This is a life-style designed for those who wish to feel more certain about their health and more in control of what the present and future will bring them in that all-important area of existence. None of us wants to be sick. None of us relishes the idea that we may become a medical statistic. This is a simple, easy-to-follow health-style that can enable you to stack the cards very much in your favor.

Our experience is that a health-producing life-style brings us the health we all cherish. A disease-producing life-style brings the diseases we all dread. The main premise here is that **LIVING HEALTHFULLY IS NOT AN ART THAT WE MUST LEARN, IT IS AN INSTINCTIVE WAY OF LIFE TO WHICH WE MUST RETURN.** The pages of this book will, in commonsense, layman's terms, make that premise apparent!

Yes, what we have to say *is* different! Yes, it is a new approach. Yes, it contradicts many of the doctrines of the day, but it reaps a multitude of benefits for people, of that there is no doubt. It may not be the answer for everyone, but it is already affecting millions in a positive way, so there is certainly the chance it can benefit you also. It is something that you should at least be aware of, so that you recognize the option that is open to you. And that is precisely what it is, an *option*. We hope you have not put up a wall against change because of too many past disappointments, because the same wall that keeps out disappointment also keeps out that which can genuinely help you and is worthy of your consideration.

No one has *all* the answers. Not us. Not anyone. **What we are offering you is AN OPPORTUNITY FOR A NEW WAY OF LIVING.** This then is our vital message: **EVERYTHING WE NEED TO BE HEALTHY OR TO RESTORE OUR HEALTH HAS BEEN PROVIDED FOR US BY NATURE.** We offer you no program of treatment, but rather an intelligent plan of living that conforms to the laws and normal conditions of life and will not only preserve health but will also enable the sick to restore themselves to health. We present you an option of understanding, indeed, an *outrageous probability:* that **YOU CAN BE IN COM-PLETE CONTROL OF YOUR HEALTH!** It will always be up to *you* whether or not you wish to embrace it.

Explore that option and see for yourself if it can benefit you the way it is benefiting so many others. What a shame it would be if you were to miss out on something that could dramatically increase the length and quality of your life simply because you did not investigate it and give it the opportunity to prove its worthiness to you.

We all wish to be happy and healthy. We all wish happiness and health for those we love. That is our common truth. We lovingly and respectfully offer you this blueprint for living as our contribution to your effort to become a shining, joyous, real-life example of living health!

INTRODUCTION

HARVEY AND MARILYN:

If you read our first book, **Fit for Life**, you may be making the often heard statement, "Aha, they had a big hit, and now they are trying to capitalize on their success with another book that is just more of the same with a different title." Although this is certainly the case in some instances, **Living Health** does not happen to be one of them. In fact, this is the book we wanted to write *first*, but we had to test the waters, so to speak, before we could present it to you.

Fit for Life is merely one thread from a tapestry in the science of Natural Hygiene, which addresses itself to every aspect of building and nurturing health and preventing disease. Natural Hygiene maintains that **HEALTH IS NOT THE ABSENCE OF DISEASE, BUT RATHER AN OPTIMUM STATE OF BODY FUNCTION.** What Natural Hygiene does for us is bring us to that optimum state.

Before writing this book we had to be sure that people were ready for an approach to health care using a body of nontraditional life-style principles never before widely discussed. So we decided first to write a book not on the entire vast subject of health care, but on the one area that seemed to be so important to so many people: weight loss. If we could be successful with an approach that was *not* a diet but gave people total control over their weight, that was easy to implement, sensible in its application, provided delicious food, *and worked*, surely they would be open to related information on all other aspects of health care.

Well, we received our answer and our highest expectations were exceeded. Indeed, America *was* ready! *Fit for Life* has so far sold more than 2 million copies in hardcover, has been on the best-seller lists for well over a year, and is in print in fourteen other countries. We have received thousands of letters from all over the world, so many that we have now created a bimonthly newsletter to enable people to share their wonderful stories with each other. People have lost weight and are feeling wonderful about their newfound well-being. What made this possible?

Who could be more jaded than someone who has gone on every fad diet imaginable only to look for yet another program to take the weight off and *keep* it off. The approach in **Fit for Life** successfully put an end to that need to diet for hundreds of thousands of those people. As a result it opened the door for us to introduce much more of the same system, Natural Hygiene, to show how it can lead to exuberant health and freedom from a host of maladies that otherwise beset people. For as sure as the sun is hot, applying the principles of Natural Hygiene works just as successfully for those with more serious problems as for those who are overweight. Here is an all-encompassing approach that enables the individual to reach his or her fullest potential, the highest state of well-being. By applying the principles in this book, you can easily adopt a new health life-style, improving your health so much that every day of your life will be a joy and a pleasure to live, free of diseases, nagging ailments, and discomforts. More-over, you'll be free of the *fear* of suffering from them. Remember, if the pathway to health were to be pictured as a tapestry of many threads, **Fit for Life** would represent only one. This book details much more of the tapestry.

Now that there is persuasive evidence that **Fit for Life** is ef-fective in dealing with one of America's major preoccupations, losing weight, it is time to pull the other threads together. If our first book was an eye opener for you, then you'd better sit down when you read this one. Much of what we present here is pro-vocative and controversial. But just as **Fit for Life** shows that you can take control of your weight and no longer have to feel like a hapless victim in that area, this book will show you how to take control of your health. With the *same* confidence, you can assure yourself a pain-free, disease-free existence.

These are exciting times. More and more people are striving to be healthy and fit and are doing what is necessary to enhance and maintain that fitness. The information is here and available to help you. With a desire to succeed and with an open mind, *nothing* will stand in the way of your reaching the high level of vigorous health that is **YOUR BIRTHRIGHT**. After all, **VIBRANT, GLOWING HEALTH IS OUR NATURAL STATE OF BEING, AND HEALING IS A BIOLOGICAL PROCESS OF THE BODY NOT AN ART DONE TO THE BODY.** Health should be the norm. The fact that so many people have at least some health complaints may lead you to the false conclusion that some pain, discomfort, and ill health are the norm. Don't you believe it! No one will ever convince us that the God who, in his infinite, incomprehensible wisdom, created us and this spectacular planet, established as part of the grand scheme of things a plan of chronic physical suffering from the cradle to the grave.

We are not trying to imply that we have some magical formula. We do not! There is more than one path to the top of the mountain; this is merely one of them. It is based on the idea that **HEALTH IS FREE AND IT IS OURS TO EMBRACE**. We, and thousands like us, have found this path to be simple, safe, and reliable. So may you. Given the chance, the path of Natural Hygiene can get you to your destination.

PART

I

Then
and Now

CHAPTER 1
New Information

HARVEY:

Let's talk about something really exciting. In fact, let's talk about what is without doubt the most exciting subject there is to discuss: *new information*. ''What!'' you say. ''New information?'' Skiing on a powder base is exciting. The seventh game of the World Series is exciting. Watching fireworks on the Fourth of July is exciting. But next to the discovery of new information, these pale in comparison. If you doubt this, merely try to envision a world devoid of new information. If not for the fact that new information is *always* replacing old, we would still be afraid to sail our ships too far for fear of falling off the edge of the planet.

Look around you at anything you like—television, automobiles, lights, telephones, pens, computers, books, stoves, you name it. Without new information, none of these would exist. Imagine, if you will, what the world would become if, as of today, not one scrap of new information were to come into being. In a very short time, life would become stale, unpleasant, and unbearably boring. Monotony would be the order of the day. Life would be woefully uninteresting.

For centuries, people dreamed of flying, but until the Wright brothers made flying a reality at Kitty Hawk, it was only that, a dream. Their flying machine was cumbersome and unsophisticated, but their contribution would lead to a flying machine so sophisticated that it would travel 17,000 miles an hour and go to the moon and back.

Alexander Graham Bell talked on a machine from one room to

another, which led to talking from one continent to another. Consider Thomas Edison's experiments with electricity. Try to envision a world without electricity. So much of what we do depends on it that if it were somehow to disappear, we would hardly be able to function. An astronomical amount of new information was necessary to create what we now have, an electrified world.

The point is this: Life would be an ordeal without new information coming to light on a regular basis. We thrive on it. We need it. We depend on it. We *demand* it! Consider the scientist in any branch of science. A scientist's reason for research is the daily hope of discovering new information. Without the prospect of coming up with new information, there would be no scientists. Knowing all of this to be true, knowing that new information is impatiently looked forward to, eagerly anticipated, anxiously awaited by practically everyone (whether they are consciously aware of it or not), *it is mind-boggling that all through history, new information has been met with negativity, hostility, and sometimes violent opposition*.

"But why?" you may ask. Hey, great question. If you discover a reasonable answer, let us know. We humans are a strange breed. We resist what we most desire. It's as if anything new must be rejected before it can be accepted, even when it makes no sense to resist. We clamor for improvements, then persecute the very people who bring them to us. We are like an audience cheering and stomping wildly for an encore by an actor who has just given a smashing performance, only to pelt him with rotten eggs when he reappears onstage. As certain as the earth is round, new information *will* inevitably replace old. Nevertheless, whenever the new makes its debut, it is invariably resisted.

Three hundred years ago, Galileo, using one of the first telescopes, proved the Copernican premise that the sun did not rise and set or move across the sky. Rather, it was the earth spinning on its own axis that created the *illusion* of the sun moving. Did this most valuable and momentous piece of new information bring Galileo world fame and admiration? No, it earned him a stay in the slammer, where he had time to rub the knots on his head received from people throwing rocks at him for his blasphemous statements. And yet there are precious few people today who do not acknowledge the truth of his observation.

A hundred years ago, Ignaz Semmelweis, a medical doctor, made public his concern that medical practitioners were adding undue risks and presenting a danger to their patients by failing to wash their hands prior to surgery or the delivering of babies. Even immediately after performing autopsies on diseased corpses, surgeons would go directly to another room to assist in childbirth, without so much as rinsing off their hands. How was this new information received? Dr. Semmelweis was condemned and vilified mercilessly by his colleagues, who hounded him out of his chosen profession. He died in a mental institution, dishonored and destroyed. Anyone know if surgeons are presently washing their hands prior to surgery?

More often than not, new information is attacked for no other reason than that it is different. It upsets lazy minds, especially if they have a vested interest in old ways. Learning something that is different seems a forbidding effort for many. What really stuns the intellect, however, is that the field that purportedly most aggressively seeks new information most violently *resists* new information! Doesn't it seem odd that the group most explicitly devoted to fresh knowledge and new information also puts up the biggest battle against it and the changes that it heralds? This group goes under the general title of "the sciences." Marilyn and I have had some very personal experience of this.

When **Fit for Life** first came out, it was a heavy dose of new information—not that it was newly *dis*covered, but it was newly *un*covered. True to history, there were rumblings of discontent. Disapproval came from a small group on the fringe of established medicine, the nutritionists and dietitians. Fortunately, many members of the medical profession who were having a great deal of success with the program were more supportive. Medical professionals are often the first to admit that diet has not been given the emphasis it deserves in medical schools. Of the 127 medical schools in the United States, only one-third even *offer* nutrition, and only one-half of those require attendance. Nevertheless, a small segment of nutritionists and dietitians, fancying themselves keepers of the Holy Grail when it comes to how to eat, rejected out of hand the new information revealed in **Fit for Life**—not because it was not viable, but because it was new and different from what they had learned. They persisted in mouthing the same old nutritional hooey they have been trying to stuff down the public's throat for the last several decades.

Could it be possible that nutrition is the only area of study that should *not* change, that should *not* benefit from new information?

Hardly! Yet new information in nutrition is routinely attacked by some nutritionists and dietitians *simply because it has not emanated from their ranks*.

The plight of new information all too frequently falls into the scenario described by the sixteenth-century French philosopher Montaigne. In his words, "Whenever a new discovery is reported to the scientific world, they say first, 'It is probably not true.' Thereafter, when the truth of the new proposition has been demonstrated beyond question, they say, 'Yes, it may be true, but it is not important.' Finally, when sufficient time has elapsed to fully evidence its importance they say, 'Yes, surely it is important, but it is no longer new.' "

In the case of **Fit for Life**, these antagonists have backed off somewhat because they hear the testimonies of great numbers of people. When great numbers of people are feeling better as a result of the use of newly available information, you're unlikely to be taken seriously when you try to tell them it won't work.

All anyone in *any* field of endeavor asks from others is a fair hearing. When new and perhaps difficult-to-accept information comes along that attacks established belief systems, the first impulse may be to discard it. But *all* new information deserves to be looked at with an eye for what may be of value in it. It should be scrutinized, *intensely* scrutinized. But condemnation without investigation is ignorance and arrogance of the highest order. As an illustration of this, let me quote a passage from a book written in 1912 by a medical doctor, Isaac Peeples.

> A fair minded person believes what he does because he believes firmly it is the truth and as such is willing to discuss it with any other fair minded one. He is willing for it to be sifted and tested to the uttermost, for he does not want to believe what is untrue and he knows the truth will stand any real tests, and too, the more it is tested, the more it can be seen to be the truth. He is willing to concede that those who differ from him are sincere until the opposite is disclosed and this disclosure of insincerity will not be his defeat in argument. If he is defeated in arguments, he will not try to relieve himself of his defeat by slandering his opponent, but he will thank him for enabling him to see his weakness and the faultiness of his belief.

Oh, what a blessing it would be if we could count on all health professionals to assume such a stance of integrity.

Now, let us clearly state the point of all this talk about new information and all these examples from history showing what a difficult birth new information so often experiences. The point is this: **A GREAT DEAL OF WHAT IS PRESENTED IN THIS BOOK IS NEWLY UNCOVERED INFORMATION.** Many of the ideas, when contrasted with conventional thinking, are provocative and controversial. **THE IDEAS HERE ARE INTENDED TO STIMULATE THOUGHT AND INVESTIGATION.** In the words of Herbert M. Shelton, one of the greatest thinkers in the field of Natural Hygiene, "Every advance that the human race has made has had to meet and overcome the old order. Because the old order was part and parcel of the makeup of the minds of the period, advance could come only through a mental revolution. People had to be taught to see things differently. They had to learn that progress does not mean the destruction of the universe. They had to acquire a new view of things." In the words of Russell T. Trall, M.D., one of the fathers of Natural Hygiene, "It has always been one of the most difficult practical problems in the world how to present new truths so as not to offend old errors; for persons are very apt to regard arguments directed against their opinions as attacks upon their persons; and many there are who mistake their own ingrained prejudices for established principles."

Once again, as in **Fit for Life**, the faculties we have all been endowed with at birth will be called upon to help direct us in our endeavor to grasp new information: namely our instincts, sense of logic, and, most importantly, our good old common sense. These inborn traits are with us throughout our lives. They help us and give us direction. If one authority says one thing and another authority says the opposite, where does that leave the lay person who just wants to feel better and not become a medical statistic? By using the tools that God saw fit to give you and allowing yourself to listen to what you feel and sense is in your best interest, you can start to recapture your natural ability to guide yourself in the direction that will most benefit your health and longevity.

You don't need a "board certified expert" to tell you that you feel better. *You* can tell the expert when you feel better. If you make use of certain new information and you start to feel progressively better, will any amount of intimidation or efforts to discourage you by any so-called authority persuade you to abandon your new approach and revert to whatever it was you were doing that made you feel worse? I should certainly hope not! There is no better proof of something's value than its success. If you make use of something and it works for you, what other proof of its effectiveness do you need?

If you eat differently for a period of time and chronic digestive ailments you have suffered with for years go away and stay away, would you stop eating that way if you were shown a piece of paper that said eating that way was not effective in relieving digestive ailments? Would you stop if some television MD or dietitian sponsored by the drug industries that manufacture digestive aids tried to scare you away from your new way of eating so you would continue to support that two-billion dollar industry? We've all been so conditioned to rely on others for their advice on how we should care for our bodies that we are afraid to trust our own instincts. But you have far more ability in that area than you realize or are given credit for. If you can get back in tune with your own body, it will tell you what it wants. One way of doing that is to start to have more faith and confidence in your own instincts, logic, and common sense.

As I am writing this, I am filled with immense gratitude that I was fortunate enough to learn this lesson and utilize it in my life to recapture my own health. I am equally filled with an overwhelming desire to help others discover that they, too, can have control and power over their own health. To illustrate one's ability to come from a place of virtually no knowledge of how the body works or how to properly care for oneself to a point of understanding how to acquire and maintain a consistently high level of health, I would like to relate to you the journey I traveled—from a sickly, uninformed individual *afraid* of my own body to someone totally confident of the fact that if I want to live a long, pain-free, disease-free life, *I can*!

CHAPTER 2
Looking Back

HARVEY:

I was born coughing. As a tiny infant, I lay coughing in my hospital crib, suffering from serious ill health that unfortunately would get worse before it got better. Three short weeks into life, I was rushed back to the hospital for emergency treatment. I had acute symptoms of *starvation*! The infant formula I had been prescribed in the hospital was severely deficient, and as a result, at three weeks of age, I almost lost my life! Not a very auspicious beginning.

From the time I was a very young child until I was twenty-five years old, I suffered from the most intense kinds of stomach pains whenever I ate. It was something so much a part of my life that I just figured it was simply part of the eating experience. I would eat dinner, have dessert, get my stomachache, and bear the pain until I fell asleep. As a child I would frequently wake up in the middle of the night from the pain and go sleep in the bathroom with my pillow on my lap. In the morning one of my four brothers would find me and exclaim, ''Harv slept in the bathroom again.'' More often than not I would not tell anyone that my stomach hurt, because otherwise I would be treated to some Pepto Bismol, which I came to call Pepto Abysmal. Pepto Bismol appealed to me about as much as walking naked through the tsetse fly country of Africa. I never knew which was more unpleasant, the stomachache or the Pepto Bismol.

In addition, I always had colds—three, four, sometimes six colds a year. I was always blowing my nose. I'm sure I personally raised Kleenex stock two points. These were not the minor colds where you sneeze and cough for a few days, blow your nose, and it's over. These were more like "My God, I'm *dying*!" Perhaps you know the kind of cold I'm referring to—you feel like screaming if you cough one more of those rasping coughs that feels like hot sandpaper stripping away the insides of your throat. Each time you cough it feels like someone hit you on the side of the head with a two-by-four.

I remember taking so much medication that I could hardly walk—something for the cough, something else for the stuffy feeling, something else to ease the headache, something else for "all around relief," and all that topped off with enough Nyquil to stop a water buffalo in its tracks. Between the cold and the medication, I felt like I'd been run over by a truck.

As a youngster, I was pathetically skinny. I don't just mean thin; I mean not enough meat on my bones to pinch. When a wind came up I had to grab hold of the nearest stationary object. During those years, I never *dreamed* I would ever have to struggle with a weight problem.

From age eighteen to twenty-two, I served in the United States Air Force. My last year of duty was spent in Vietnam, where a lot of the food that was available to eat was left over from World War II—literally. In fact, for someone like me, whose love for eating could be attributed only to having known what it feels like to have nearly starved to death as a child, these "leftovers" were worse than standing guard duty in the middle of the night. Frequently, meals were C rations. If you have never eaten pound cake, scrambled powdered eggs, and "assorted ground meats" from cans marked "Packed in 1944," you were born under a lucky star. Give thanks.

Upon my release from the service, because of the depression I suffered from seeing some of the horrors of war and eating meatloaf out of little green tin cans that were packed before I was even born, I took to eating as if I had been told, "Today is the last day you will ever get to eat." I ate absolutely anything and everything I could fit into my mouth, and I started to gain weight faster than a sumo wrestler. The once pathetically skinny kid now weighed 202 pounds. And then I couldn't get the weight back off! I could hardly believe it, but **I WAS FAT!** *Me!* The kid strangers would give food to because they thought I hadn't eaten in a week.

I *hated* being fat. All of my weight was between my navel and my knees. I looked like a giant pear with arms and legs. It was embarrassing. When I walked my thighs were like two whales colliding. Like so many other millions of frustrated Americans, I joined the dieting merry-go-round—starve it off and then gorge it back on. Between my daily stomachaches, my frequent colds, and my excess tonnage, I was not exactly the happiest person in the world.

Then, a new awareness as a result of a catastrophic event in my late teens catapulted me to a quest for help from which no force on earth could keep me: my father's death. It was not only the fact that he died, it was *how*! After several years of complaining about violent stomachaches, he died of stomach cancer. He was only fifty-seven.

Quite honestly, I never had the good relationship with my father that I would have liked. We were frequently at odds with one another. However, you can be absolutely certain I loved him dearly. Unfortunately, I never told him so. I had joined the Air Force several months before he died, and just prior to his death I was called home on emergency leave. I had not seen him since I joined. On the flight home, knowing it would be the last time I ever saw him alive, I was filled with an overwhelming need to express my love for him. I went over in my mind a thousand times what I would say: "Dad, I love you. I know I've never told you that before, but I'm telling you now. No matter what has ever transpired between us, I love you deeply and completely." As I arrived at the hospital, along with my sadness, I experienced a feeling of relief and even joy at the prospect of relating my innermost feelings of love to my father. By the time I was at his door I was actually excited. I was going to lay to rest years of misunderstanding and frustration. I was going to pour out uninhibited love—embrace him and make up for the years of miscommunication between us and share with him, even if it could only be briefly, some honest, devoted feelings.

Upon entering his room, my heart pounding and emotions welling up from inside me, I could not have been more shocked than if the devil himself had been standing there, arms raised and ready to plunge his burning pitchfork into my chest. I simply was not prepared for the sight that confronted me. You see, I had been thinking only of the positive aspects of our reunion. I had not known what had been done to my father in the months since I had enlisted. All three of the only "proven" scientific methods of treatment had been *tried* on my father. Between the surgery, which had removed his stomach and much of his intestines, the radiation treatments, which had blistered his skin, and the drugs he was bombarded with to quell the excruciating pain of chemotherapy, he had been reduced to a discolored, disfigured, hollow shell of a man, unable to hear, see, or speak.

I stood there in total shock and disbelief, while my mother literally yelled in his ear, "Irving, Harvey is here; Harvey has come to see you." It hit me like a tidal wave that I was not ever going to get to utter those three words that I was so looking forward to saying to him. The sight of his broken, tortured body made me instantly sick to my very core. I ran from the room crying and throwing up. It was the last time I ever saw my father. Cancer took his life. The treatment took his dignity, and he was gone. That final sight of him has been seared into my memory forever as if with a branding iron.

Over the next few years, many a time I awoke in the middle of the night with a jolt, in a pool of sweat, my heart pounding in my throat, racked with fear, seeing again my dad on his deathbed, convinced that I was to suffer the same fate. Why not? I had all the symptoms. Imagine how I felt. My father complained of violent stomachaches before dying of stomach cancer, and I had violent stomachaches *every single day*. There I was, only twenty-five years old, and instead of thinking about a career or marriage, my thoughts centered around cancer and pain and suffering. Plus, I had ballooned up to over 200 pounds, so I had that to think about just in case there were ever a few hours that my stomach didn't hurt.

But something happened. I don't even know what exactly. It was nothing specific. All of a sudden, instead of feeling like a helpless victim waiting for things to get worse, I got angry, angry at the whole mess—my stomachaches, colds, constant weight loss diets, and the specter of cancer. I had had it. If I was indeed to become a cancer statistic, it wasn't going to be without a fight. In fact, I made a commitment to the universe that *I wasn't going to allow it to happen*. I would do whatever had to be done to prevent my gradual deterioration and demise. I severed myself from all existing responsibilities to devote myself entirely to the study of health. I started getting excited. I knew it was going to be a long haul, but already I began to feel more positive. My stomach still hurt but my attitude was transforming. Thoughts of becoming a medical doctor, conquering cancer, and saving millions of lives seemed like a good place to start.

I started to research at various institutions to see what school I should attend, what direction of study I should take. I *wanted* health, so I wanted *to study* health, just as if I wanted to be rich, I would certainly not study the poor to see how to become so. But as I went from one school to another, asking where the best course on the subject of health could be found, I was told over and over again that it was the study of *disease* I would have to take up. Curricula invariably had many courses on pathology (disease) but *none* on health! I couldn't grasp it. "You mean there is a word for the study of disease but no such word for the study of something as important as health? **WHY?**"

Some of my enthusiasm was starting to wane. In fact, I was beginning to get downright disillusioned. What *really* made me start to feel life was playing a perverted joke on me were occasions when I had doctor's appointments to get advice on how to care for myself to improve my health. Frequently my appointment was with someone who was easily as overweight as I. Many were also bald, had pasty skin, and even *smoked!* When I asked if they were following their own advice, I was told, "I'm not the patient here, you are." Ah yes, I see. It became apparent to me that the traditional approach to healing was perhaps not the road I wanted to travel. But it wasn't as though I could look up schools in the Yellow Pages under "Alternative Health Care." Not that such places did not exist, but whoever heard of them? My spirits were a bit dampened, but not my commitment. I felt a dramatic and forceful course of action had to be taken.

I decided to "take my quest on the road." Something told me that if I traveled and kept my eyes, ears, and *mind* open, perhaps what I was looking for would find *me*. It worked. After logging thousands of miles around the United States, my travels brought me to Santa Barbara, only ninety miles from where I had started. It was so pretty there and I had such a good feeling about the place. Even though it was a place where I could easily just have relaxed and languished in the sun, the pain in my stomach reminded me why I was there. It was shortly after my arrival in Santa Barbara that I met the most shining example of living health that I had ever encountered in my life, and that incredible person introduced me to a philosophy of health care that would change my life forever for the better. That philosophy is called Natural Hygiene. If you're like me you may be thinking, "Right, Natural Hygiene. Brush your teeth, wash behind your ears, right?" Not exactly. I found out that it is so very much more than that.

We've given the history and background of Natural Hygiene in **Fit for Life**, all in the context of weight loss and energy enhancement. But Natural Hygiene is so very much more. This approach to living also supplies a coherent, simple, and sensible formula for a vigorous long life by addressing itself to every aspect of life as it relates to our health and well-being. In every area of health, Natural Hygiene gives a pertinent, understandable, verifiable explanation and course of action to undertake to bring about a high level of personal well-being.

I knew my prayers had been answered and that I had found something that would be momentous in my life. I knew because the person who introduced me to the subject *looked like health* personified: clear eyes, lustrous hair, nearly translucent skin, no excess weight, and an excitement for life that I had not come across in a long time. The clincher for me was when I asked him if he ever had stomachaches. His answer was a simple *"Never!"*

I explained that I had been suffering from piercing stomachaches every day for *over twenty years*, that my father had had the same difficulty and had indeed died of stomach cancer, and that I was certain the same end awaited me. He gave me *one* simple principle (proper food combining) to employ to see if any measure of relief could be realized. That was the last day I ever had a stomachache. Yes, you read correctly and, no, I am not exaggerating. In one day, twenty years of pain and suffering ended. I couldn't believe it. I kept waiting for the pain to recur. It never did. Then, as I began reading more about the subject and applying other hygienic principles, in a short period of time I stopped having headaches and colds and lost fifty pounds, *eating all the while*! Nirvana at last.

That was in 1970. Since then I have not suffered from these problems, nor have I gained back any of the weight. I am beginning to believe that it works. You can't possibly imagine the joy and excitement that filled me, nor the fervor with which I studied and learned all I possibly could about Natural Hygiene. Of course, I wanted to know where one went to study the subject formally. I was told that although Natural Hygiene had a 150-year written history and probably more books on the subject had been written than I could possibly ever read, there was *nowhere* to go that offered it as a course of study. I couldn't believe it! It was like being told the location of a treasure chest laden with a king's ransom in precious jewels and then being told that there is no way to get to it. How could there be an approach to health that was so effective and so universal in its application and yet so unknown that there wasn't even a place to learn about it? How could this knowledge, as precious as life itself, have been kept secret all this time?

So I studied Natural Hygiene on my own, reading every book I could get my hands on pertaining to the subject and involving myself with people in Santa Barbara who had incorporated its principles into their life-styles. Three years later, I established myself in Los Angeles, continuing my studies while I counseled people informally on Natural Hygiene.

NATURAL HYGIENE: THE HEALTH SCIENCE THAT WOULD NOT DIE

I *was* fortunate enough to discover Natural Hygiene for myself, notwithstanding efforts over the years by established medicine to discredit and repress it. After eight years of independent study much to my excitement and delight, a complete course based on Natural Hygiene principles finally became available in 1978.

The American College of Health Science was founded in the late 1970s. The college is *not* "accredited."

Do you know why schools that offer alternative health curricula are *not* accredited? In the early 1900s the Rockefeller and Carnegie Foundations became heavily involved in philanthropic grants to medical schools. Their goal was to create a "respectable" male, upper class medical profession, which based its philosophy on drug therapy. (Coincidentally, at that time the Rockefellers were already in the business of selling drugs.) At that point in history there was a great deal of diversity of health care, with drugs being used mostly by a wealthy elite and more natural approaches to health care being supported by a large segment of the population. In 1909 the Carnegie Foundation sent Abraham Flexner on a national tour of all schools that offered training in health care, from the largest right down to the most humble. It was up to Flexner, *one man* representing only one philosophy, to determine which schools would receive philanthropic funding in order to become more established and which would not. Flexner selected as recipients for generous grants only the larger, wealthier schools that were willing to conform to the medical model of drug therapy preferred by the Carnegies and Rockefellers. For smaller schools and those with more natural approaches, the message was clear: "Conform to the medical model or close." As far as Flexner was concerned these schools were not worth saving. The desire of the population for freedom of choice was not even considered.

The now infamous *Flexner Report* of 1910 put the nails in the coffin of health care diversity in this country. Alternative schools closed by the score, including six of America's eight black medical schools and all the medical schools admitting women. Those who fought closure were vandalized and destroyed by goon squads. The new medical elite sanctioned by the Rockefeller and Carnegie foundations had no desire to share the health care field with anyone whose philosophies might be different than theirs, and they had no intention of making their costly training available to blacks, women, or lay healers. (In his report Flexner had actually complained that as a result of popular pressure in the previous century, any "crude boy" was able to seek medical training.) Now the doors were closed to all but white middle and upper class males.

As a result of the legislative clout that the Rockefeller and Carnegie foundations possessed, tough state and federal licensing laws and regulations were passed limiting official recognition to the favored medical approach. This was done with the expressed intent of precluding diverse philosophies of health care being made available to the public, in effect guaranteeing a monopoly on health treatment. The following remarks by Dr. W. A. Evans, Commissioner of Health of Chicago, which appeared in the September 16, 1911, *Journal of the American Medical Association*, make that clear: "As I see it, the wise thing for the medical profession to do is to get right into and man every great health movement. Man health departments, tuberculosis societies, child and infant welfare societies, housing societies, etc. The future of the profession depends on keeping matters, so that when the public mind thinks of these things, it automatically thinks of physicians and not of sociologists or sanitary engineers [his name for Natural Hygienists]. The profession cannot afford to have these places occupied by other than medical men." *The profession cannot afford to have these places occupied by other than medical men?*

In the ensuing decades all forms of health treatment other than medical treatment were outlawed or driven into hiding. Homeopathy and midwifery were outlawed. Natural Hygiene was outlawed. Chiropractic was discredited to the point of nearly being outlawed. Now, thank goodness, we see a great movement toward liberalization and freedom of choice. What was outlawed is now legal in *some* states. And though nonmedical health care schools are still unable to receive government funding or medical accreditation (obviously), they are presently flourishing nonetheless as people aggressively search for new answers to problems that have not been solved by "established" medical solutions. With all of the free flow of nonmedical information now evident, we are clearly in the midst of a popular health reform movement; freedom of speech and freedom of choice are finally being extended to the area of health care.

The alternatives didn't resurface out of nowhere. The public demanded them, and over the last thirty years men and women of conviction have withstood harassment and even the threat of imprisonment to meet the public demand. (Hygienists like Dr. Herbert Shelton, Dr. William Benesh, and Dr. Gian-Cursio were actually imprisoned for extending successful treatment to cancer victims who had previously been treated and given no chance for recovery by the medical establishment.)

I received my Ph.D. in nutritional science from the American College of Health Science in February 1983. No, it's not "accredited"—today's Abraham Flexners have seen to that—but it is the one and only institution *anywhere* in the United States that even has a course of study in Natural Hygiene.

This brings me to a subject that must be addressed and laid to rest: *credentials*.

When it finally became apparent to some of the dietitians and nutritionists that their attempts to malign the information in **Fit for Life** were simply an exercise in futility due to the huge numbers of people obviously benefiting from it, they decided to attack *me* instead, asserting that I had no credentials—if you don't like the message, attack the messenger. This, of course, is a typical half truth used extensively by those not secure with their own status. They left out one word. It's not that I don't have credentials, it's that I don't have *their* credentials. With *their* credentials I would blithely be spouting the same stale, antiquated myths about eating and "the basic four food groups" they insist on ramming down our collective throats, thereby aiding and abetting the spread of disease and suffering that plagues America today. *Truth is not established by credentials!*

The American Dietetic Association (ADA), which has failed miserably to present to the American people a simple, workable approach to eating that brings healthful results, is very threatened by and antagonistic toward those who succeed where they have failed. They have become expert at throwing up smoke screens to mask their own shortcomings, muddle the work of others, and distract attention from the real issue, their own ineffectiveness. Their goal seems to be to maintain a level of public confusion that makes it difficult for people to embrace and stay with any innovative eating program that differs from what the ADA is pushing.

It appears to me that the people most interested in credentials are those who have them and nothing else—they have no innovative ideas, they have no new information to impart, they have nothing of practical value, but they *do* have their certificates. What is the ADA? In the early part of this century there were several nutritional philosophies. A group of private citizens with similar views got together, *issued themselves* certificates and took on the official sounding title, American Dietetic Association. From that time until today they have been trying to stifle all other philosophies in the vast field of nutritional study. No legislative body appointed them. The people did not elect them. They simply designated themselves as authorities and now claim to have the last word in nutrition. They like to stand around congratulating each other for being credentialed and attack with a vengeance *anyone* they have not admitted to their club.

If credentialed dietitians had all the answers, would 90 percent of the people of this country consider themselves overweight? Would millions of people be so anxious to rush to the bookstore for new answers every time a book on diet comes out? How absurd it is that such a closed-minded, self-serving organization as the American Dietetic Association should think it is in charge of deciding who should and should not be ''certified'' to impart nutritional information. It is virtually the same as asking someone who has never successfully sailed on the open seas to judge whether a ship is worthy to sail around the world.

The dietitians' all-time favorite smoke screen, the issue of credentials, should not even be the issue. The real issue is truth. **HAVING ''CREDENTIALS'' DOES NOT MAKE THE**

**TRUTH MORE THE TRUTH, AND NOT HAVING "CRE-
DENTIALS" DOES NOT MAKE THE TRUTH LESS THE
TRUTH.** The truth is the truth no matter who utters it. If a man
who never went beyond the fourth grade tells you that gravity will
destroy your body if you jump from the top of the World Trade
Center, will you jump anyway because he has no Ph.D. in physics?
Would someone with a degree in physics but no belief in gravity
be spared?

What exactly does it mean to be "accredited"?

John Bear has a Ph.D. in education. He has taught at major
universities (Iowa, Berkeley, Michigan State). He was Research
Director for Bell & Howell's Education Division, Director of San
Francisco's Center for the Gifted Child, and has been a consultant
to large organizations such as General Motors, Xerox, and En-
cyclopaedia Brittanica. Since 1974 Dr. Bear has investigated and
written about nontraditional education. His book *Bear's Guide to
Non-Traditional College Degrees* is considered the standard text
in searching out alternative education.

Introducing a statement made by the Carnegie Commission on
Higher Education on the relationship between accreditation and
nontraditional approaches, Dr. Bear said, "One of the frequent
complaints leveled against the recognized accrediting agencies is
that they have, in general, been slow to acknowledge the major
trend to alternative or nontraditional education." No kidding!

In the *ninth* edition of Dr. Bear's book, his latest, he critiques
the curriculum at the American College of Health Science. He
notes that he was initially suspicious of the college but after reviewing much of the material found it to be "comprehensive and
undoubtedly of value."

He is not alone in recognizing the college's worth. The University of Paris School of Medicine, one of the most prestigious
medical schools in all of Europe, has translated and incorporated
this "unaccredited" approach into its curriculum to be taught to
its medical students. Interesting that instruction in Natural Hygiene
would be worthy of acceptance from such a reputable institution
of higher learning but not from the "dietetic establishment" in
the United States.

Detractors can attempt to divert attention away from the true
issues by denigrating our credentials all they want. It will do
nothing to deter people from seeking out and utilizing valuable,
pertinent information on a subject far too important to be monop-

olized by the select few who have *declared themselves* exclusively qualified to impart nutritional information by virtue of their self-proclaimed "superior" credentials.

What are the credentials that really count? A piece of paper on the wall? Or results in people's lives? The success of **Fit for Life** in improving the lives of hundreds of thousands of people is a matter of record. *Those are our credentials*—positive results in people's lives. They are the *only* credentials to which we will ever aspire.

I once asked Mr. T. C. Fry, the founder of the American College of Health Science, if he resented being told his college could not be accredited despite the monumental effort he had put into developing a viable and important course of study. His answer indicates the kind of special person he is, a man interested in truth, not accolades. Without blinking an eye, he said, "On the day of reckoning, I doubt we will be judged by what certificates we have on the wall, but rather by the scars incurred in the battle for humanity." That's T. C. Fry in a sentence. He could not care less that he is not accepted by today's "authorities." He simply does his work and lets his results speak for themselves.

In the early years of my studies, I used to become upset when Natural Hygiene was attacked by dietitians and nutritionists for not being a "bona fide" field. Today, of course, because of the phenomenal success of **Fit for Life**, they have to pursue a different tack. After all, you can look mighty silly telling hundreds of thousands of people that the information they are using to feel better and improve their health isn't viable and only because the dietitians don't agree with it. With the fantastic results that so many people are experiencing, one would think the dietitians would investigate the field in earnest to see what, if anything, they might have missed. Perish the thought! Rather than see the benefits that people are obtaining in applying Natural Hygiene principles, the dietitians are actively trying to have it **outlawed**, to have non-ADA practitioners jailed and fined if they don't toe the establishment line. That's right! They want Natural Hygiene banned, not because it has nothing to offer—certainly the opposite has been dramatically demonstrated—but because *they don't agree with it!* Yes, right here in the enlightened, technologically advanced 1980s, we see followers of one field of study vigorously attempting to ban another field of study so as to remain unchallenged on their self-constructed pedestal. I guess they feel that the inscription on our two-cent stamp, "Freedom To Speak Out— A Root of Democracy," does not apply to nutritional and dietary matters. Can you imagine one baseball team having another team prohibited from playing because the latter had a better chance of winning the World Series?

And it's not as if the dietitians are so in tune with the body's requirements that their approach can't use some improvement. If you want to see how much the dietitians in this country know about what we should be eating, visit your nearest hospital and gaze on what's being offered to the sick. It looks like a plot to keep them there, food easily surpassed in quality at any fourth-rate restaurant in the country. I personally don't have any recollection of people coming out of a hospital and remarking, "Wow, the food! It would be almost worth going back for." Hospital food is the handiwork of the very dietitians who are trying to get every other field that offers nutritional advice *banned*! In 1984 and 1985 the American Dietetic Association lobbied for passage of bills proposed by Representative Claude Pepper (HR-6049, HR-6050, and HR-6051) that would have made it illegal even to *suggest* that a person dying of thirst should drink a glass of water—illegal unless you were a member of the American Dietetic Association or designated "acceptable" by the ADA. The bills died in Congress due to an overwhelming outpouring of outrage by the public and the dedicated and tireless work of health reformers like Maureen Kennedy-Salaman, president of the National Health Federation in California. Ms. Salaman went to Washington, lobbied, and brought to people's attention the travesty that was being perpetrated against them. She even talked to Representative Pepper, who promised not to introduce the bills again. These bills, disguised as "anti-quackery" bills to prevent fraud against the elderly, have provisions that would have resulted in people like T. C. Fry, Ms. Salaman, myself, and thousands of others being fined and sent to prison for long terms simply for sharing health information that we found to be true—*not* because it wasn't true, but because the members of the American Dietetic Association deemed it unworthy.

Undeterred in their attempt to control *all* nutritional information in the United States because of mere public outrage, the American Dietetic Association has convinced Representative Pepper to introduce a new bill, HR-1581, which would give them virtually the same power they hoped to win via the other three bills.

Part of the ADA's strategy for gaining absolute control over the entire field of nutrition is to attack any work that differs from theirs.

Consider this: The food our children are eating in schools all across the United States is so overloaded with fat that you can squeeze the grease right out of it. These school lunches are approved by the ADA, indeed they are *formulated* by the ADA. Practically every school has vending machines dispensing sodas, candy bars, and other valueless junk foods. Why hasn't the ADA attacked the industries responsible for this assault against our children? Why, instead, have they decided to attack a program that has helped millions of people eat more fruit and vegetables; cut back on salt, sugar, and processed foods; and reduce fat and cholesterol—all of which is right in line with the dietary recommendations of the National Cancer Institute, the American Heart Association, and the National Academy of Sciences? It's simply because they are more concerned with protecting their powerful position than with protecting people. And for that reason they will continue to lash out at anyone who has not been admitted into their closed circle of elitists, whether the person being attacked has information of value or not.

Be assured of one thing: That the American Dietetic Association is not happy with our work could not concern us in the least. We have given them ample opportunity to indicate that they are concerned with people, not power. They have proven that they are not. We did not write our books for the ADA, we wrote them for the people who have most emphatically demonstrated their delight and gratitude. The ADA can stay busy trying to insure themselves a monopoly of power, we will stay busy undoing the damage *caused* by the ADA, and helping people.

That there is controversy raging over who should or should not be "permitted" to dispense nutritional advice is clearly evident, but where does that leave you while all the authorities are bickering?

It is vital that the public be free in its choice among health care alternatives. This freedom of choice *must* exist. It's not a profession obsessed with its "official" position and determined to preserve itself from reproach that we are attempting to convince. It is the public we are determined to reach, people contending with everyday concerns about health. We've found them more than willing to hear the simple truths that are the message of Natural

Hygiene, which they can personally verify for themselves. *The public should have a right to choose what works for them*. We are totally confident that the principles in this book can withstand the most intense scrutiny and will prove themselves to be every bit as relevant and exceptional as we suggest they are.

Unlike other systems, Natural Hygiene does not seek to veil its simple message behind mysterious and incomprehensible terms. It has nothing to conceal. It is open, clear, and easily understood. There are no secret potions to offer, no panaceas to sell in bottles, and no wonder drugs to produce health where health cannot logically exist. We merely point to the laws of nature, which enable us all to attain and maintain the most glorious health. All we hope is that the information contained in this book makes sense to *you*, that you will simply put it to the test and see for yourself if it assists you in experiencing a higher level of well-being. Any body of knowledge, no matter how great, will have its detractors, and we certainly do not expect to escape that fate. But that which is truly good will withstand the test of time and prove its value, if given the opportunity. Natural Hygiene asks for nothing more— and nothing less—than to have that opportunity to demonstrate its value to you.

All of the effort I put into this field of study was rewarded in the best way possible. I've enjoyed a well-being that at one time seemed beyond reach. I've seen others awaken to the *living health* that nature makes possible for us all. And crowning it all, the universe sent me the "light of my life" in the form of the most beautiful, sensitive, and loving person I have ever met—Marilyn. For years we swam against the current together, fighting to be heard by a mammoth system that refused to acknowledge the validity of information that had literally saved both our lives. Now we see the tide turning. The public's eyes are increasingly open to the fact that Natural Hygiene has passed the only real test of science: *It works!*

CHAPTER 3
Why Do We Do
This Work?

<u>MARILYN:</u>

When I finally got the opportunity in 1975, at the age of thirty-one, to sit on the grass in front of the local health food store in Venice, California, and talk to Harvey, I was ill and desperate. For over two decades I had suffered with a spastic digestive tract. I can vividly remember burning, piercing pains below my diaphragm, so debilitating in my teens that frequently, on a date or at a school dance, I would have to excuse myself, go to the girls' room, and *lie down on the floor* because I could no longer deal with the distress in my body. In college this constant physical suffering kept me from participating in much of the spontaneous social activity that others enjoyed. It made me irritable and tense, and my relationships suffered. Finally, at the age of twenty, I entered the hospital for surgery, not on my stomach or digestive tract, as you might expect, but on chronically dislocating knees. On the standard American diet (SAD) which included plenty of meat, dairy, and eggs, my knees became so calcium-deficient that both required surgery.

What that surgery did was give me a personal experience of hospital care. In a public hospital funded by New York City—a *teaching* hospital for an important New York medical school—I saw scenes of suffering, the impressions of which I still carry with me. The surgeon who was to operate on me was a knee specialist from South Africa, not licensed to perform surgery in any other hospital. But for that fact, I never would have had the opportunity to see what people who cannot afford private hospitals go through, and that opportunity probably did more to shape my future than any other. In this public facility patients were lined up in beds so close that they could practically reach out and touch one another. The rooms were dismal and stuffy. The insufficient personnel, overworked and past caring, answered pleas for assistance with sedatives, laxatives, pain-killers, and tranquilizers. Patients who were not actually bedridden frequently had to assist bringing bed-pans and removing them for others because there was not enough personnel to do this job. I felt drugged in, trapped in a nightmarish room with glaring overhead lights, tiny barred windows, and PAIN.

And the *food*! It was thrown at us much the way mail must be distributed in the army. It would have been better if they had kept it. It consisted of greasy, watery-thin gravies on powdered mashed potatoes, stiff, grayish meat, white bread and margarine, watery canned vegetables, canned fruit, and stale sugary desserts. (Thank you, American Dietetic Association.) How could anyone be expected to "get well" on such a regimen? I nearly starved to death! When my doctor finally decided that I wasn't getting the kind of care that I needed to help me recuperate, I was sent home. There I spent the next three weeks in bed, convalescing from my surgery *and* my hospital stay.

That experience was a turning point in my life. I never again felt right about a system of health care that permitted so much negligence with regard to the basic, human needs of the sick. Unconsciously, I had already begun my search for nonmedical alternatives.

The surgery did repair my diet-damaged knees, but the pain in my stomach continued. Somehow I managed to keep going, but by my mid-twenties (I was married, with two children), that pain was like a knife. And then it spread to my back. At times it felt as if the middle of my body were on fire! The only relief I could get was by taking Valium, which I took regularly for five years. I also regularly mixed the Valium with cocktails, wine, and other pain-killing drugs.

In 1971 I had the opportunity to move from New York to Los Angeles. There I began to become conscious of new ideas about health. I started to change my life-style; I used whole grains, cut down on alcohol, and became very uncomfortable with my dependency on Valium. I stopped taking the drug, not realizing that

I was about to experience some very stressful drug detoxification symptoms. I became extremely disoriented and depressed, and the stomach pain was now more than I could live with.

When I sat on the grass with Harvey that day in 1975, looking into the clearest blue eyes I had ever seen, I was in the worst shape of my life. My body was breaking down physically; emotionally and psychologically I was a wreck. What I saw in Harvey's eyes and in his smooth tanned skin was a clear radiance that I had never seen before. He was so vibrant. He seemed so *clean!* And there was a lightness and joy in him that conveyed an ease with life that I had never known. This "health" that I was witnessing was so foreign to me that I felt overwhelmed and intimidated by it. It beckoned nonetheless, and I knew I had to go for it.

I wanted then more than anything in my life to learn what Harvey had learned. I wanted to shine with the same inner glow of confident health that I saw in him. I knew he had the answers for me. We began to spend nearly all our time together, and I began to learn that I could control my health. Two months later Harvey and I were married in the produce store where we had met and where he worked. It was an early morning candlelight ceremony, with dewy fresh fruits and vegetables surrounding us.

The location of that ceremony was a clear indication to me of what our life together would bring! Even so, the early years were frequently a painful trial of our strength and endurance. During the first year my body underwent a natural detoxification from the drugs I had been taking for much of my adult life. We were both taken by surprise by the extreme symptoms I experienced, which were very difficult to understand. At the time it was not known that these were symptoms of Valium withdrawal. Harvey's steadfastness during the ups and downs of my recovery never ceased to amaze me, but now that I know who he is, I realize that that steadfastness is Harvey's dedication to people's health. At the time, Natural Hygiene was still repressed and could not be publicly practiced, but Harvey pursued his profession anyway, giving his knowledge away to anyone who was interested. Those were lean years, but Harvey always said that if he just kept sharing what he knew and helping people, ultimately we would be taken care of.

The best part was that as we worked to develop the **Fit for Life** program and I moved toward vegetarianism, my lifelong stomach pain went away! By the time three years had passed, I felt strong enough to have a baby.

Our son was born at home, in one hour and twenty minutes, in the most natural way possible. I couldn't believe the energy I had during that pregnancy on our program. I wrote and completely illustrated a children's book. In the week prior to his birth, I worked night and day at the sewing machine, piecing together a new quilt cover for our bed, which was soon to welcome our precious little newcomer. I felt so great that forty-five minutes after he was born I was able to get up and bathe him myself. For someone whose health had been impaired for decades, this was an outstanding personal validation that health had been restored. It was also a validation of how well and strong a pregnant woman would feel on a hygienic diet.

People have asked me why we do this work. I was given a second chance at a whole new life of health, and that is why I do what I do. To be sick and drug dependent, in pain and out of control, is a living nightmare. No one who has been as unhealthy as I once was and who has been blessed enough to find the right answers could resist the call to share those answers with others. I really don't like knowing that people are suffering unnecessarily. That is why I do this work. Harvey *is* this work. That's why he does it.

CHAPTER 4
Review of the Principles

HARVEY:

The best way to demonstrate the value of something, *anything*, is to see it work. I mean *really* work. The real beauty of this information is that you don't have to take our word for any of it. In fact, *please don't!* You can easily prove for yourself how effective Natural Hygiene is. Because it is not complicated, because it is simple, because it is right in line with how your body works physiologically, you can easily verify for yourself how much it can benefit you. Regardless of what you are trying to achieve in the area of your health, certain fundamental principles can be used. The most basic of these deserve mentioning.

   Although these principles are described in detail in **Fit for Life**, it is important at least to review them. The approach to eating suggested by and described in **Fit for Life** is designed to accomplish the vital function of keeping the inside of your body clean and in tip-top working condition. When everything is fine on the inside, it is reflected on the outside. Even though **Fit for Life** addresses itself to energy enhancement and weight loss, its underlying goal is to cleanse the body. Keep in mind that your body, like anything else, can become dirty. If the inner workings of your car become all sludged up, it will not operate well until it is cleaned out. The same holds true for your body. Your insides can be impeded in their operations by uneliminated metabolic waste. You can either clean it out or ignore it. Of course, ignoring it, which in effect is allowing it to become cumulatively worse, makes about as much sense as jumping in front of a speeding truck.

How does your body become clogged up? By what is called a metabolic imbalance, or toxemia. Metabolism is the sum total of all the processes of the body in taking in food, using what it can, and getting rid of all the rest. Stated a little differently, metabolism is the building up (anabolism) and the breaking down (catabolism) of tissue in the body. When waste builds up faster than the body can eliminate it, you become toxic (or poisoned). The more toxic you are, the sicker you can become.

Every day your body breaks down somewhere between 300 and 800 *billion* cells. *Every day!* They *must* be eliminated. Why? Because, besides being no longer of use to the body, they are in fact toxic or poisonous to the body, which is where the word *toxemia* comes in. Spent cells are *dead*. If they are allowed to build and build at a faster rate than the body can eliminate them, then you will reach a point where they begin to poison the body and start damaging its internal organs. The breaking down of cells is not the only source of toxic material. There is another contributor to the level of toxemia with which the body must contend. *Food!* That's right, our old friend that we all know and love.

The people of the United States have a diet that has more than its fair share of highly processed and overcooked food. Because the body absorbs nonusable debris and toxic additives from the intestinal tract, there is a slow buildup of food residue and additives (which are toxic) that cannot be used by the body. This waste matter coupled with the toxic debris generated by the breaking down of cells is what creates a metabolic imbalance or toxemia.

You want to have a system as clean and free of toxic waste as possible. The key to living a long, disease-free, pain-free life lies in understanding and minimizing your level of toxemia.

Dr. John H. Tilden, who discovered the phenomenon of toxemia in the early 1920s, first laid out his findings in his landmark book *Toxemia Explained*. Dr. Tilden was a practicing physician who became disillusioned with the drugging approach to healing and turned to Natural Hygiene. The success he had employing the principles of Natural Hygiene with his patients totally convinced him of the worthiness and excellence of this field of science. He described the extent to which toxemia is the root cause of the many ailments we humans suffer. He demonstrated dramatically that, more often than not, **WHAT WE CALL DISEASE IS NOTHING MORE THAN THE BODY'S OWN EFFORT TO CLEANSE ITSELF OF TOXINS**.

Of course, the different problems are given different names, depending on the area of the body used for the elimination of this waste, creating the illusion that there are thousands of separate maladies when, in fact, most of them are one and the same, toxemia. To think that every single malady is a distinct and different problem is like thinking that water, dew, ice, frost, and snow all have a distinct and different essence. Envision a huge dike holding back a large body of water. This dike is made from bricks and mortar. Because of a prolonged rainstorm, the body of water becomes larger and larger, putting more and more pressure on the dike. Ultimately, the dike starts to succumb to the ever growing body of water. First, some of the mortar loosens and water starts to trickle through. Then some bricks pop out and water starts to come through those openings. With the breach, some of the structure itself starts to crack and crumble, and finally the foundation starts to erode, with the result that some of the structure collapses. Finally, the water level becomes so great that water simply surges right over the entire dike and floods it under.

The problem here is *not* the bricks or the mortar or the foundation or the structure itself. The problem is the ever increasing, vast amount of water that ultimately became more than the dike could withstand. There were not four problems, there was one: an overload of water.

To understand what happens with toxemia, imagine that your body is the dike and that the water is your level of toxemia. No matter how strong you are, no matter what measures you take to remain strong, an ever increasing level of toxemia will in time take its toll. It will overwhelm you and lay you low with some malady. This is why I say that the secret to longevity is in keeping your level of toxemia as low as possible.

When eating in accordance with the principles of **Fit for Life**, three crucially important objectives are achieved: (1) The eating experience remains a joyous one—you eat truly scrumptious food and do not have to follow any dogmatic, hard-to-live-with regimen; (2) a minimum of toxic food residue is generated in the system; (3) existing toxic waste is continuously expelled from the body. The principles are wonderfully easy to incorporate and almost immediately verify their effectiveness. One reason they work so well is that they are right in line with your natural body cycles, or what are called circadian rhythms. *Circadian* means "around the day.'' Circadian rhythms are the rhythmic occurrences of different functions of the body at certain times during each twenty-four-hour period. That these rhythms exist is disputed by no one. There have been hundreds of studies on them; a look at the index file at any medical library will list literally hundreds of books on circadian rhythms. In his studies on body rhythms, Dr. Charles Czeisler at Harvard Medical School has shown conclusively that **EVERY PHYSIOLOGICAL FUNCTION OF THE BODY OPERATES UNDER CERTAIN CLEARLY DEFINED CYCLES**.

In terms of the body's utilization of food, there are three distinct, approximately eight-hour cycles every twenty-four hours: appropriation (eating and digestion); assimilation (absorption and use); and elimination (of body wastes and food debris). These processes are not all exclusive of each other; all may occur simultaneously. However, one or another of them is predominant at different times.

In the 1940s, a Swedish scientist by the name of Are Waerland first laid out what hours of the day correspond with each cycle. He did this by determining the timing of the elimination cycle. By knowing when the elimination cycle is dominant, it is an easy matter to determine when the others in turn dominate, because they follow a natural order. Thus, the assimilation cycle must follow the appropriation cycle. If a blood test were to be taken every hour on the hour for twenty-four hours, it would show that the bloodstream is most heavily burdened with the by-products of metabolism during the hours between 4:00 A.M and 12:00 noon, indicating the stepped-up elimination cycle, because it is the blood that carries waste material to the four channels of elimination: the bowels, bladder, lungs, and skin. So the three cycles and their respective times are:

Appropriation cycle: 12:00 noon to 8:00 P.M.

Assimilation cycle: 8:00 P.M. to 4:00 A.M.

Elimination cycle: 4:00 A.M. to 12:00 noon

Although each of these three processes is always going on to some extent, the function of each is heightened during certain hours of the day. The appropriation cycle is the time of day when the body is most capable of efficiently taking in and digesting food. Assimilation is more intense while we are asleep, and it is during this cycle that the nutrients extracted from food and absorbed from the digestive tract are most heavily utilized. The elimination cycle is when the body has accomplished its other chores and rids itself of waste. *Elimination is not merely one bowel movement, it's the overall elimination of waste from all of the cells and tissues of the body.*

When you awaken in the morning with what is called "morning breath" or with a coated tongue, you are witnessing firsthand the effects of the elimination cycle. The elimination cycle is without question your greatest ally in the preservation of health and prevention of disease. This is a bold statement, I know. Nonetheless it is an accurate one. If the toxic waste that regularly builds up in your body can be effectively removed just as regularly, your system will remain clean, and health, rather than disease, will build. **THE PURPOSE OF THE ELIMINATION CYCLE IS TO REMOVE TOXIC WASTE FROM THE BODY.** It is literally your body's built-in mechanism for cleaning itself, and it proceeds daily, *automatically.* You don't have to force it into action or take something to get it to work any more than you have to force yourself to breathe or to blink your eyes. Your only obligation is to allow this cycle to function freely and not thwart it in any way. Interfering with its operations is tantamount to *asking to become sick.* Ways to help it or to hinder it will be made clear to you shortly.

As stated earlier, the **Fit for Life** principles take into consideration these physiological cycles and are designed to facilitate their optimum operation. There are only three principles that relate to eating.

1. THE PRINCIPLE OF HIGH-WATER-CONTENT FOOD

The hygienic approach to eating is designed to cleanse the inside of your body of accumulated waste matter. Your body needs to be cleaned with the same substance you would use to clean anything else, be it your car, your clothes, your garbage can or your driveway—**WATER!** Without water, you would have a tough time cleaning any of these things. (Try cleaning your car with a slice of pizza.)

The water found in all fruits and vegetables has a unique quality.

Unlike plain drinking water, the water in fruits and vegetables fulfills a two-part role that is of incalculable importance. First, it is a transport medium for nutrients. All of the vitamins and minerals and other elements inherent in fruits and vegetables are extracted from the cellulose and fiber and carried by the water into the intestines, where they are absorbed and utilized by the body. Second, this same water, after dropping off the nutrients, picks up waste matter and flushes it from the body. Because of the extreme importance of this twofold operation of bringing in nutrients and taking out waste, the importance of consuming a sufficient amount of high-water-content foods (fruits and vegetables) is self-evident. Your diet does not have to be exclusively high-water-content foods, but certainly there must be a fair share of those. The person whose diet is mostly high-water-content food, as opposed to food that has had much or all of its water removed by processing or cooking or both, is undoubtedly creating the environment for health and longevity, far more so than the individual whose diet is predominately low-water-content food.

The inside of your body deserves no less attention than the outside. Most people I have met take a bath or a shower every day, or at least every other day. Imagine if you will the effluvia that would emanate from the body of a person who had not washed in, oh, let's say six months. You know that the odor would be so foul, so offensive, that you would not be able to approach within six feet without becoming nauseated. Bring this person into a closed room and it's "gas masks all around, thank you." Well, my dear friends, there are great numbers of people living in this country right now who have not washed the *inside* of their bodies in *decades!* Small wonder that 4000 people die *every day* in the United States from cancer and heart disease. Their inner bodies are so dirty and overladen with waste matter that has accumulated over a period of years that they simply cease to be able to function. But don't panic if you are one of those who have neglected to wash out the inner body regularly, because it is *never* too late to do the right thing. Given the opportunity, your body is ever alert to cleanse, repair, and maintain itself.

In the pages of this book, you will be presented with the tools to help you do just that. One of those tools, and a critical one at that, is the consumption of a sufficient amount of high-water-content foods, fresh fruits and vegetables.

2. THE PRINCIPLE OF PROPER FOOD COMBINING

Eating foods in combinations that are compatible in digestive chemistry is mandatory for optimum health. Combining foods properly works, and that can be proven by *anyone* in a short period of time merely by giving it a try. There are those—mostly people who have *never* tried it—who say this principle is not scientific, which is bullfish. As a result of the Flexner Report and medical monopoly at the turn of this century, science in health care was overnight defined as anything "medical" and relating to drug therapy. How can that be? The proponents of one philosophy in a given subject simply cannot *grab* the word "science" and make it their own simply because of political and economic clout! **SCI-ENCE IS THAT WHICH WORKS!** Of course, this simple, commonsense definition of science may be too obvious for the overeducated or those educated beyond their intelligence. Never-theless, proper food combining *is* scientific because *it works*, and there is not a soul on earth who can demonstrate otherwise. Food combining, it is true, has *nothing* to do with *medical* science which is based on drug therapy, but it is an important principle in the science of Natural Hygiene. The same people today who are claim-ing that food combining is unscientific, ten years ago protested that a high fiber diet could cause liver cancer. Ten years from now they'll be telling you to combine your foods properly. Why are the "experts" always the last to catch on? After suffering from excruciating digestive pains for more than two decades, proper food combining eliminated them in twenty-four hours for me per-sonally, and since the publication of **Fit for Life** in June 1985, we have received thousands of unsolicited letters of testimony from people all across the United States describing similar positive re-sults. If you have not succumbed to the art of complication, you too can start to reap (if you have not already) the many rewards of combining your foods according to the way your digestive tract works rather than according to the four basic food lobbies.

Have you ever felt tired after eating? Do birds fly? Is water wet? Ever notice that the bigger the meal, the more tired you are af-terwards? Remember as a kid being told that you must not go swimming after lunch or you would get cramps?

The reason you are tired after eating is because the digestion of conventional food takes such a tremendous amount of energy to accomplish. In fact, it takes more energy than *anything* else you can do. The way the stomach is designed, food is to remain there approximately three hours for digestion before proceeding on to the small intestine. Proper food combining is a means of ensuring that the food you eat does not stay in the stomach any longer than it should.

Just like anything else, the digestive tract has certain limitations. I wouldn't ask you to jump off a three-story building, because you could severely damage yourself. I wouldn't ask you to drive a car over 200 miles an hour into an embankment, because you could get killed. A friend of mine, working on a construction site, fell three stories and landed on the edge of a pool and got up and walked away. Shirley Muldowney, a professional race car driver, slammed into a wall at 220 miles an hour in 1985, and a year later she was preparing to go back to racing. The body does have the ability to survive punishment, but why push it? How many falls and how many crashes can one expect to live through? Yes, people can still function even though they eat practically anything in any combination as long as it fits into their mouths. But, *is it appropriate*? Let's examine that.

The archaic notion that we need to eat from each of the four basic food groups at every meal is probably responsible for more digestive difficulties than any other dietary habit we have. If you look at any other animal living in nature, in the wild, you will see that there are very few "seven-course meals." In fact, none! We are the only species on earth to so complicate our meals. Elsewhere in nature, meals are very simple—usually only *one* food at a time. Ever see a rabbit reaching for Rolaids? Ever see a tiger with Tums? A giraffe with Gelusil? Or a Panda with Pepto Bismol? Ridiculous, isn't it?

Why is it that the people of the United States spend over $2 billion a year on digestive aids? *Why?* Could it possibly be that the food in those anguished digestive tracts is contributing to the problem? *Could it be anything else?* If a hundred balloons were blown up beyond their capacity and all exploded, would you attribute that to anything other than too much air? If you took ten perfectly running cars and started to run them on kerosene instead of gasoline until every one of them became inoperable, would you recognize it was because the wrong type of fuel was used?

Since the primary function of the human digestive system is to deal with the food (at least 50 tons over the average lifetime) that is taken into the body on a regular basis and most chronic digestive ailments occur *after* the consumption of food, how much sense does it take to realize that it is the *food* that is the problem? However, more often than not, it isn't so much the food itself as the *combination* of various food groups, thrown together haphazardly and indiscriminately in the stomach at the same time, that is the cause of the difficulty.

Here's why.

Most digestion of food occurs in the stomach by digestive juices. The type of digestive juice secreted for the digestion of one type of food is of no value in digesting another type of food. In fact, some digestive juices cancel each other out when forced into contact with each other. Sadly, the traditional way of eating in this country almost always puts food together in combinations that guarantee digestive difficulties—for example, meat and potatoes, fish and rice, chicken and noodles, eggs and toast, cheese and bread, cereal and milk.

Right about now you may very well be saying, "What do you mean? I've eaten those foods together all my life." So did I when I walked around feeling as if a red-hot knife were permanently imbedded in my gut. Here's the simple reason why: Every one of the examples listed above is a protein and starch combination, and **PROTEINS AND STARCHES CANNOT DIGEST EFFICIENTLY IN THE STOMACH AT THE SAME TIME**. Protein, including all flesh foods (meaning beef, chicken, fish, pork, lamb, or *any* other animal), dairy products, and nuts demand a digestive juice that is acidic in its nature. Starches such as breads, pastas, grains, potatoes (cooked), and cereals demand a digestive juice that is alkaline in its nature. Anyone with the most elementary knowledge of chemistry will tell you that an acid and an alkali in combination will neutralize each other. When you eat meat and potatoes simultaneously and they enter your stomach together, acid is secreted to break down the steak and alkali is secreted to break down the potatoes.* The food is in the stomach for the purpose of digestion, but with the acid and alkali cancelling each other out, *there are no working digestive juices available to do the job*.

So what happens to the food? Remember that the way the human

---

*Actually, only a small amount of alkali is secreted in the stomach. However, when chewing a starch in the mouth, the saliva saturates the starch with an alkali that is then swallowed to come into contact with the acid.

stomach is designed, food is to remain there approximately three hours before being passed on to the small intestine. However, if the food is not broken down, it sits and, unfortunately, it spoils. Ever eat a meal and six, seven, or eight hours later still have that "heavy" feeling in the stomach? That is because the food was not digested, due to one incompatible combination or another, usually a protein being eaten with a starch. This creates a mess in the stomach so foul that you certainly would not want to be there. Undigested protein putrefies and undigested starch ferments, resulting in acid indigestion, gas, flatulence, heartburn, upset stomach . . . and voilà! Bring on the Rolaids, Tums, Gelusil, Pepto Bismol, Digel, Alka Seltzer, Bromo Seltzer, Gaviscon, Gas-X, Tempo, Mylanta, milk of magnesia, Maalox, Maalox-Plus, Riopan, Amphogel, Simeco, etc., etc.

All of the digestive complaints that prompt taking any of those drugs to quell the pain result from food rotting and fermenting in the stomach. Now, for some reason, all the dietitians and nutritionists with stomachs full of rotting food can't stand to hear that their food *can* rot in there. They dislike hearing this so much that some of them insist (in a tone that would imply they actually know what they are talking about) that "food *can't* rot in the stomach." Of course, this includes only those who have had their common sense surgically removed, as it were. (I do not mean to imply that all dietitians and nutritionists have rejected physiological truth. In fact, many have contacted us to report how successful applying this new information has been in their practices.)

Anyone who makes the statement that food can't rot in the stomach is guilty of the most abysmal, unforgivable ignorance of physiology. It would be one thing for such a statement to be made by someone in a field that doesn't require a knowledge of the workings of the human body, but for a supposed authority on diet and nutrition, such drivel is unpardonable. I wonder if any of these "experts" have ever thrown up. Now, even a dietitian knows that regurgitated food is expelled from the stomach—not the bowels or intestines or esophagus, but the stomach. And when food (which should have passed out of the stomach in approximately three hours) is thrown up six, eight, or even ten hours after being eaten, something is very wrong. And how does this thrown-up food smell? Pleasant or vile? Appetizing or *rotten*? It smells rotten because it *is* rotten. Unappealing, I know, but *true*!

Incredibly, even the evidence of food rejected by the body isn't enough to convince the more hardheaded of these "authorities." A case in point too classical not to relate comes from a panel debate I was involved in. One of the participants who didn't think food could rot in the stomach was questioning the validity of food combining and stated that there was no scientific evidence to back it up. I pointed out that there was an abundance of scientific evidence to back it up, starting with Dr. Ivan Pavlov, one of the greatest research scientists who ever lived, a Nobel laureate no less, who did groundbreaking research in this area, backing up our information on food combining. This was immediately dismissed as irrelevant, even though the "expert" admitted having no knowledge of it—a classic example of "my mind is made up, don't confuse me with the facts."

What data was this rejection based on? It didn't happen to jibe with what the "expert" *wanted* to be true! And yet, to this day, Dr. Pavlov's work has *never* been disproven.

It was very difficult to take seriously anything this person had to say after that. I mean, how seriously would you take a person who had never even *seen* a baseball game, telling Reggie Jackson that his batting stance was all wrong? The point is that some people, no matter what, insist on holding on to their cherished beliefs regardless of indisputable evidence showing the contrary to be true. But you know what? There are still people who insist that the world is flat. There are people who insist that the Holocaust never happened. And there are people who insist that food cannot rot in the stomach. Fine. Someone has to shell out those billions of dollars to support the antacid industry. Just don't let yourself be one of them. Let the "experts" who do not believe in food combining have the stomachaches.

But what about those who regularly eat these undesirable combinations with no recognizable manifestations of digestive discomfort? Well, the human body *is* remarkably adaptable. It has the ability to overcome quite a bit of abuse and still function with apparent ease. But do these people ever experience other discomforts? Headaches? Lethargy? Skin eruptions? Backaches? Colds? Sleeplessness? These can also be the result of impaired and inefficient digestion. The effect of indiscriminately combining foods, which is contrary to the way the digestive tract is designed to operate, is taking its toll on the American population. Both the nonprescription and prescription drug industries attest to that. But the entire situation can be avoided with ease and simplicity. Moreover, you can have obvious evidence of the effectiveness of proper food combining in a short period of time.

Simply *try* combining correctly. If you wish to have a steak or piece of chicken or fish, merely forego having a starch (potato, rice, bread, pasta) at *that* meal. Combine with the meat an assortment of well-prepared vegetables—steamed, sautéed, grilled, baked, or however you like them—and complement this with a nice mixed salad. There is no need to go hungry or not enjoy the foods you like. Just do not eat them all at the same time. If it is potatoes you desire, great! Have a baked potato or yam *as a main course*, with an assortment of vegetables and a salad. Or perhaps you want a nice pasta dish. No problem. Have it with a vegetable sauce and a salad. If you are anything like me, then you just love mashed potatoes with gravy and biscuits. Oh yes! But, you say, that is *so-o-o-o-o* fattening. Wrong! It is fattening only when eaten with roast beef or some other protein. That's what makes it a problem. Eaten with vegetables and a salad instead of the traditional meat, you can enjoy "forbidden" favorites like these and *not* sabotage your health and longevity by contributing to the toxic load in your body. (And make it a vegetable gravy, for which we have included a recipe, of course.) Food that spoils in your digestive tract supplies no nutrition; it only increases your level of toxemia.

Food combining works, of that you can be absolutely certain. But please, **DON'T BELIEVE US**. We are not asking anyone to believe anything. **PROVE IT TO YOURSELF.** It is extremely easy to do so. Eat all your meals for one week the traditional way. In other words, mix all the food groups together at each meal just as some dietitians and nutritionists advocate. Then for one week follow the suggestion of not mixing a protein and a starch at the same meal. (Not even the most backward-thinking dietitian would suggest that there is danger in not having a potato *with* your steak.) At the end of that second week, you will know without any possible doubt what proper food combining has to offer. If you really want to confirm how effective food combining is, after one week of properly combining meals go back to mixing proteins and starches at your meals. That will be the clincher.

You see, this has nothing to do with belief. It is physiology, plain and simple. It is how your body works, and as soon as you start to respect its efforts, rather than thwart them, health and vitality are the result.

Does food combining work for everyone? Yes. Absolutely everyone. Human beings have what is called a species-specific digestive tract. The inner working of all species of animals are identical in operation within their species. The digestive tracts of all bees anywhere in the world are exactly the same. The digestive tracts of all giraffes, horses, kangaroos, wombats, gorillas, or humans operate exactly like all others of their species. Nowhere will you find any college text on physiology that teaches that humans have digestive faculties naturally different from each other. Nowhere will you find one iota of evidence that humans differ in their biological equipment. What goes on in the stomach of one person is identical to what goes on in the stomach of any other person anywhere on earth. This is why I say it has nothing to do with belief. Even if you refuse to believe in food combining, it will still work for you, in spite of your skepticism. It will even work for those dietitians and nutritionists who have been educated so far beyond their competence level that they know a whole lot that is not so (even though some would rather be mauled by a wild animal than admit it).

Proper food combining *cannot* be disproved, and I challenge anyone to do so.

Here, in the final analysis, is the crucial point. It does you no good to hear the experts argue up and down about who's right. It is the easiest thing in the world to have one say, ''I think it's true,'' and find someone else to say, ''No, it's not.'' How do *you* know what's right? Prove it for yourself in the greatest laboratory on earth: your body. If you properly combine your foods for one week and feel enormously better and are able to throw away your medication for digestive ailments, will any expert with any amount of data convince you to return to the habits that were causing you pain? We ask for nothing more than your honest evaluation of a simple one-week test that can be carried out with the greatest of ease.* Remember, **SCIENCE IS THAT WHICH WORKS!**

---

*Please check in the back of this book to see how you can obtain the **Fit for Life** Proper Food Combining Chart.

3. THE PRINCIPLE OF
THE CORRECT CONSUMPTION OF FRUIT

Upon reading this, you may ask, "What do you mean the *correct* consumption of fruit? Correct is, you put it in your mouth and chew it up."

That's true enough, but it is also imperative that you understand the way your digestive tract operates. There are very specific body conditions in which fruit can be most effectively and efficiently utilized. Fruit has a totally unique quality with respect to its digestion.

As I pointed out in the description of proper food combining, food needs to remain in the stomach approximately three hours. There is one exception: fruit. Fruit is the *only* food on earth that requires *no* digestion in the stomach. It contains its own digestive enzymes and, when ripe, is virtually predigested, requiring only about twenty to thirty minutes in the stomach before passing on to the intestines, where its nutrients are absorbed and utilized by the body.

Be aware of the fact that fruit contains *all* of the necessary nutrients required by your body for sustaining life. That includes glucose from carbohydrates for energy and vitamins, minerals, fatty acids, and amino acids for the building of protein. This is where the word *correct* comes into play. For these building blocks of life to be made available for use by the body, two essential prerequisites must be met. First, because of fruit's rather delicate nature, it must be consumed only in its fresh, ripe state. Whether it is fruit juice or the whole food, fresh is the *only* way it can be of significant value to the body. Canned or cooked fruit or pasteurized juice (such as juice made from concentrate) will ferment in your stomach, turning to acid and actually contributing to the body's toxic load, whereas *fresh* fruit and fruit juices have the effect of assisting the body in *cleansing* itself of toxic residue.

Second, in order for it to pass quickly through the stomach as required by the body, **FRUIT SHOULD BE EATEN ALONE ON AN EMPTY STOMACH, NOT WITH ANYTHING OR IMMEDIATELY FOLLOWING ANYTHING.** The traditional habit of eating fruit with a meal or having it as a dessert is precisely why people have so many misconceptions about fruit being fattening, acid-forming, too high in calories, or detrimental to hypoglycemics. If fruit is forced to remain in the stomach with other longer-digesting foods, it quickly ferments and interferes with the digestion of the other foods in the stomach. Under these circumstances, fruit does indeed have negative repercussions. However, eaten correctly, meaning *alone on an empty stomach*, fresh fruits and juices can only have a positive effect on your health.

Prove this for yourself. Eat several meals including fruit at the end of each meal, and then eat several meals eating the fruit first and allowing twenty to thirty minutes to elapse before eating the remainder of the meal. See if there is not a recognizable difference in the way you feel.

Here is where fruit performs its greatest service to your health and longevity. If you have not already read **Fit for Life**, you're in for a shocker. I'll just come right out with it: **EATING A TRADITIONAL BREAKFAST IS ONE OF THE MOST UN-HEALTHFUL DIETARY HABITS IN EXISTENCE IN THIS COUNTRY.** All that propaganda about breakfast being the most important meal of the day is a bunch of commercial hooey. This propaganda is swallowed hook, line, and sinker by everyone not having an understanding of human physiology. It serves commercial interests. Even the dietitians and nutritionists, who one would expect to know better, have fallen victim to the ploy perpetrated by the cereal producers in the early part of this century to bamboozle people into eating their products every day upon awakening in the morning. Breakfast is the most important meal of the day *to skip!* Your own common sense, a commodity sorely lacking in today's "experts," will bear out the validity of this statement.

You will recall our pointing out how much energy is required for the digestion of conventional foods. Remember, *digestion takes more body energy than any other function*. Food put into the stomach becomes the number-one priority, and the body must proceed with digestion immediately. It takes a huge amount of energy, as evidenced by the tradition of afternoon siestas and the warnings not to go swimming after lunch so energy won't have to be divided between digestion and physical activity.

What is *your* usual inclination after eating? To rest or to run around? Perhaps you remember last Thanksgiving? After somehow finding a way to get just "one more bite down," did you feel like doing jumping jacks or like communing with the couch? When you wake up in the morning, you have at your beck and call more energy right then than at any other time of day. If you eat a "hearty breakfast," you are going to use up a huge quantity of your available energy. That is where the all-American coffee break comes in. After eating a traditional breakfast, which is a slap in the face to the principle of proper food combining, the body is working so hard dealing with it, using up its energy, that it's straight to the coffee machine for that "pick me up." The tragedy here is that the energy called upon to digest the breakfast is the energy that was to be used to fuel the elimination cycle. It is diverted to the stomach instead, thus severely impeding the all-important daily cleansing cycle. If this scenario is played out every day, that means this critical cycle is *never* allowed to perform its health-producing functions. Ill health is the only possible consequence.

By regularly thwarting the elimination cycle you lay the foundation for and guarantee diminished health. Enter fruit, the one food that demands practically *no digestive energy*. It is the perfect food to eat in the morning. It is the *only* food that should be eaten in the morning. If you wish your elimination cycle to properly cleanse your body—and why wouldn't you—**THE SINGLE MOST BENEFICIAL HABIT YOU CAN POSSIBLY CULTIVATE IS THE HABIT OF CONSUMING EXCLUSIVELY *FRESH* FRUIT AND *FRESH* FRUIT JUICE FROM THE TIME YOU AWAKEN IN THE MORNING UNTIL 12:00 NOON.** Exclusively! Anything else will stay in your stomach and hamper the elimination cycle.

Of course, this does not mean that if on occasion you don't adhere to this strategy, all is wasted. No, no! However, the less often you violate this principle, the better. Even if you eat fruits in the morning only two or three times a week, that is better than nothing. But before accepting or rejecting any of this, try it! As we've said, it's the easiest thing in the world to verify for yourself. Don't believe us. Simply try it for a week and see if you don't feel better. Do it for one week, then don't do it for the next week. You'll see! You don't need an expert to tell you that you feel better. You'll know! Nothing succeeds like success, and there is no better proof of something's worthiness than good results.

The reason for reviewing the three body cycles and these three eating principles is that they are an integral part of understanding and utilizing the elements of health. When you look at a brick building, you don't notice without closer scrutiny the mortar between each brick holding the structure together. The above described principles are to Natural Hygiene and the elements of health what mortar is to brick. For a more in-depth description of these principles, please refer to **Fit for Life**.

PART

II

The Elements of Health

CHAPTER 5

Introducing the Elements of Health

HARVEY:

Isn't life glorious? Consider for a moment the beauty and perfection of nature. Think about the constant tendency of life toward what is best for it, in both the plant and animal kingdoms. All around us are examples of the indescribable wisdom and power of Creation, and at the very apex of Creation stands a glowing tribute to the Infinite Designer—*the* masterpiece of Creation, the human body.

A marvel of tireless performance, the human body was constructed for health and happiness. The ultimate achievement of life on earth, the most praiseworthy accomplishment possible, is to live a life of joy and robust vitality—a life filled with enthusiasm, well-being, boundless energy, and a zest for living that is constant and unshakable. It is living totally in tune with life's grand symphony! What a delight!

Is it possible? Is it possible for children to go through their childhood without being tormented by every problem imaginable, from ear infections to colds, from skin rashes to stomach distress? Is it possible for them to be free of tantrums? Is it possible for adolescents to enter adulthood without first suffering from headaches, stomachaches, splotchy skin, and excess weight? Is it possible for them to be well balanced and spared the all-too-common emotional roller coaster? Is it possible to reach maturity and enjoy seniorship free from the hundreds of aches and pains that appear to be inevitable and unavoidable? Is it possible to live a pain-free, stress-free, and disease-free existence filled with loving relationships?

It is possible! Without question. And **WE ALL CAN DO IT!**

MARILYN:

The human species has been on this planet for many millions of years. Recorded history only extends back 6000 years, and the recorded history of health care is only 3000 years old. If anyone tells you that all we've ever known about our health is encompassed in the brief 3000-year history that modern medicine claims as its own, believe it if you wish, but it's not true. We once knew much more about survival than we know now. Our ancestors made it through all those millions of years without *any* of the "advancements" we now "enjoy." That they were strong and able to endure is not open to debate. That was no weakling who tamed the first horse! If they had kept coming up against the challenge of Nature and losing, *how would we be here?* They lived in harmony with Nature, not at odds with it. They possessed a wealth of *instinctive* knowledge that allowed them to survive, reproduce, and raise their young.

What was that instinctive body of knowledge? We can begin to have a sense of it when we consider how the ancients lived: in fresh air and sunshine, drinking pure water, resting and sleeping when the sun set, relying on the foods Nature provided, living physically active lives, living in interdependence and community.

All of these natural elements determined the instinctive way of life of our species. We are heir to that great body of instinctive knowledge from that way of life, and even though civilization has placed between us and Nature a huge mass of unintelligible technology, we still have this knowledge deep within us. We have been drawn further and further from our natural endowment and innate understanding of how to live, but, despite it all, our inherent nature as a species has always survived in the sometimes resonant, sometimes weakened voices of the few who, luckily for us, refused to surrender the ancient memory. Today, the voices are resonant and we can all hear them if we choose.

In Greece, around 1500 B.C., we find the temples of Asklepios, the great Greek healer. The temples were run by priests. They were beautiful, airy structures, distinguished by their healthful locations, situated on hillsides overlooking the sea, in groves, or near mineral hot springs. These "hospitals of the day" served hundreds of thousands of Greeks for nearly 1500 years. They give us great insight into the care and treatment received by the sick at the height of one of the greatest civilizations in recorded history. Many historical descriptions remain to give us a clear picture of the effective health care measures utilized by the perfect Greek bodies, once living beings, who are now immortalized for us in stone. Victor W. Robinson, M.D., tells us in *The Story of Medicine* that the temples were located in such beautiful surroundings that "the sight alone often served to bring the first smile of hope to the weary invalid."

Like our ancient ancestors, the priests knew to rely on what nature provides. They understood that the natural biological needs of life that are part of our species's heritage—fresh air, water, sunshine, food, rest and sleep, peaceful and beautiful surroundings, exercise, and a loving, supportive emotional environment—had to be met in order for the ailing to recover. That we in the present have forgotten this is aptly described by Dr. Herbert M. Shelton, one of the resonant voices for health reform in this century, in his book *Rubies in the Sand*.

> During the last century we located our hospitals amid the tan yards and slaughter pens and other places that emitted foul stenches. Today we locate them in crowded cities on busy streets where exists the greatest concentration of carbon monoxide and traffic noise, and they are as noisy inside as out. A modern hospital is like Grand Central Station, all noise and hubbub, and is filled with smoking physicians, nurses, orderlies, patients and visitors. Soft drinks are sold on each floor and everybody guzzles those popular poisons. The stench of chemicals offends the nose while tranquilizers substitute for quietness. It is to the eternal credit of the priests that they provided the pleasing perfumes of flowers instead of the foul stenches of drugs and melody of music instead of the roar of the buffing machines in the halls.

From the decline of the Asklepian temples in 400 A.D., we plunged into a progressively darker and darker age during which our bodies were regarded more and more as our enemies. We were taught to focus on the afterlife rather than this one. After millions of years of survival with *only nature* to rely on, in sickness and in health, through the greatest civilization in history with its understanding of *nature's role* in healing, it was during this dark era when we came to accept poisons of all kinds as healing agents. We overruled our instincts and emotionally and intellectually began to trust that poisons administered to us as medicines were somehow magically transformed into miraculous healing agents. Three hundred years ago, in order to restore health, we swallowed bats' blood, cow and horse dung, bees, eels, spiders, snakes, mice, the urine of bulls and goats, powdered mummy, wood lice, animal intestines, human saliva, afterbirth, menstrual blood, human excrement and urine, skulls, brains, hair, blood, earwax, finger- and toenails, and mothers' milk. We are still doing it today! Such substances as putrefied monkey kidneys, animal glands and livers, pig or cow hormones, urine from pregnant mares, pus from infected horses and cows, infant foreskins, amniotic fluid, placentas, Spanish flies, snake venom, and mustard gas, have been used recently and are used presently in vaccines, serums, ''health'' supplements, drugs, cosmetic rejuvenators, and in chemotherapy. We still use *anything* that is poisonous as experimental cures on the sick, and all too often the side-effects of these ''cures'' produce illnesses that are worse than the original disease.

Clearly, some pretty amazing things have been done to our bodies in the name of health care. For centuries, bleeding was the most popular healing technique. Leeches were applied to *restore* health! In the last century, medical doctors withheld water from the sick, thinking it would harm them. Fresh air was feared. (Hygienic doctors campaigned against this ignorance and finally won, notwithstanding that they were viciously attacked as quacks by the doctors who disagreed with them.) Dr. Oliver Wendell Holmes, commenting on the stupidity of treatment prescribed by his fellow doctors, once wrote, ''God gave his creatures light and air and water flowing from the skies. Man locks them in a stifling lair and wonders why his brother dies.'' Because some doctors believed fruits and vegetables *caused* disease, they were *banned* at the turn of the century. Today the deadliest and most feared substance in our society, radiation, is used on those who are sickest. Instinctively, we recoil. Intellectually, we are asked to accept.

In the United States we have more hospitals and more doctors than in any other country in the world. Yet our workers lead the world in the degenerative diseases! Twelve percent of our children are born with birth defects. Our old people are drugged with an average of *thirteen* prescription drugs annually. We're transplanting organs like we would transplant trees in our gardens.

HARVEY:

When one reflects on the fact that nearly *half a trillion* dollars are spent annually on health care in the United States and, despite this, heart disease and cancer still take 4000 lives *every single day*, one begins to wonder where we have gone wrong. When you add to this the fact that millions of people suffer from arthritis, diabetes, emotional breakdowns, and diseases of the skin, digestive tract, kidneys, liver, prostate—in fact, every area of the anatomy—it is doubly hard to accept. Unfortunately, we have come to look upon impaired health as normal. It is not! *Health is normal* and should be so. That it isn't is a sad commentary upon the status of our species. For such a low state of health to be tolerated and declared normal is an insult to our intelligence.

Good health is our birthright! If we do not possess it, it is not the fault of our bodies or the laws governing them. **THE TRUE CAUSE OF IMPAIRED HEALTH LIES IN OUR FAILURE TO COMPLY WITH THE LAWS AND REQUIREMENTS OF LIFE. ALL HEALTH PROBLEMS ARISE FROM THE ABUSE OF NATURAL LAWS, NOT FROM THE CORRECT USE OF THEM.** Natural laws cannot be broken. They can be abused, violated, or ignored, but not broken. To say that someone broke a law of nature is merely a convenient word form, like saying the sun rises and sets, which it does not do. If a man were to fall from a twenty-story building, he would not be *breaking* the law of gravity, he would be *illustrating* it. How you are affected by natural law depends on the conditions under which they operate—conditions that *you* create. You, therefore, can control how you are affected by natural law.

The automobile is a fantastic invention. You can either use it or abuse it. If you drive your car prudently, it can be of great service to you. If you choose to drive abusively, you can wrap it around a tree and be killed. So it is with natural laws. You can live according to the laws of reality and reap the rewards or ignore and abuse them and endure the consequences. It all depends on how you choose to interact with them.

Health is spontaneous. The organs of the body are designed to perform normally and healthfully from the start and to continue doing so throughout life. If not deranged or prevented from doing so as a result of violations of natural law, they will function with all the regularity of the sun, in a natural vigorous manner, because they cannot do otherwise. In fact, the organs of the body will perform their functions normally with less difficulty than they do abnormally. It takes fewer muscles to smile than to frown. It is not difficult to breathe or to breathe right or enough or to breathe wholesome air, but it *is* difficult to refrain from breathing or to breathe too little or to breathe polluted, noxious air.

The power and adaptability of the body is astonishing. It is often able to continue functioning in spite of being habitually abused. Even after becoming sick, it still endures the abuse and goes on year after year until one wonders how it stays alive. It requires great and long-continued abuse of the body to reduce its functions sufficiently to produce the state of impaired health known as disease.

Life is naturally healthy! Under the proper conditions of life, health is as inevitable as the rise and fall of the tide. *It is easier to have good health than it is to have poor health*. You don't just get sick. You have to work hard at it. You have to forsake the very needs of life *consistently* to get sick. However, the greatest, most powerful force on earth, natural law, is on your side to help you achieve and maintain the highest level of health possible. It would be well for us never to forget that we are a part of nature, not above it and not separate from it. There are natural laws that govern life on earth. The closer we live by these laws, the better off we are. This is just plain common sense. Were we not so conditioned, propagandized, pressured, and bulldozed into forsaking our natural inclinations, we would know *inherently* how to care for ourselves properly in order to live the joyous life of well-being we deserve.

LIVING HEALTHFULLY IS NOT AN ART THAT WE MUST LEARN, IT IS AN INSTINCTIVE WAY OF LIFE TO WHICH WE MUST RETURN! We already possess what we need. Just as a bee constructs a comb without ever having studied engineering and a cow transforms grass and grain into milk without any knowledge of chemistry, so too are we naturally equipped and able to live healthfully. A newly hatched chick, without being taught the value of corn or the danger of a fox, eats one and runs from the other. We have from birth similar instinctive apparatus to guide us on our journey through life. Deep within the human constitution lie indelible laws of nature that should guide us in the conduct of our lives. We merely have to get back in tune with them. They have existed since the beginning of time and will continue to exist as long as life lasts. Before there were physicians, before there were hospitals, before there were nutritionists or dietitians, before there were many contrasting schools of thought, there was natural law.

SCIENCE FAILS US IF IT CAN TELL US THE CAUSE OF SPOTS ON THE SUN BUT NOT EXPLAIN TO US THE LAWS OF LIFE AND THE CONSEQUENCES OF VIOLATING THEM. Laws are laws and *must* be obeyed. They govern what we need *biologically*. All species living on earth have biological needs. We humans need to understand our biological needs in order to be able to satisfy them. Otherwise we become biological outlaws and pay the penalty of the outlaw. In this case the penalty is ill health, suffering, and premature death. Understanding what our biological needs are and what we are biologically adapted to is the key to health, vitality, and longevity. Regardless of the ever changing views and systems and the coming and going of different theories, the needs of human beings as a species are permanent, exact, and unchanging.

The fact is that *ways of life that ignore the natural laws of life are the causes of poor health*, and there is no escape from this obvious conclusion. **THE WAY TO RESTORE HEALTH AND INSURE ITS PRESERVATION IS TO LIVE HEALTHFULLY.** The very same natural elements that were necessary to construct us in the first place will keep us healthy and support the restoration of our health if we lose it! They are necessary in a state of vigorous health and they are necessary in a state of impaired health, for *they are our biological needs of life!* These needs do not depend on some accidental discovery or upon something stumbled upon in blind groping or even upon the results of painstaking research. Rather they depend on something that has been with us since the beginning of existence. They are rooted in life itself. What are they? They are the same elements the ancients depended on: air, water, food, sunshine, exercise, rest and sleep, and love.

Equally important are cleanliness, pleasant surroundings, and quiet moments. The rewards for the proper use of these elements cannot be bought and hoarded by the richest person in the world, yet they can be had for free by the poorest. They are priceless. If you were drowning, you would take one more lungful of air over a treasure chest laden with diamonds, rubies, and emeralds. If you were dying of thirst and on the brink of collapse, you would take a glass of cool water over all the gold in Fort Knox. Sunshine is more prized and precious than all of the finest art the world has ever created.

When we were created everything we would need to live out our lives healthfully and happily was also created. We can either utilize what was put here for our benefit or ignore our needs and just hope for the best. Personally, I'd rather take the hope out of it and make it more of a sure thing. That becomes a possibility when one lives a healthy life-style. The fact is that many health seekers attempt to regain or improve health by using partial or incomplete measures. Instead of a *total* program they adopt only one or two elements of a health-building way of life and treat them as a hobby. So you find people who eat relatively well but never exercise, and they can't understand why they just don't feel fantastic. Or there are those who exercise a lot but then ignore the need to rest sufficiently, and they don't eat particularly well either. They feel the exercise should be enough to ensure health, just as the first group thinks diet alone will do it. That's not the case. A balance of all the elements of health is what is required in your life-style . . . *permanently*—that is, if you wish to be *permanently* healthy.

Full health requires—no, demands—a *full* program of healthful living, and that means more than just diet or just exercise or just mental equilibrium. None of the needs for a healthy life should be neglected, nor should they be overindulged. Common sense reveals this to be so and, as we have said and will repeat again, common sense, logic, and instinct are tools we must never cease to rely on. These tools must never be considered mere relics to be thrown onto the junk heap of the past, to be discussed but not utilized. They may have been suppressed, but they have not been extinguished. One should not expect to harvest figs from a thistle bush. If thistles are planted, then thistles will grow. Nor should one expect to harvest watermelons after planting a briar patch. If vibrant health is your desire, then *that must be what you cultivate.*

Living healthfully today ensures a healthy tomorrow. If by the daily avoidance of the elements of health only the seeds of ill health are cultivated, then ill health is the *only* possible consequence. **HEALTH WILL AUTOMATICALLY FOLLOW IN THE WAKE OF A HEALTHY LIFE-STYLE!**

Far too many people assume that their bodies can be pushed to the very brink of disaster and then be resurrected with a pill or a shot or some other magic potion to rescue them from the inevitable damage from their negative living habits. But it's a simple matter of logic: If you want health, then you must nurture health. Listen to your instincts. You know poisons cannot make you healthy. There is no bigger fool than the fool who fools himself. And surely there is nothing more foolhardy than to think you can consistently forsake the elements of health for years and then try to force health into existence with drugs or some other unwholesome measure. Would you take radiation treatments when you are feeling fine? Then why do it when you are sick?

We must recapture control of our health. We seem to be a species that refuses to take responsibility for our problems. We'll look under every rock, behind every tree, and in any dark corner for something to blame our ills on. We have a victim mentality, as though the body is just a helpless, hapless victim of unfortunate events, a convenient playground at the mercy of every malevolent entity that happens by. A victim of circumstances? Wrong! There is plenty we can do to determine our destiny as it relates to our health, and we should speedily make it our business to do so.

Become familiar with your biological needs and you will have gone a *long* way in accomplishing that. Rely on nature's grand elements to strengthen yourself. Every way that you interact with your environment affects your health. Elements like food, air, and water obviously receive most of the attention, because without them you would literally perish. Although the neglect of the other elements does not have such immediate negative ramifications, that neglect *will* take its toll over the long term if these elements are not acknowledged, nurtured, and utilized as well. We'll take a close-up look at these elements of health and see not only how they effect us individually but also how, in concert with one another, they supply what is needed to build a powerful foundation for health that is both dynamic and lasting.

As you read through the description of these elements of health and how to use them in your life, you are bound to be struck by their extreme simplicity. In fact, some are so simple that your initial reaction may be to discount the possibility of such small effort resulting in such huge benefits. However, that is the beauty of Nature's gifts: simple but powerful. We have been so conditioned to expect changes to be hard and complicated that when we are actually presented with ones which aren't we tend to be skeptical. What you will come to realize is this: each of the recommendations we suggest to you is on its own quite simple, but using them *together* is what makes the difference. Their interaction with one another is what makes them so powerful. What seems insignificant on its own becomes greatly magnified when in the presence of the others. This will become apparent to you as you start to use them in your life.

ENERGY—THE ESSENCE OF LIFE

MARILYN:

Once we understand the elements of health, we can incorporate them into a comprehensive life-style program to recapture control of how our energy is spent. Why would we want to do that? Because, dear reader, **ENERGY IS THE ESSENCE OF YOUR LIFE.** Abundant energy, great life. No energy, no life. Every body process depends on energy. Every activity of life requires it. The activity that requires it the most and which frequently gets none is the *natural healing process* of the body.

The truth of the matter and the fundamental premise upon which *all* of Natural Hygiene is based is that **HEALING IS A BIO-LOGICAL PROCESS OF THE BODY, NOT AN ART DONE TO THE BODY.** Your body had the ability and intelligence to grow, *unassisted*, from a single fertilized ovum to a full-grown adult. All that needed to be accomplished in that growth was accomplished with no outside intervention and only the elements of health utilized as raw materials. You know that is how it is. The body grows according to its own innate intelligence, which far surpasses our own. Even with a minimum of some of the elements—and certainly with some of them in very inferior form—the body grows. If we are raised with plenty of good air, water, food, rest, sunshine, exercise; if we are taught to keep ourselves clean, given a supportive environment, treated with love, allowed to live in peace, we grow better than if we are deprived. But even if we are deprived, the body still grows. Given its ability to self-generate is it even imaginable that it would be unable to self-repair? How could it possibly possess such intelligence as to be able to grow and then be left at the mercy of some outside "healing agent" if it breaks down? When you cut yourself, doesn't your body close the wound? You can practically watch the skin cells form to close the opening. Once a broken bone is set, does not the body do the rest?

Whatever the problem, the body will fix it. I know that sounds hard to accept, given our national tendency to "treat" illness with drugs, surgery, and all kinds of other therapies, but the truth is **YOUR BODY IS A SELF-MAINTAINING ORGANISM.** Just as a plant, deprived of light, will reach out with all its might toward whatever light source is available, **YOUR BODY IS ALWAYS STRIVING TOWARD HEALTH.** The reason this doesn't appear to be the case is *us. We get in the way!* We interfere, we second-guess, we do all sorts of things to *try* to get better, and our life-styles burn up so much energy that our bodies never have any energy left to heal themselves.

Disease is an energy crisis of the body. We deprive ourselves of the elements of health in the disease-producing life-styles that we live. And then we wonder why we get sick. A cancer-producing life-style causes cancer. An AIDS-producing life-style causes AIDS. No mystery there! Want to be well? Choose your life-style. **YOUR BODY IS TOTALLY ABLE TO KEEP ITSELF HEALTHY, IF YOU LET IT!** It all comes down to energy. Without energy, our bodies cease to function. The good functioning of every one of our organs depends on ample energy.

We can compare ourselves to the automobile, which, just like our bodies, is made up of many related parts. In the automobile we find a battery. From it runs a cable and many wires that go to the various parts of the car—the sparkplugs, lights, starter, horn, lighter, radio, and so on. When the battery is well charged, the car runs well. When we turn the ignition, the engine starts. The lights burn brightly. The horn honks when you push it. The radio plays well. If the battery is low, the engine may turn over, but it may not start. The horn is weak, the lights are dim, and the radio plays feebly. Without the electrical energy supplied by the battery, the "organs" of the car cease to operate.

Our bodies are similar. Nerve energy starts in the brain, and the spinal cord and nerves feed it to all the parts of the body. If nerve energy is abundant, the organs work well. Digestion is good, respiration proceeds normally, circulation is maintained at the needed level, and absorption, assimilation, and elimination all proceed efficiently. The tissues and fluids of the body are sweet and clean. The cells are nourished and we are healthy. But if our energy supply is permitted to run low, if our "battery" is drained, all the functions of the body are impaired. Digestion is poor; absorption, assimilation, and elimination drag; circulation is below normal; respiration is inefficient. And guess what? All the tissues and fluids of the body turn from sweet to sour. The cells are no longer nourished, and we feel unwell. Our health declines. We're sick!

So what seems to be the most important commodity here? Nerve energy! And what is nerve energy? Nobody really understands its essential nature, but nobody knows exactly what electricity is either and we use it just the same. We understand (or electrical engineers do) the *laws* governing electricity, however, so even without knowing what it is, we are able to make great use of it. And even though we do not know what the vital force within our bodies called energy is, by understanding the *laws* that govern it, we can still make use of it. In particular, we must understand the laws governing its dissipation—how it is used up. If we understand these laws, we can control the energy in our bodies as intelligently as the electrical engineer controls electricity. When we control the energy in our bodies, we are controlling our health. When we have the awareness to control how our energy is being spent, we are embarking on a health life-style.

First, let's look at how energy is used. How do we run out? Nerve energy in the human body is spent on all the work the body does to maintain itself. All the processes of life—from blinking to breathing to digesting food—use nerve energy. Hearing, seeing, eating, circulating the blood, thinking, using muscles, talking, and experiencing emotions *all* use nerve energy.

How then is nerve energy built or generated? *Through rest and sleep*. Only when we are not at work, only when we are passive or inactive can our bodies recoup their energy supply. Now, here's a simple, even obvious mathematical law pertaining to energy. When the amount of nerve energy we spend is greater than the amount we build, there is a lowering of the nerve energy supply in our bodies. This produces a state that is all too common and one we need to understand and avoid. This state is called *enervation*. When we are enervated, all body processes run below par. The organs cease to function efficiently and a very sluggish state of affairs is created. When you are enervated, you enter into a state of "self-poisoning."

How is that possible? It's really quite simple. Since nerve energy is in short supply, nothing works well. Elimination, wherein toxic end products of metabolism are collected and expelled from the body, is depressed. Toxic wastes start to accumulate because there is insufficient nerve energy to get rid of them. They are poisonous and they sour the body. At the same time, other processes are also depressed or even checked because there is no longer sufficient nerve energy to carry them forward. Thus we have poor digestion, poor assimilation . . . and a compounding of the self-poisoning as the body absorbs food that has spoiled in a sluggish digestive tract.

Can you see how enervation leads to our *not* feeling well? As all the body functions drag along, we become more and more poisoned or toxic. Finally, that toxic state causes a real body breakdown. We become diseased. Whichever part of our body is genetically weakest or has been abused the most is the area in which the disease manifests.

How can we keep from being enervated, then, since enervation seems to be the cause of our not feeling as well as we would like to feel and ultimately of disease? As I mentioned above, nerve energy is expended on activity—*all* activities—the activity of the body in maintaining itself and the activity pursued as part of daily living.

Living requires expenditure. This does not mean that we should cease this expenditure. Not at all! It only means that you should be aware of how you spend your precious energy. Energy is not a limitless commodity. If you run out, you feel sluggish and lethargic and you may get sick. Hence, try not to spend energy excessively or unwisely. If you have a week of heavy work demands, that is the time to eat right; get regular exercise, fresh air, and plenty of sleep; and maintain your emotional poise. It's not a time to party, indulge in alcohol, get in the middle of your sister's marital problems, or become upset with an assistant who is one hour late to work. The secret is to learn how to live your life so that you don't spend more nerve energy each day than you can earn back each night. The trick is to avoid the "overs"—

overwork, overindulgence, overeating, overdoing—and the "excesses"—sexual excess, emotional excesses, excess thrills, and excess worries. Just as you scrupulously avoid leaving your car lights on overnight so that you don't awaken to a dead battery in the morning, you must remember the importance of turning off your own energy drainers to prevent having dead batteries.

Enervation can be chronic. You will run on high for a while, feeling great, and then, boom, you've overdone it. You're worn out. You don't look or feel well. Your body is toxic and dragging. Luckily, it is easy to restore normal nerve energy. Just stop all the leaks.

Take an inventory of the elements of health in your life. Are you getting fresh air, enough pure water, pure food, enough exercise, rest and sleep, sunshine, peace, lovingness? Is your nest in order? Are these elements in balance? If not, it is up to you to do what must be done. No one can do it for you the way it needs to be done. The era of going to someone else to passively "get health" is coming to an end. **HEALTH *ONLY* COMES FROM HEALTHFUL LIVING.**

Many of the habits of daily living that we take for granted drain far more energy than we realize. For example, many people think they are getting relaxation in front of a television. But that is debatable. Much of television can be very enervating, both mentally and emotionally. The content of the nightly news can contribute to enervation. Who can deny that? The continuous talking that is so much a part of most television programming can be excessive in an already noisy society. Ever watch a sports fan "relax" while his favorite team is losing? Most children's programs, too, are enervating, what with their dissonant soundtracks and abrasive narratives. Commercials are a drain, for sure.

The point is to be aware of what we do in the periods of relative inactivity when we can be recharging our batteries. Peace and quiet are the backdrop for rest and sleep, and rest and sleep are the states during which we recoup our nerve energy. It is erroneous to think that you *gain* nerve energy from any activity, because *any* activity requires a nerve energy *expenditure*.

We'll talk more about rest and sleep and peace and quiet in later chapters. For now, understand that the best way to avoid enervation, the low, unwell feeling that results from it, and its acute state (disease), is to adopt an intelligent plan of living that will keep your energy level high enough so that you are consistently in a very good state of health. That intelligent plan of living is what this book is about.

Now that you understand how much your well-being is affected by energy, let's move on to consider the elements of health and how they all, in one way or another, affect your energy.

CHAPTER 6
Air

HARVEY:

We might as well start off with the element we can least afford to do without. There is no arguing its importance. Air is an indispensable need of the living body under *all* conditions of existence. It is possible to go weeks without food and days without water, but six minutes without air and you're a corpse.

Want to hear a real screamer? Until about seventy-five years ago, many doctors of the day considered fresh air to be dangerous to the sick! Air was actually *feared*, especially night air. Windows were kept closed tight and all air holes were plugged to prevent any fresh air from entering. Honest! The Natural Hygienists of the day (called sanitary engineers) who tried to explain that fresh air should be sought, not avoided, were considered loony for espousing such "unscientific" views. As we've noted before, new information doesn't usually have an easy time of it, and that includes even something as obvious as the need for fresh air! Luckily, today not even the most backward thinking "expert" would demand experiments to prove that you need fresh air or insist on tests to prove that fresh air is superior to foul, so we are making some progress.

Even though air is our most urgent need, necessary every moment whether we are awake or asleep, we take it totally for granted. When we awaken in the morning, we assume that we will be able to take a nice deep breath of life-giving air. It's not as if we wake up with thoughts like, "Oh, I sure hope there's enough air to go around today. I really have a busy schedule." Seldom, if ever, do we contemplate the immeasurable importance of the air we breathe, and although almost all life on earth is supported by a layer of air less than two miles thick, we are not apt to run out. Right now, we have about 6000 billion tons of air on this planet, so quantity is not something that we need to be concerned about. But quality could sure use some regular attention. It's been said that all of the world's air has been contaminated to some extent. Even penguins at the South Pole have been found to be somewhat contaminated.

You know why air is so important? Oxygen. Your blood and the trillions of cells that make up your body and perform the functions of life must be oxygenated regularly or death occurs. Cut off someone's air for a very short period of time and he or she starts to turn blue. About 21 percent of air is made up of oxygen, and we receive our supply of oxygen by extracting it from the air we breathe into our lungs. This is called respiration. A normal pair of lungs contains about a billion tiny air sacs. Here blood is purified, supplied with oxygen, and sent on its way to the rest of the body. When we breathe out we exhale carbon dioxide gas and a lot of other waste materials.

Merely to say that carbon dioxide is deadly is like saying the Grand Canyon is a crack in the earth. If you were to breathe air with only 3 percent carbon dioxide, you would become noticeably drowsy. Breathe in amounts larger than that and you will be ushered to your grave. Every twenty-four hours the amount of carbon dioxide eliminated from your lungs is equal to a lump of charcoal weighing eight ounces.

Guess what? All charged drinks, including soda, seltzer, and beer, have carbon dioxide present in them. Of course, I can just hear a representative from the soft drink or brewing industry explaining that you would have to drink 100,000 gallons to get enough carbon dioxide just to make you yawn. Right-o. To me that's like someone saying, "Let me punch you in the face *real easy*, you'll hardly feel it. I'd have to punch you ten times in the same spot for you to even turn a little black and blue." Thanks pal, but no. Keep your punches in the face *and* your carbon dioxide. **WHAT'S NOT GOOD IS NOT GOOD IN ANY AMOUNT.**

When you consider the almost unbelievable fact that we consume more weight in air than in food and water *combined*, it becomes quite evident why people become so devitalized by polluted air and why we simply *must* take what measures are in our control to supply our lungs with the finest air possible. The air in most cities contains enough pollutants to read like a chemical soup: carbon monoxide, sulfuric acid, hydrochloric acid, nitric acid, hydrocyanic acid, benzene, methane, ammonia, and more.

Considering the extreme importance of air, good air being foremost, I suggest three measures you can take to help you get the best and help you *make the best use of* the air you breathe.

1. GO WHERE THE BEST AIR IS

Even though it is practically impossible to have really pure air in this day and age, we certainly can place ourselves in situations where we have the purest air possible. There is no insurance that we will have the best air possible no matter what we do or where we go, but it doesn't take much to realize that the air outdoors and farthest from civilization is the best offered. Luckily for us, Nature has her own defense mechanism and is constantly purifying and cleansing the air. Rain cleans air. Plants convert carbon dioxide into oxygen, and the oceans constantly recirculate and cleanse the air all over the planet.

We have choices, and to live a healthy life-style and ensure our own well-being, it's important to make some good choices for ourselves. Example: Where do you feel better? Scurrying around the city and freeways sucking up the exhaust from thousands of autos belching out their carbon monoxide or strolling down a country lane. No need to answer. That's like asking if you'd rather vacation in a tropical isle or hike barefoot in Siberia. The reason one always feels more relaxed and renewed after a walk in the woods is because of the splendor, intelligence, and wonder of Mother Nature's grand system of symbiosis between the plant and animal kingdoms.

Country air is fresh because plants and trees growing there absorb our carbon dioxide and expel oxygen. Plant life and animal life are constantly supplying each other with the needs of life. The waste product of one is a *necessity* for the other. That is too glorious for words. Whenever I reflect on something as exquisite as this, I am overwhelmed with awe at the resplendent glory, magnitude, and remarkableness of the grand scheme of things on this planet.

Compare the amount of time you spend on crowded city streets to the time you spend walking along the seashore, in the park or through the woods. Your health is simply too important for you not to think of these things. The difference in your health when fresh air is supplied to your lungs and blood is dramatic and obvious. Do it! Get out there and treat yourself and your loved ones to a gift greater than gold. You *know* how good you feel when you do it, yet too often something else manages to take precedence over what is so important.

Consider what you have read here. Consider how exceedingly crucial good air is. Consider that air is the number-one necessity for the perpetuation of life, and *please* incorporate into your life-style walks where the air is freshest. It can only increase your chances of a long, disease-free life.

Long ago, when we humans lived in harmony with Nature, surrounded by plant life, we were automatically adapted to satisfy our biological need for fresh air. Today we have been moved so far from understanding our true biological needs that, after a whole week of being in confined spaces, on our *one* day off we *voluntarily* confine ourselves inside malls where there is not a breath of fresh air. There are other, more healthful alternatives and we should utilize them.

2. EXERCISE

Exercise is another of the elements of health. We will discuss it at length later. However, it is important to mention here that exercise *greatly* assists in the oxygenation of your entire body, especially aerobic exercise, which accelerates the heart's pumping action. The point I want to stress here is that, *whenever possible*, you should try to exercise where the air is best.

The best time to walk and exercise is early in the morning. This is before all the cars have been started up and driven around, fouling the air. If you run or jog, find a route near a beach or park or trail or at least on side streets. When I see runners running along thoroughfares, not five feet from a steady flow of traffic, I cringe. I'm flabbergasted that so many people could be so removed from their common sense as to run and take in all those deep breaths of carbon monoxide directly from the cars' exhaust pipes. What could they be thinking? It's like finding out you've won an all-expense-paid trip to Europe and, when asked where you would like to sit on the plane, instead of choosing to sit in the first class section you choose the cargo hold.

Make the smart choice. If you're already making the commitment to exercise regularly, increase your benefits many times over by exercising in the purest air possible. The value of doing so is measured by your life-span.

MARILYN:

3. DEEP BREATHING

Very few people in Western society have an understanding of the impact of breathing on every aspect of our lives. We tend to ignore our breathing, to act as if we are separate from it. Yet, our breath *is* us; *it is our life force*, moving in and out of the body. When breathing stops, life is over. When breathing is deep and even, life is strong. If it is shallow and alarmed, life itself is diminished and threatened.

Breathing supplies us with the fuel that keeps us alive. How we breathe affects how we absorb oxygen into our bodies. The oxygen feeds the brain, the nervous system, and every cell of the body. However, this vital body function that affects our very being is horribly mistreated in Western culture. It is interfered with from birth and, in most cases, severely harmed by our traditional medical birthing procedures.

When an infant is born, it has not yet had the opportunity to use its lungs. The infant has been fed all the oxygen it required through the umbilical tube that attached it to its mother. At birth the lungs are not immediately ready to be used. There is a critically important transition period of about forty-five minutes during which time the infant *must* be allowed to adapt to breathing through its lungs on its own and during which time the umbilical cord must *never* be cut. Until the infant can breathe entirely on its own, it is still relying on the oxygen coming through from its mother. During this interval, the infant should be placed on its mother's stomach, head near the familiar heartbeat, and allowed to rest quietly as it slowly begins to breathe on its own. Only then, after milking the umbilical cord of all the remaining oxygen-rich fluids, is it appropriate to cut the cord. This is an understanding and procedure common among most midwives. *This procedure establishes the foundation for correct breathing*.

What do we see on the other hand in our hospitals? We routinely see treatment of the newborn infant that is sickeningly ignorant of the mechanism of the life-giving function of breathing. In case after case, we find haste, *speed of delivery*, to be the criterion that takes precedence over all others. The infant is pulled out of the birth canal as quickly as possible, and what happens next sets up the dysfunction that interferes with its health for the rest of its life. Instead of the infant being allowed to make the transition to breathing on its own, the umbilical cord is immediately severed. The infant, unable to breathe on its own with its tiny lungs, is held upside down and whacked on the behind, *forced*, as it were, to gasp for air. Indeed, the first breath of life is a gasp. Cold air (remember, all elements of the infant's life have so far been supplied at 98.6° Fahrenheit, the temperature of its mother's body) streams into its raw, unprepared lungs. This is a contributing factor to asthma and other respiratory impairments later on in life. Furthermore, the ignorant whack of the physician breaks blood vessels in the spine, and that contributes to sudden infant death syndrome in too many cases. It causes severe emotional damage to the child, who is biologically poised to be treated with the utmost tenderness and gentleness at the moment of birth, not smacked! In the animal kingdom you never see such roughness. Animals, at birth, demonstrate the tender, loving, instinctive behavior that we "superior" human beings have lost.

This harsh treatment affects our breathing for the rest of our lives. Our first breath is a gasp and, for most of us, every breath thereafter is shallow and gasping. What *should* our breathing be? Since so many of us are prevented by our birth experiences from breathing *normally*, the way we are intended to as a species, we must actually "learn how to breathe" later in life as we become aware that we are breathing improperly and suffering greatly as a result. In order to improve our breathing, Harvey and I have studied with Alan Finger at his Yogaworks Studios in Santa Monica, CA and New York City. The following explanation on correct breathing and the exercises provided are based on Alan's teachings.

Normally, we should breath abdominally. An abdominal breath is a *full, complete* breath. Typically, we breathe quickly from our upper chest. We do not use our whole breathing mechanism and therefore must breathe faster to get sufficient air in. The more quickly we breathe, the more tense we are. This can easily be verified. If you are frightened or angry, your breath comes fast and from your upper chest only. If you receive a shock, you actually gasp—a shallow throat breath. If you are lying in the sun, relaxing, or getting a massage, your breathing is slower and deeper.

Your breathing directly affects your mind. If you breathe quickly and shallowly, your mind races and your body tenses. If you breathe slowly and deeply, your mind is tranquil and your body is relaxed. Since so many of us can thank our birth experiences for the inability to breathe normally, we must now as adults *learn* how to do what we should be doing instinctively. We must acquire an intellectual understanding first of something that *should* be happening but cannot happen automatically.

Once you have the intellectual understanding of the mechanism of breathing normally, you can begin to practice doing so. After years of incorrect breathing, you are going to realize an enormous difference in the way you feel when you begin to breathe normally. There are enormous benefits that accompany breathing the way your body is designed to breathe. *Your whole life* is going to be affected by it, because breathing *is* life, and if you think life is already wonderful, just wait! It is going to get immeasurably better once you learn how to breathe more deeply and fully into your lungs.

This is how proper breathing actually works: The activity initiates in the abdomen. Your diaphragm muscle cuts across your midsection, inside the chest cavity, just beneath your lungs. When you breathe in, the diaphragm muscle, which is dome-shaped, has to pull down. In order for it to do so, the stomach and digestive organs have to shift out of the way. The abdominal muscles have to push out in order to make room for the stomach and digestive organs to move down. So when you breathe in, the abdomen moves out, the stomach moves down, and the diaphragm pulls down to create suction in the chest cavity. The suction in the chest cavity causes a vacuum, which forces the lungs, which have no muscle, to swell up with air. This happens basically in the bottom half of the lung, which absorbs about 80 percent of the oxygen. The top half, which absorbs 20 percent, is only used when there is extra exertion, when the nervous system is in stress, or when you are thrown into a fight-or-flight response. In other words, you only need to use the top half of your lungs when you need to attack or run away from something or when there is extreme physical exertion. But that is *in addition* to using your remaining lung capacity. If you were to try to carry out those special requirements without using *all* of your breathing apparatus and only use the top half (as most of us do) you would probably have a very difficult time of it. When you are in a regular state, however, you should be breathing abdominally, working the lower half of the lungs only, which will feed you the 80 percent of the air you need for normal living.

Due to the stressful births we have undergone and the breathing habits we have developed as a result, we tend to gasp our way through life, forcing ourselves to survive on shallower and shallower breathing. Furthermore, for many of us existence is full of the additional shocks and stresses that constantly bombard us from modern life. Thus, because of our shallow breathing, which stresses our bodies, *and* the stressful assault from the outside, we live our lives *stressed*. Most people today breathe totally from the chest. They never use the abdomen, and therefore their lungs never fill in the lower portion, which should be supplying 80 percent of the oxygen to their bodies. They exist in a state of semisuffocation as the norm in their lives! They are hyped up, stressed, anxious, and many live on tranquilizers when *all they really need is air!* The moment they learn how to breathe deeply from their abdomen and thereby get air into the *lower* half of their lung, the stress in their lives is dramatically reduced. Stress may continue on the outside, but because everything is peaceful on the inside, they cope with it more easily. That's what makes it possible for some to float cheerfully through the madness of modern living while others tear their hair out. Breathing and your state of mind are directly connected. If your breath is short and shallow, your mind races. As you slow your breathing down and deepen it, your mind becomes more peaceful. Your entire awareness changes. Instead of a frenetic, disconnected state of being that results from the racing of the mind, you become more conscious of yourself, more able to separate yourself in a positive way from the pressure around you. People frequently find that when they focus more on breathing correctly, the pressure and turmoil dissipate entirely and they realize that their mind was creating those stresses all along.

The interesting thing to add here is that the clear, tranquil mind you develop from abdominal breathing will not make you less aware or less active. On the contrary, it will make you more active, but your activity will be more precise and relevant. Abdominal breathing clears your mind and relaxes you. It doesn't space you out. It balances you. Abdominal breathing is the key to relaxation and to the correct oxygenation of your body. Without it, the tension and the oxygen deprivation that results set the stage for disease and pain in the body.

Another benefit, as if you need more, relates to your heart. The heart is located between the lungs, and when you shallow-breathe in the chest, the pressure constricts inward and almost strangulates your heart, since your body is not designed to breathe that way. Abdominal breathing takes the pressure off the heart, which shows once more the extent to which breathing properly is an amazing key to our existence.

Abdominal breathing, as well as de-stressing and relaxing us and taking undue pressure off the heart, also has an amazing effect on the nervous system. Breathing is an involuntary function of the autonomic nervous system, and it is the *only* function of that system that we can actually use to override the system voluntarily. You can't say to your sweat glands, "Stop perspiring." They'll ignore you. And you can't say to your intestines, "Stop digesting." You can't control these functions of the autonomic nervous system. But you *can*, by changing your breathing, *voluntarily* unwind and gain mastery over the autonomic nervous system. In Western culture, we call this involuntary set of functions the autonomic, or "automatic," nervous system because we generally assume that we are unable to control it. However, the yogis have known for thousands of years that we in fact have *total* control over it via our breathing. By deep abdominal breathing we can slow down all of the so-called "autonomic" functions of our bodies.

Now that we have explored intellectually the mechanism and benefits of abdominal breathing, let's take a practical look at how you can begin (immediately) to reap the benefits. Unfortunately, simply knowing that abdominal breathing is normal and unquestionably beneficial does not automatically make it happen in our bodies. *We have to make it happen*, and in the beginning we have to concentrate on this goal in order to break our habit of incorrect breathing. Basically, what we want to have happen is the following:

We want the abdomen to expand as we breathe in, and then we want the air to move up into the chest as high as is necessary or comfortable. This may not be very high at all, since when one is relaxed and breathing normally one does not need as much air. (You'll notice the same thing happening when you eat only living food. You get so much nourishment from it that you don't need to eat as much. See the introduction to the **Living Health Cook-**

book, page 353.) What we are striving for is to keep our breathing abdominal and not allow it to become shallow.

There are two little exercises you can do to practice this and, if possible, you should do them every day. Remember, *breathing is life*. In doing these exercises, you are investing a few minutes in your life. So *do* these exercises. They may feel awkward at first, but practice makes perfect and the benefits are indescribable.

ABDOMINAL BREATHING EXERCISE

This can be done either sitting or lying down. If you practice it sitting, you should keep your spine erect, so sit in a chair with a straight back or cross-legged on the floor with your back against the wall. Place your hands on your abdomen, one above the navel and one on it, as you breathe in. Feel the navel swell out first, and then feel the breath slowly rise up into the chest. As you breathe out, the hand positioned above the navel will "sink in," followed by the lower hand. In this way, you can actually feel the abdominal breathing taking place. Breathe comfortably like this for at least two minutes, and gradually work the exercise up to five minutes a day. As you breathe in, count to four, hold for two, and then release the breath for four counts.

A second way to practice this exercise is to lie on your back on the floor, and this works particularly well if you have bad posture, a lot of tension and stress, or have been through some shock or developed some fear that keeps your breath "locked" in your chest. Roll a bath towel up the long way and place it under your spine from your waist to the top of your head. This will force your chest to press up and expand as you lie on the towel. This position will also automatically pull the breath down into the abdomen. Place your hands on your stomach as indicated above, and breathe slowly and comfortably for two minutes; work up to five minutes if you can.

This is by far the most powerful, deep abdominal breathing exercise you can practice. As you do it, you will find that you become conscious of how you should actually be breathing *all the time*, and this awareness will begin to filter into your daily life. You will begin to notice when you are *not* breathing normally and when your breaths are coming in short gasps from the chest and your mind is racing. You will automatically begin abdominal breathing, which will immediately relax you and calm your mind.

ALTERNATE NOSTRIL BREATHING

This second breathing exercise can be used as a highly effective tool to balance your nervous system. In each of our nostrils there are nerves that lead into the center of the brain. The brain has two sides. The right side is creative, inspirational, and relaxing. The left side is mechanical and calculating. The yogis have found that there is a body rhythm in which every hour and twenty-eight minutes the sides of the brain alternate dominance. The nostrils reflect this. One nostril will also be dominant during that period. If the right side of the brain—the healing, resting side—is dominant, the left nostril will also be dominant. If the left side of the brain—the mechanical calculator—is dominant, the right nostril will be dominant.

In our typical fast-paced Western life-style, most of our time is spent employing the mechanical and calculating activity of the left brain. It is difficult in our society to structure one's life for the creative, inspirational, healing, and relaxing activities of the right brain. These do not harmonize with the frenetic qualities of the American life-style, especially in the cities. Our very life-style forces an imbalance between the two sides of the brain, which creates a great deal of tension in our lives. By understanding that each nostril connects to the opposite side of the brain and using this information in a breathing exercise, you can actually balance the two sides of the brain, and the result is an amazing sense of equilibrium.

Sit in a chair or comfortably on the floor with your back straight. Essentially, what you will be doing in this exercise is breathing in one nostril and out the other, then in the second nostril and out the first. In other words, you will breathe in the left nostril to the count of six, using your finger to hold the right nostril closed. Hold the breath for three counts. Then release the right nostril and breathe out to the count of six, closing off the left nostril with your finger, and breathing back in the right nostril for six counts. Hold for three counts. Then release the left nostril and breathe out to the count of six. By alternating the flow of air through your nostrils six times, you will experience an unbelievable sense of relaxation, and the balancing effect this will have on your brain will be miraculously tranquilizing. A tremendous peace and harmony will come into your being.

You can do this exercise as often as you wish, but you should try to do it at least once a day. It is especially helpful before a meeting or in preparation for a stressful and emotionally charged event.

Both the abdominal breathing exercise and the alternate nostril breathing exercise are extraordinary tools in today's high-pressured society. Try them, remembering that breath is life and life warrants a few minutes of your time each day. It is really a disservice to the benefits you will reap to try to describe them for you here. They must be experienced to be believed and you certainly deserve to experience them.

HARVEY:

There is another situation in which you must have fresh air, and you would be stunned at how many people, not being aware of it, actually force themselves to breathe foul, used air. It's when you are sleeping. I frequently ask people if the room in which they sleep has a window open and more often than not the answer is *no!*

This is one of those simple little measures that you can take to effect an *enormous* change for the better. Remember, with every breath you exhale you are breathing out poisonous carbon dioxide as well as other poisonous wastes. If you are sleeping in a closed room for six, seven, or eight hours, that carbon dioxide builds up and you start to breathe some of it back in. Further, each successive breath has less oxygen in it. Although many of the body's functions are at rest when you are sleeping, many others are in operation. For one thing, that is when the assimilation processes are at work, absorbing and utilizing nutrients. The assimilation cycle's effectiveness is considerably diminished when the sleeping body is deprived of fresh air.

One of the major reasons people wake up groggy in the morning is because their lungs have had to contend with stale air all night instead of fresh. And if there are two people sleeping in the room, the air is made stale twice as fast. Hey, I have a good idea—*open a window!* If it is a chilly time of year, only open the window an inch or two and throw on an extra blanket if necessary. Please don't take this suggestion lightly. You will notice a marked improvement in your vitality *immediately* once you perform this simple, yet enormously beneficial act. Again, it's plain common sense. *Whenever* fresh air is to be had, take advantage of it.

Life is a precious gift. All who have been fortunate enough to receive it wish to be healthy. No one wants to be sick or unhappy or racked with pain or to meet a premature death. To knowingly place your life in danger, to intentionally jeopardize your well-being by deliberately participating in dangerous habits that are *known* to kill has to rank with the most senseless of activities. Life is simply too special to waste. Since we know without question that air is at the top of the list of biological necessities for life and that our lungs are the apparatus used for transforming air into life, why, *why* would anyone with an ounce of gray matter in his or her head knowingly, willfully damage his or her own lungs? Of this you can be certain: Any interference with the function of your lungs will bring about a corresponding depletion of your vitality and the shortening of your life.

SMOKING AND HEALTH

There is no way to discuss the importance of air and your lungs without discussing the vile, stinking, filthy, offensive, hurtful, anti-life, anti-natural habit of smoking, as emotionally, creatively, intellectually, and spiritually injurious as it is physically. There are not enough nasty words in the English language to characterize this putrid, depraved habit appropriately. Strong language? Not to me. There is no language too strong to condemn this habit of self-destruction, suffering, and premature death. How has something so inherently bad, so horrendously harmful, so completely and totally devoid of *any* value whatsoever become such a common addiction for so many millions of people? This is a human tragedy of monumental proportions. How sad that such a deadly practice should be so pervasive among the populations of the world. Are people so disgusted with themselves that they would deliberately destroy their own bodies?

Our Creator saw fit to bestow the precious gift of life. Is it an appropriate showing of gratitude to inflict such hellish ravages on that gift? A thousand people die of tobacco-related illnesses every day in the United States alone. That is more than seven times as many people as die in motor vehicle crashes. More people die *every year* because of tobacco than the total number of Americans killed in World War I, World War II, and the Vietnam War *combined!* I don't know about you, but that shocks me to the core. Worldwide 2 to 2.5 million people die a year. That's more than 6000 people a day! In an editorial in their journal in 1986, the American Medical Association opened a scathing attack on tobacco companies, calling them "vultures seeking to create addicts hooked on their products." (The American Lung Association calls them "merchants of death.") If spreading this addiction is the goal of these "vultures," they should be real proud of themselves. Former President Jimmy Carter, referring to cigarettes as *the greatest* menace to public health, stated, "I think there is a deliberate commitment on the part of the tobacco industry to cause death for profit."*

There are now some *54 million* smokers in the United States, some 75 percent of whom are considered to be addicted to this vile narcotic.** Of course, when people hear the word *addicted*, they tend to think of heroin or alcohol or some other dangerous drug. According to Dr. William Poland, the director of the National Institute on Drug Abuse, *tobacco has far worse addictive potential than alcohol or heroin*. In fact, he says that tobacco may be as much as eight times deadlier than excessive use of alcohol and is far more resistant to successful treatment than heroin addiction, which is also less likely to be fatal than tobacco use. Dr. Poland has called for recognition of tobacco use as far deadlier than *any other* dangerous drug.

Los Angeles Times, September 30, 1986.
**Until its latest issue, *Taber's Medical Dictionary* consistently described tobacco as a narcotic.

Heaven only knows to what extent disease and ill health can be attributed to smoking. But what is known reads like a horror story—a *horrible* horror story: cancer, heart disease, emphysema, bronchitis, spontaneous abortions, fetal death, birth defects, ulcers, damage to DNA, high blood sugar, high blood pressure, infertility in women, impotence in men, dried up testicles, pathological increase in the heart rate and subsequent damage to the heart, constriction and even total collapse of blood vessels, numbness of hands and arms, marked increase in stomach acidity, crippling of taste buds, and massive destruction of vital cells from the lips to the lungs. Tobacco smoke is much hotter than hot food. It wipes out cells and taste buds wholesale. Ever notice how much salt and pepper smokers use? It's because they can't taste their food. These condiments further irritate the lining of the mouth, lips, tongue, gums, cheeks, throat. *The latest findings suggest that smoking may even contribute to Alzheimer's disease in people as young as forty-eight.* Sound inviting?

The tobacco companies pull in more than $20 billion a year selling a product that causes incalculable pain, suffering, anguish, and death. No wonder the AMA calls them "vultures." And to think that less than seventy-five years ago many physicians did not consider smoking harmful. Note this statement made by a Brooklyn medical doctor in 1913: "The history of human experience as well as exhaustive investigations conducted by men highly trained in scientific research point to the fact that the moderate use of smoking tobacco is not harmful to either the body or the mind." Compare this to the open-eyed realism of Dr. Russell T. Trall, a medical doctor turned Natural Hygienist, who, recognizing the extreme danger of tobacco, dedicated the entirety of one of the books he wrote to assailing its use. (This was in 1857.)

Cigarette smoke contains more than 3000 chemical substances, and a few of them deserve mentioning:

● **ACROLEIN**—a toxic, colorless liquid with irritating cancerous vapors

● **CARBON MONOXIDE**—a highly toxic, flammable gas used in the manufacture of numerous chemical products. Inhalation of carbon monoxide interferes with the transportation of oxygen from the lungs to the tissues, where it is required.

● **NICOTINE**—a poisonous alkaloid that is the chief addictive substance in tobacco. It is also used as an insecticide and to kill parasitic worms in animals. *One pack of cigarettes a day, inhaled, gives you enough nicotine to kill you outright if you were to receive it all in one dose.*

● **AMMONIA**—a gaseous alkaline compound of nitrogen and hydrogen used as a coolant in refrigerating and air conditioning equipment and in explosives, artificial fertilizers, and disinfectants

● **FORMIC ACID**—a pungent liquid gas used in processing textiles and leather. Exposure to the acid irritates the mucous membranes and causes blistering.

● **HYDROGEN CYANIDE**—an extremely poisonous liquid used in many chemical processes including fumigation, and in the case-hardening of iron and steel. Hydrogen cyanide gas is used as the lethal agent in *capital punishment.*

● **NITROUS OXIDE**—a group of irritating and sometimes poisonous gases that combine with hydrocarbons to produce smog. Nitrogen dioxide can weaken bodily tissues and increase susceptibility to respiratory ailments.

● **FORMALDEHYDE**—a pungent gas used primarily as a disinfectant and preservative. It is extremely irritating to the mucous membranes.

● **PHENOL**—a caustic, poisonous acidic compound present in coal and wood tar and used in disinfectants

● **ACETALDEHYDE**—a highly toxic, flammable liquid that irritates the eyes and mucous membranes and accelerates the action of the heart. Prolonged exposure causes blood pressure to rise and causes proliferation of white and red blood cells.

● **HYDROGEN SULFIDE**—a poisonous gas produced naturally from putrefying matter and used extensively in chemical laboratories

● **PYRIDYNE**—a flammable liquid used in pharmaceuticals, water repellents, bactericides, and herbicides

● **METHYL CHLORIDE**—a toxic gas used in the production of rubber and paint remover and as an antiknock agent in gasoline

● **ACETONITRILE**—a toxic compound found in coal tar and molasses residue and used in the production of plastics, rubber, acrylic fiber, insecticides, and perfumes

● **PROPIONALDEHYDE**—a colorless liquid with a suffocating odor, used as a chemical disinfectant and preservative as well as in plastic and rubber

● **METHANOL**—a poisonous liquid alcohol used in automotive antifreezes, rocket fuels, synthetic dye stuffs, resins, drugs and perfumes

. . . AND! Let's not forget arsenic.

All these chemicals in the body create untold dangers. Dr. Paul Erlich, Professor of Biological Science at Stanford University, has stated that almost half a million tests would have to be conducted just to determine the effect of any *two* chemicals in conjunction with each other in the body.* Technology capable of determining the harm of sixteen at one time doesn't exist.

Ever notice some of the ads the tobacco industry uses to hook more women into smoking? It's always a picture of some superchic, ultrasvelte beauty having the absolute time of her life. (For obvious reasons, they won't show a picture of someone in the middle of a coughing spasm hacking up a chunk of diseased lung.) Ever notice that the ads *never* show the evil weed on her lips? She's always holding it ever so delicately, as if it were some cherished possession. Know why? Because the sight of a cigarette dangling off a woman's lip is so offensive that the advertising rule is *not to show it*. For some reason however, to show it dangling off a man's lips is supposed to be "macho" . . . that is, until he's had his voicebox removed and has to talk through a tube stuck in his throat.

One sight never ceases to amaze me. It's usually in an airport. I see a very, *very* well dressed, beautifully turned-out woman, impeccably stylish, with hair and makeup done flawlessly—ob-

Los Angeles Times, June 2, 1978.

viously a lot of time and effort went into looking just so. And you know those standing ashtrays that are all over airports? They're about two feet high, round, about ten inches across, with a big hole in the top in which to deposit ashes and butts. Remember the smell when you get close enough? Right. We're talking about one of the foulest stenches possible—something like a dead goat that has been decomposing for a couple of weeks. This exquisitely turned out woman goes over to one of these things and pulls it over to her so she can flick the ashes from the cigarette she just lit up.

So pretty on the *outside*, with not even one hair in her eyebrow turning in the wrong direction, and she voluntarily drags one of these foul, stinking containers full of filth over to her. It is like stopping on the highway to pick up a dead skunk that has been run over and then stuffing it down your shirt. Hours spent being sure the exterior is perfect while assaulting the inside with cancerous poisons. I have seen this scene played out hundreds of times, but each time I cannot help but experience disbelief and sadness at the situation.

I find it hard to swallow that the Department of Health and Human Services spends millions of dollars in taxes a year in an effort to combat smoking, and another arm of the same government, the Department of Agriculture, spends hundreds of millions of dollars of our tax monies to subsidize the industry. Think about that. Out of one side of the government's mouth it's, "Better stop smoking; you're going to die of cancer," and out of the other side of the mouth it's, "Here, let me pay you to grow tobacco." Does this strike you as strange? Do you know that if a farmer's crop cannot be sold on the market at a fixed price, a federally supervised corporation buys the tobacco with money borrowed from the government, then holds on to it to sell later when the price is better? *You* can be dead-set against smoking, but *your* tax money can be used to subsidize the tobacco you deplore. Charming.

SIDESTREAM SMOKE

I know there will be people reading this who say, "Hey, if I want to smoke, it's *my* business." True enough. You can also stick a knife in your chest, set your hair on fire, or jump off a cliff. And as foolhardy as those actions would be, at least they would not hurt anyone else.

This brings up what I find to be the most outrageously objectionable issue about smoking: secondhand, or sidestream, smoke —the smoke that winds up in the lungs of an innocent bystander.

People may have the inalienable right to poison them*selves*, but they certainly have *no* right to poison you or your child. If you were in a store shopping and someone came up and slapped your kid in the face, what would you do? You could have that person arrested. But let that same person blow malodorous filthy smoke from his or her cancerous lungs into your child's face and lungs and you're supposed to "realize that smokers have rights, too." Well, that's a real interesting concept. Because people have the insane, perverted habit of poisoning themselves, they expect the *sane* segment of the population to stand idly by while they impose their perversion on others.

Let's take it a step further. Does the person who loves to get drunk have the right to run down a kid on a bike? Does a gun enthusiast have the right to shoot someone in the head?

You may say, "Wait a minute, you're getting a little carried away."

Am I? Let me tell you about sidestream smoke.

I did not have a great deal of information about sidestream smoke when I began research for this book, although my common sense and natural aversion to it told me what to suspect. I contacted Action on Smoking and Health (ASH) in Washington, D.C., a highly visible, highly respected organization started twenty years ago by a distinguished body of physicians, attorneys, and other prominent citizens to use the law to fight back against the might of the tobacco companies. I called and asked for whatever they could send me on sidestream smoke.

What I received stunned me. I knew that sidestream smoke was harmful, but I never realized just *how* harmful. Over the last fifteen years there have been literally thousands of studies on sidestream smoke, and they are reported in the most prestigious medical journals in the world, including the *Journal of the American Medical Association, The New England Journal of Medicine, Lancet, British Medical Journal,* and many others. The results are depressingly discouraging. The unquestionable, irrefutable fact is that tobacco smoke exposes nonsmokers to potent, killing carcinogens. The question is not whether sidestream smoke poses a cancer risk to nonsmokers, it's the magnitude of the risk.

Consider this the next time someone exercises his or her "rights" and causes a plume of smoke to waft into your face: Three of the most poisonous elements in smoke are tar, nicotine, and carbon monoxide. Carbon monoxide is the most deadly of them. Sidestream smoke has been shown to contain *twice* the tar, *twice* the nicotine, and *five times* as much carbon monoxide as mainstream smoke. *Plus!* . . . In an article in the *Los Angeles Times* dated August 15, 1986, there was reference to a new study finding: "People sitting in a room filled with cigarette smoke retain the dangerous chemicals (end product of nicotine) they inhale more than twice as long as people doing the smoking." Marvelous! So perhaps the next time you're in a restaurant eating a nice meal (or trying to) and the people next to you exercise their "rights," bear in mind that they are inflicting on your lungs probably the most potent pollutant in the environment.

One fourteen-year study in Japan showed that wives of smokers have a much higher risk of developing lung cancer than the wives of nonsmokers. This was attributed to sidestream smoke. One Environmental Protection Agency report based on a dozen studies from several countries and reported in major medical journals concludes that as many as 5000 nonsmokers may die each year from lung cancer caused solely by breathing other people's tobacco smoke. Any allergist at a major hospital will tell you about people among the estimated 30 to 40 million Americans who have conditions such as asthma, hay fever, or sinusitis and can be sensitive to the point that exposure to tobacco smoke in everyday situations makes them so ill they require medical attention, sometimes hospitalization.

To me, the most despicable, unforgivable outrage is the damage that sidestream smoke inflicts on children. In a study of the correlation between respiratory infection in children and the smoking habits of their families, it was shown that the percentage of children with these diseases rose in direct relation to the level of family members' smoking. The incidence of pneumonia and bronchitis in infants examined over the first three years of life showed a definite relationship between these diseases and parents' smoking habits. It was lowest when both parents were nonsmokers, highest when both smoked, and lay between these two levels when only one parent smoked. Within the first year of life, exposure to cigarette smoke generated by parents' smoking doubles the risk for the infant of an attack of pneumonia or bronchitis.

Do you have children? Do you smoke? Do them a favor—step outside!

Medical literature reports numerous studies performed to discover what effect passive smoking has on the development of the most innocent nonsmoker of all, the fetus. It is not good. Aside from depriving the fetus of air (which is tantamount to strangling it!), smoking can reduce birth weight by up to 10 percent below normal. Lack of oxygen in the developing fetus causes brain damage.*

ADVERTISING ILL HEALTH?

Poisoning oneself has actually become commonplace in our society. If you saw a man standing on a corner hitting himself in the head with a brick, you would be shocked. You would try to help him, wouldn't you? But you see people everywhere, all the time, poisoning themselves with *proven*, cancer-causing substances and do not even bat an eyelash. These substances are even *advertised* for sale, for heaven's sake! And that when it's been proved that tobacco use is deadlier than any other dangerous drug, including heroin.

Since tobacco can legally be advertised, should we also allow full-page ads exploiting the soothing virtues of heroin? Ridiculous, isn't it? **BUT TOBACCO IS WORSE!**

Why is it okay to sell tobacco out of magazines and from billboards all over the country? The tobacco industry spends $2 billion a year to get you and your teenagers hooked. Perhaps you've seen some of the full-page ads that one tobacco company has been placing to try and combat our people's trend toward health. You would think that a company making its fortune on the suffering, pain, and death of millions of people would keep as low a profile as possible. Forget it! Consider the arrogance required to actually try glossing over absolute, indisputable, irrefutable evidence of

---

*Should you be interested in receiving any of the information I have discussed, or should you like to read some of the studies, contact ASH, 2013 H Street, N.W., Washington, D.C. 20006; telephone number: (202) 659-4310.

harm, trying to make it appear that they are just simple folk working to make a living.

One ad states: "We deplore the actions of those who try to manipulate public opinion through scare tactics." Guess what they're referring to—the medical community trying to warn people to stay as far from sidestream smoke as possible because it can be harmful. The tobacco company deplores that. What they really deplore is decreased profits.

There is a Yiddish word, *chutzpah*. The best illustration of chutzpah that I have ever come across is the story of the man who killed his parents and at his trial pleaded for mercy because he was an orphan. But the tobacco companies should win the all-time grand prize for chutzpah. They've taken it to heights never before imagined. For a tobacco company, which makes its money on people's misery, to deplore trying to *save* people's lives as a "scare tactic" is like the terrorists who blew up the Rome airport deploring the work of the ambulance drivers who came to pick up the injured.

Tobacco companies can say whatever they want. *Healthful habits don't cause suffering and death.* The obituary columns are not filled with the names of those who died from the effects of pure air!

If you've never heard of the Tobacco Institute, allow me to introduce you. The Tobacco Institute is located in a fashionable downtown Washington office building not far from Capitol Hill. It has about eighty employees and lobbyists there, and about twenty or so others are deployed around the country. What does the Tobacco Institute do? Well, the best way to describe what they do is to use an analogy. Imagine Adolf Hitler using a P.R. firm to convince people that "Adolf isn't really such a bad ol' guy. He's just trying to exercise his right as a human being to express himself in his own peculiar way."

That's what the Tobacco Institute attempts to do for the tobacco industry. Its employees have placards on their desks that say cute things like "Thank you for not breathing while I'm smoking" and "Kiss my butt," and the Institute's spokespeople talk about surveys *they* conducted that point out that in *96 percent* of the instances when people were coughing indoors where smoking was going on it was *not* due to the cigarette smoke. "It was fungus in the air causing people to have allergic reactions they were blaming on tobacco smoke."

I love that one. That makes as much sense as saying that a

person killed by a drunk driver was not killed by the car or the driver. Rather, death was caused by the *paint* that happened to be spread on the three tons of speeding steel being erratically driven by a drunkard.

The Tobacco Institute *very* adamantly points out that it is not defending smoking per se, it is defending *"rights."* It frequently hires its own medical "experts" and flies them in to testify at hearings where legislation to restrict smoking is under discussion ("Have Credentials—Will Travel").

One thing of which the people at the Institute are very proud is that *anyone* in their employ, from the president on down to the office clerks, can at any time go into a death-rattling coughing spasm where you think their eyeballs are going to pop out of their head and no one will pay the slightest attention. No frowning glances of pity, scorn, or alarm. That's the kind of warm hearted acceptance and camaraderie the Tobacco Institute is really proud of. And its representatives will not sleep at night until that kind of democratic freedom is everywhere to be found. They won't rest until every man, woman, and child *knows* that he or she can go to any street corner, grab hold of a lamppost, and go into a convulsion of coughing that makes you think they're going to hack a lung right up into the street without some wild-eyed antismoking fanatic making a sarcastic crack like, "Hey, you all right?" According to the Tobacco Institute, a certain acceptable etiquette has to be displayed when you come upon someone who, veins bulging out of his or her neck, explodes into a coughing seizure that splatters saliva on everything and everyone within ten feet. Your response should be something like, "Excuse me, did you see the Lakers game last night?"

Attempting to take the Tobacco Institute seriously is like trying to take seriously someone's contention that war is fun. It's hopeless. If you listen to them, only about one out of every 2 million smokers ever even coughs and when that person does it's because of some beastie in the air. According to the Institute, there's less chance of dying of a smoking-related death than there is of being stepped on by a dinosaur.

Fortunately, fewer and fewer people are allowing themselves to be duped by such bunk. There's a movement against smoking that is truly encouraging. Since 1979, cigarette sales have been declining regularly. All surveys show that 60 to 90 percent of smokers would very much like to cut down or quit. Thirty-nine states and numerous localities now have ordinances against smoking. In March 1986, New York City Mayor Ed Koch proposed what he described as the most stringent antismoking regulations in the United States. The law would forbid smoking in *any and all* closed public spaces. In September 1986, Los Angeles County banned smoking in all public hospitals. Think of it. Smoking in hospitals has to be *legislated* out of existence! One might logically expect that the one place where you would *not* find people smoking would be our hospitals. Go into any hospital in this country (except in Los Angeles County), and you will find "health" professionals sitting around puffing away on their "cancer sticks." *Doctors and nurses!* Lord help us.

I think a Nobel Prize for health should be given to Dr. C. Everett Koop, the United States Surgeon General. Dr. Koop, a vehemently outspoken critic of smoking, calls cigarettes one of the most destructive substances in our environment and the chief preventable cause of death in our society. It is his lofty goal to make the United States a smoke-free society by the year 2000. My kind of guy.

You must be clear on something. Your body has 96,000 miles of blood vessels. With every puff of smoke that is inhaled, every one of those blood vessels constricts. That is why smokers frequently complain of cold hands and feet. Their extremities are not receiving sufficient blood. More alarming is the fact that every organ in your body is dependent upon fresh oxygenated blood. When you regularly force the organs of your body to be deprived of their fair share of blood you are inviting more trouble than you ever imagined. Understand that *everything* is prevented from operating optimally. Your liver, kidneys, heart, stomach, thyroid, brain, eyesight, hearing, skin, **EVERYTHING!**

There is no finer, no more noble undertaking than making an effort to give up smoking. We have been fortunate enough to see many people literally transform their lives by doing so. It is truly a marvelous sight to witness the ecstatic feelings people radiate once they successfully throw off this ruinous habit. If you are a smoker, you, too, will bless the day you finally free yourself from its deadly grip.

Let's go on the premise that you definitely want to give up smoking but could use a little help. You have two ways to go: Either just give it up for good in one sudden burst of resolve or eliminate it slowly. In either case, there are things that you can expect to happen and there are tools you can use to help you achieve your goal. Keep in mind that you are dealing with an addiction, and as with any other addiction, there may be some withdrawal symptoms. They may be uncomfortable, but they *can* be minimized. That you may experience headaches, discomforts, and/or edginess is understandable. After all, your system has been saturated with highly toxic substances, and when that stuff starts to be eliminated it can be rather uncomfortable.

Over the years, we have seen hundreds of people give up smoking, and their symptoms of withdrawal ranged from nothing whatsoever, even among those who went ''cold turkey,'' to extreme discomfort in individuals who only tried to cut down slowly. There is no norm, no set rule stating what you will or will not experience. You simply have to be prepared for some possible unpleasantness. If you do experience feeling out of sorts, please do not become discouraged. Rather, take comfort in the fact that you are on the road to making your body more fit and your life more enjoyable.

Keep in mind that we are an alkaline species. Our bodies are slightly alkaline.* If we overindulge in habits that are acid-forming, it lessens our alkaline balance; our bodies suffer and we pay the price. I can think of nothing more acid-producing than smoking. Remember our explanation of food combining. There we pointed out that when an acid and an alkali are mixed, both are neutralized. You can use this bit of physiological knowledge to your benefit to effectively minimize potential negative ramifications of giving up smoking. Unfortunately, the nicotine, tar, and other nasties in cigarettes saturate your tissues, and when the body starts to get rid of them, this acid is stirred up, which is what creates the discomfort.

A lot of people find that the minute they give up smoking they gain weight. Some of this is obviously due to increased food consumption, but there is another factor involved that you should understand. The body is infinitely wise. Nicotine and tar released from the tissues are dangerously poisonous, so the body does the only thing it can to offset the threat: It retains water to dilute the poison until it can be flushed out through the normal channels of elimination. This contributes to the weight gain and lasts for as long as is necessary for the body to eliminate all of the accumulated

*The alkaline/acid (pH) balance ranges from totally acid, 0, to totally alkaline, 14; 7 is neutral. Our blood pH range is from 7.35 to 7.4.

tar and nicotine. The longer one has smoked, the longer this water retention usually lasts. Fear not. The detoxification process can be hastened by dietary changes, especially by a dietary focus on fruits and vegetables, which promote elimination.

There are other things that you can do. First, since it is acid that you are trying to get rid of, it simply makes good sense to minimize the amount of acid you add to your system at this time. The most acid-forming elements in the average diet are animal products (all flesh, dairy products, and eggs), salt, cereals, coffee, sodas, and alcohol. It is not necessary to eliminate these items entirely. Rather, *reduce them as much as you comfortably can*, during this time of cleansing your body of the acid by-products of cigarette smoking. Does that not make all the sense in the world to you? If you want to get rid of acid, why add more? If you were trying to put out a fire, would you throw kerosene on it? If you were in a rowboat that was sinking, would you bring more water into the boat? It's the same thing. To whatever extent you decrease the amount of acid you add to your system, to that extent you will hasten ridding yourself of what is already in your system. The sooner you cleanse these poisons from your body, the sooner any cravings you have will disappear.

The second step you can use to reduce the acid in your body is to *neutralize it with alkaline foods*. All foods that you eat are either acidic or alkaline in the body, except fats, which are neutral. If you cut down on the acidic foods mentioned above and simultaneously consume certain foods that are highly alkaline, you can *greatly* reduce both the acid in your body and your craving for cigarettes. We have seen this work numerous times.

I'll bet I know your next question: What foods are alkaline? Good question. Actually, when eaten raw and properly combined, *all* fruits and vegetables are alkaline. So what that means is that if you follow either the program laid out in **Fit for Life** or the three-day Detoxification Menu in chapter 17, you will automatically be eating a diet that lowers acid intake while increasing alkali consumption.

Interestingly enough, one of the most alkaline foods you can eat is celery. I've known people who, because of some dietary indiscretions (a polite way of saying they "blew it"), had severe heartburn or burning in the stomach and, upon eating a couple of stalks of celery, totally neutralized the acid and ended the pain.

It's practically impossible to ill-combine celery. You can have it whenever you wish. Celery works before, during, or after meals. I have found it to be especially useful when, about an hour or so after a meal, I feel like having something else or I am thirsty and it's too soon to drink water. Because of its high water content, celery is a real thirst quencher.

There are other vegetables that serve this same role: cucumbers, red or green bell peppers, or lettuce leaves. The sweet inside leaves of romaine lettuce are highly alkaline, sweet and tasty, very high in water, and a fabulous thirst quencher. This is a way to intelligently use some of the foods that ordinarily do not receive a great deal of attention and that also help us make up for occasional indiscretions.

You may be thinking, "But, hey, I just don't stand around eating lettuce leaves." I got it. I said that very thing when it was first recommended to me. I can't help thinking of Woody Allen's jab at the "health food nuts" when, in *Annie Hall*, he went into a restaurant for lunch and ordered the "alfalfa sprouts with mashed yeast." I know that suggesting to some people that they eat lettuce leaves or celery is like telling them to stick their finger in a live socket. But I'll tell you what: It's a lot better than it may sound, and it is a classic example of using a good habit to crowd out a bad one. Plus, as an added bonus, munching celery and lettuce, which are zero calorie foods (meaning they *take* more calories from your body as it breaks them down than they give it), will help combat the weight gain that so frequently accompanies an attempt to break the smoking habit. All I ask is that you give it a try. You may surprise yourself. There are no magic formulas, but when you are trying to free yourself from the grasp of something as malevolent and damaging as smoking, even the simplest measures that can help should be explored.

Air is your most basic and elemental biological need. Your lungs were developed to utilize the freshest air the planet has to offer. Nurturing an awareness of this fact and holding it in your consciousness can only *improve* your health. Of this there can be no doubt. Whatever effort you make to get the best air you can, whenever you can, will reap benefits for you far greater than the effort you make. The body can do a lot with a little. Even a small effort brings big rewards.

I have always felt that if people had even a smattering of information about the actual physical needs of their bodies, they would do whatever was necessary to fulfill those needs if they possibly could. I don't think most health professionals give people enough credit. People have been put in the position of relying on the "experts" for practically every decision, good or bad. They are ready to take charge of their own lives. At last they are ready to rely more on themselves and their own inborn ability to direct their lives correctly.

As you develop self-confidence, you'll enjoy a positive outlook that then affects all aspects of your life, your work, your relationships, everything. If you decide to utilize some of the simple guidelines offered in this chapter to improve the air in your life and the vitality of your lungs, you will experience firsthand precisely what I am talking about. Personally, I hope you make the effort. You are worth it.

MARILYN:

For many people, smoking is an almost involuntary habit. Ask them if they smoke, and they reluctantly apologize rather than boast enthusiastically that they do. Many people overtly or secretly hate the fact that they smoke. They want to be free of cigarettes, but they can't seem to break the addiction.

It is a hard situation but not a hopeless one by any means. Many people have been hooked on cigarettes, and many have been able to quit. That is something to remember. If *one* can quit, *all* can quit. I know that firsthand, because between the ages of seventeen and thirty I was addicted to cigarettes, and yet I was able to quit.

I remember vividly what it was like to smoke. My whole stomach and digestive tract would tighten up in a sick, nauseated feeling as I pulled the first inhalation of smoke into my lungs. By the time I had finished a cigarette, there would be a spacey feeling in my head, which I now understand resulted from oxygen deprivation to the brain. I would become irritable, a further effect of oxygen deprivation. I hated the taste of smoke, as well as the smell of it on my hands and breath, and I was always self-conscious when I held a cigarette, as if I were doing something that no one else should witness. (I guess that makes sense, since suicide, even gradual suicide, is not really something one wants to do in public.) I remember my son Greg, who was very young when I smoked, *begging* me to not "light that cigarette," because he couldn't breathe when I did. But like so many other smokers, my addiction deafened me to others' needs, *even to those of my child!*

When I finally realized that I was able to quit, I began to separate myself from the act of smoking and analyze it objectively. What I became aware of was that, for me, smoking was usually a way to distract myself from very negative thoughts about myself and my life. Alone or with others, idle or in some kind of activity (usually social), a familiar, depressing thought would surface, usually a thought related to some negative emotion like envy or jealousy or to my insecurity about myself. In the midst of that thought, I would reach for a cigarette. While "killing myself" emotionally and intellectually with self-demolishing thoughts, I completed the process by going through the motions of killing myself physically little by little. As I grew stronger and closer to quitting, I began to notice what types of situations and what kinds of people prompted me to reach for a cigarette, and I realized that those situations and people probably were not so good for me and should be avoided.

I also began to realize that I was the master of my thoughts. Rather than allowing my brain to act like an out-of-control projector running negative tapes at my own expense, I would take charge. I could become the producer of my own "sound track," and when my brain spontaneously and out of habit went to the negative, I could say, "Down, girl!" and tap into something positive. Once I learned that little trick, the psychological environment that used to support smoking became less and less a part of me. Once I knew that I didn't have to smoke, my feelings about myself as a person completely changed. I had a sense of my own strength and ability. I felt freer. I certainly felt healthier.

Smoking coarsens the entire body. It deprives the body of oxygen, causing the cells all to mass together more tightly so the skin looks thicker, coarser, and much older. When I stopped smoking, the first change that I noticed, other than a great increase in happiness, was that my skin became more translucent and glowing. I have since noticed that same change in friends who have quit. Now whenever I see young kids smoking, especially innocent young girls, I wish they realized what they are doing to their natural beauty. *Nothing* will wipe it out faster than smoking.

Visualize the act of smoking. Smoke coming out of our mouths? Now, where do we see images of people with smoke coming out of their mouths? Certainly not in representations of souls in Paradise! When we smoke, are we in fact creating our own little hell on earth?

If you smoke and wish to stop, first **REALIZE THAT YOU ARE NOT A SMOKER.** The human species, of which you are a member, is not naturally intended to have smoke in its lungs. That is why you'll never find any of us loitering in burning buildings! You may have developed the habit of taking smoke into your lungs unnaturally, but that does not mean that you are naturally a smoker. If you have a single martini or a glass of wine, that does not make you an alcoholic, does it? Starting today, **THINK OF YOURSELF AS NOT BEING A SMOKER.** Can you do that? Even as you reach for a cigarette, **KNOW THAT YOU ARE NOT A SMOKER!** Continuously remind yourself of that and it will be harder and harder for you to reach for a cigarette. **YOU CAN STOP SMOKING. MILLIONS OF PEOPLE ALREADY HAVE.** You are as strong as they are. You certainly have my loving support in your effort to do so, and I'm sure you have the loving support of all the millions of people who know that *our air is our life*.

CHAPTER 7
Water

HARVEY:

When you have something in tremendous abundance, its presence everywhere so plentiful that you could never exhaust its supply, you cannot help but take it for granted. Such is the case with water. You would, however, become intensely aware of just how precious it is if you were parched with thirst. If you were stuck in a desert, dehydrating and in danger of dying of thirst, if you could barely swallow and were on the brink of collapse, you would rather have a glass of cool water than all the gold and diamonds in the world. Despite the unbelievable, immeasurable importance of water, I wonder how many people truly realize and appreciate the profound significance of its role in their lives.

Despite its not bearing the immediacy to life that air does, water nevertheless deserves equal treatment. In fact, inasmuch as breathing is an automatic process and drinking is a consciously directed process, water deserves perhaps more attention.

Deprived of water, plants droop and wither. Without water animals thirst and die. Water is the essence of life. Without it there is no life. No seed could germinate. No plant could grow. No animal could live. Without water this planet would forever have remained one vast barren rock, a lifeless desert.

Water has often been worshiped and revered as a source of life. The Egyptians worshiped the Nile. The Hindus worship the Ganges. The natural springs of Greece were chosen as sites for temples. And, of course, baptisms are performed in water.

Without water our bodies would be reduced to a few pounds of dust. There is not one function of the body that is not dependent on water. Seventy percent of your body is water. *Seventy percent!* The following table gives the percentage of water in various body parts:

Teeth	10%	Lungs	80%
Bones	13%	Brain	80.5%
Cartilage	55%	Bile	86%
Red blood		Plasma	90%
corpuscles	68.7%	Blood	90.7%
Liver	71.5%	Lymph	94%
Muscle tissues	75%	Saliva	95.5%
Spleen	75.5%	Gastric juice	95.5%

When you reflect on how extensively water is involved in the functioning of the body, you can't help but be held in awe. Consider some of the more important functions of water in the body:

1. Water supports all of the nutritive processes, from digestion and absorption to utilization and excretion. From the moment food enters your mouth, *every* process necessary to transform it from a food to blood, bone, muscle, and tissue—no small feat—depends on water. Some people say they have never seen a miracle. What then is the process that turns an apple into blood and bone? You see how we take things for granted? A deficiency of water anywhere along the chain of processes that create these miracles of life soon manifests itself in disturbances of these operations.

2. Water holds nutrients in solution and transports all food necessary for life to the various parts of the body. Have you ever wondered how, after eating, the nutrients in the food wind up at just the right place to supply each organ, indeed *each cell*, with what it needs to carry on its duties? We all know that our food contains vitamins, minerals, proteins (amino acids), carbohydrates, fats, and the other basic nutrients of life. But how are they extracted and distributed? You guessed it—by water! The body employs water to extract them, carry them all to the proper place, and drop them off in the exact amounts needed at exactly the right time. Perfection unsurpassed. Society should reflect the same synergy and exactness. There would be a lot less stress and strife, I'd wager.

3. Water holds wastes and toxins that it picks up from the cells and carries them to the organs of elimination. We've already described the process by which toxins are produced in the body as the by-products of food decomposition and as cellular wastes. We've emphasized the importance of getting rid of them as soon as possible. Carbon dioxide, nitrogen from protein metabolism, urea, and ammonia are but a few of the toxic substances that must be collected, diluted, and expelled from the body. Water carries them to the four organs of elimination—bowels, bladder, lungs, and skin—for disposal. What an exquisite arrangement. At one and the same time, water brings in what we need and carries out what we don't.

4. Water is an essential constituent of all cells and tissues and of all body fluids. Without sufficient water you would have no saliva. You wouldn't be able to swallow! Your tongue would stick to the inside of your mouth. You wouldn't be able to talk. Since gastric juices are practically *all* water, without it the food in your stomach couldn't digest. Your vital lifeline, the blood, is over 90 percent water. The organs that perform the functions of life are all more water than anything else.

5. Water keeps the various mucous membranes of the body soft and prevents friction between tissue surfaces. Without some kind of lubricant in your body, organs would stick together and tear. Bones would grate on each other and chip rather than glide smoothly at the joints. Muscles would lose their suppleness and not function adequately. All your inner organs swim in an ocean of fluids that is mostly water.

6. Water is the chief agent in regulating body temperature, serving much as does water in the radiator of a car. One of the major reasons water balance in the body is so crucial to our health is this relationship to temperature control and regulation. An internal temperature change of only a few degrees can mean death. The body is constantly giving off water from the kidneys, bowels, lungs, and skin. Perspiration cools the skin when it evaporates. All this helps maintain body temperature.

From the foregoing, I think it's obvious that water's vital role in keeping us alive is indisputable. I'll even go out on a limb and say that there probably aren't a half dozen dietitians in the entire country who would disagree. Your body normally expels about one gallon of water every day, and that, of course, must be replaced each day as well. Given its invaluable role, consideration *must* be given to obtaining the best water available. There are three issues to consider in that connection. When should we drink water? How much should we drink? And what is the best kind to drink?

When is easy. When you're thirsty! Water needs vary with season and activity. A person engaged in active physical labor in the summer sun will obviously require far more than an office worker spending hours in air conditioning. Obviously, we need more during the summer than in the winter and more during the day than at night. The easiest rule to remember is this: **IF YOU ARE THIRSTY, DRINK.** Your body is simply too darned smart not to let you know when it needs water.

That sounds fairly simple, doesn't it? But some people actually ignore thirst when it occurs. And they tend increasingly to reach for poor-quality thirst quenchers when they do take a drink.

The people of the United States now consume more soft drinks than they do water! Even children are given sodas rather than water when they are thirsty! Biologically, my dear friends, that is a real perversion. There is no way that these chemical concoctions do us any good. In fact, they do us great harm, which you will learn more about later in this book. Where do you think we would have found streams of naturally occurring sodas over the millions of years in which our species grew in strength and endurance—until we began 6000 years of recorded degeneration? In just the last three or four decades, slick advertising using brainwashing jingles has finally turned us away from nature's fountain of life.

There is a simple formula you can use to satisfy your body's need for water and work away from a dependence on sodas at the same time. First of all, **DRINK A GLASS OF WATER WHEN YOU AWAKEN IN THE MORNING BEFORE YOU EAT OR DRINK ANYTHING ELSE.** Second, **DRINK A GLASS OF WATER TEN MINUTES BEFORE EACH MEAL.** If you begin to fade during a workout or a hike, a drink of water will pick you right up again. The water that you consume before your meals will keep you from being thirsty during or after your meals.

The one negative aspect of drinking water that deserves mention is in conjunction with mealtime. Because water leaves the stomach so quickly (five minutes), it's certainly fine to drink water before eating. It's *with* a meal or *immediately following* a meal that there is cause for concern. Digestive juices are liquid, and drinking liquid, *any* liquid, with or after the meal dilutes the digestive juices and tends to carry them right out of the stomach. This severely slows the digestive process, giving rise to many of the digestive complaints that plague so many people. Also, when drinking with meals, we tend to swallow food that is only partially masticated. Not only is it best not to drink with meals but you should wait two hours after a meal. Now, some people have a lot of resistance to waiting, so if you simply must have some water, take very small sips to minimize the adverse effects. Or have celery stalks or cucumber spears if you can. Both are very high in water content, and they won't interfere with digestion.

As to how much water to drink, there is certainly some difference of opinion on that. One thing is sure: The less you get from your food, the more you have to drink. In fact, the frequency of thirst is directly correlated to the amount of water in your food. When food has had the water either processed or cooked out of it, naturally you're going to have to obtain more water through drinking. It is because of this, no doubt, that some dunce one day came up with the lame-brained idea of drinking a minimum of eight glasses of water a day. Tall or short, male or female, physically active or sedentary, living in a hot climate or cold, young or old—*everyone* is told to drink eight glasses of water a day. This is a classic example of a nonsensical approach to a situation that just as easily could have been handled intelligently.

How much should one drink? Again, there's only one ironclad rule: Drink when thirsty. Otherwise, there are no hard and fast rules in this matter. The sensible person will not attempt to fix quantities. It is undoubtedly true that our bodies require a certain minimum of water daily. But it by no means follows that we should *all* always drink eight glasses daily. Most people get two thirds of the water they require from their diet. A moderate excess of water is passed off rather harmlessly, but heavy drinking tends to waterlog tissues, dilute fluids, and impair cellular function. Waterlogging also lowers the capacity of the blood to absorb and carry oxygen. One sweats more when drinking more, and this excessive perspiration is enervating.

Observation will readily prove that those who drink the most water suffer the most from summer heat. Of course, one might think they drink more because the heat causes them great thirst. However, when they drink somewhat less, their sweating decreases, showing that their excessive drinking, not the heat, was largely responsible for their sweating. Many times the "thirst" experienced by those who drink great quantities of water is not truly a physiological need for water. The thirst is caused by salt, spices, greasy foods, highly processed and overcooked foods, or by foods with very low water content. You can drink a *gallon* of water and not quench the thirst produced by these substances.

Overdrinking is as harmful as overeating. Drinking heavily of something as innocuous as water may *seem* harmless, but it most certainly is not. The fertilized ova of some sea animals placed in tap water are observed to increase weight by as much as a thousand times. Such growth is not normal, and the cells formed under such conditions are deficient and weak. Supersaturation of plants submerged in water weakens and even kills them. Excess water produces inferior watery vegetation, while prolonged standing in water will kill most vegetation just as surely as drought. Nothing is to be gained by excessive water drinking. There simply is no sound reason why you should drink a certain number of glasses of water a day just because someone has arbitrarily decided that everyone requires that much. People are being advised to drink these daily amounts without any consideration of the individual needs or instinctive demands of their bodies. They are advised to drink even if they are not thirsty, and to cultivate the habit of drinking a glass of water at regular intervals. There is no more good reason to encourage routine drinking than there is to encourage routine eating. Why should you drink without being thirsty? Is this any more appropriate than eating if you're not hungry?

So how much should you drink? It depends. How much should you eat or breathe or sleep? *As much as nature calls for*. And this will depend on your individual life-style, the character of your food, climate, physical activity, etc. Pay attention to body signals and you will become attuned to your body's needs. Your most praiseworthy health habits arise from being in harmony with your body.

What is the best kind of water to drink? That's easy—**PURE!** If there's anything everyone wants, it is pure water. No one wants impure water, yet most people drink anything *but* pure water. Pure water is purely water, only water, and nothing but water. You have seen water referred to by its chemical formula, H_2O. Water is hydrogen and oxygen and *that's all!* Anything in water other than these two components actually contaminates it.

Most people in this country drink the water that is most easily available to them—commercial, ''purified'' tap water. Few are aware of the many impurities and poisons that may be in the water they are drinking. Most people drink tap water without giving it a second thought, but anyone who carefully considers tap water and its contaminants will be unlikely to continue to drink it. Besides numerous chemicals added to the water at the purification plant, water that travels through an intricate web of pipelines usually picks up metallic poisons. In addition, as a result of our continual disregard for the delicate balance of our environment, almost all of the waters on earth contain chemical pollutants. DDT has even been found in the far reaches of the North Pole.

Tap water these days is more like soup, a chemical soup. Among the pollutants are soap, wood pulp, oil, sulfuric acid, copper, arsenic, paint, pesticides, radioactive wastes, agricultural fertilizers, and chemicals from industries too numerous to mention. In addition there are *in*organic minerals ranging from mildly to highly toxic—sulphur, iron, gypsum, calcium, magnesium, lime, soda ash, fluorine, chlorine, etc. Moreover, further chemical pollutants are deliberately added to water supplies, supposedly in an effort to purify the water and kill its bacteria. The only thing is, the chemicals are far more harmful than the bacteria they're supposed to kill. Water goes through many processes at the ''purification'' plants: sedimentation, filtration, coagulation, softening, chlorination, bromination, iodization, and fluoridation.

Perhaps the most important thing to remember about tap water is this: It's *more* than just water! All chemicals are unusable poisons. Dear Health Seeker, I wish there were special words I could use here to express to you the unparalleled importance of your being *fastidiously particular* and exercising the *utmost discrimination* and *ultra-selectivity* about the water you allow into the temple of your life. Please do not make the grievous mistake of relegating your drinking water to a position of secondary importance or saying something like, ''Hey, it's just water. Water is water.'' That's not true. *Water is life!* The better your water, the better your life.

If you find you forget just how crucial a role water plays in your life, just read this chapter again. Read it *every day* if that's what it takes for you to realize that the quality of water you drink is worth whatever time and effort you put into getting the best.

Since it is pure water that your body needs, there is only one type of water suitable for your body—distilled. Distilled water is *the* purest water available. It's nothing but water! When the need for water in addition to what you get naturally from the fruits and vegetables in your diet arises, distilled water is unquestionably the best. Certainly a huge controversy surrounds this issue. But there is no validity to arguments against the use of distilled water. Not one scrap of sound evidence proves anything but the need *for* distilled water.

Nature ceaselessly engages in distilling water. Were this process not in constant and eternal operation, the earth's water would long ago have become so contaminated and foul as to be unfit for life. In spite of this, all water occurring in nature is more or less impure. Some is very impure. This includes mineral water, spring water, and well water. Water from these sources has dissolved and suspended mineral matter, not the kind the body uses, but *inorganic* minerals. Even rain water contains gases and dirt it picked up in falling. Rains in some areas of the world have acid concentrations so high they destroy forests and plant life.

Distillation provides us with the purest water obtainable. Some argue that pure distilled water (other than in plant life) can't be found in nature, that our ancient ancestors had no way of getting distilled water. True. However, to the great discredit of humankind, all of our natural waters have been fouled with the toxic wastes of civilization. It is regrettable, but now we have to resort to mechanical procedures to purify water. Indisputably, the facts are clear: Without distilling there is no pure water.

WATER AND MINERALS

The major argument against distilled water is that it leaches minerals from the body. This is *partially* true, but not in the way that opponents to distilled water think. Before I explain why, it is important you understand the difference between an organic mineral and an *in*organic mineral.

Besides other vital roles that minerals perform in the body, they are necessary for metabolism. **THE BODY CAN USE ONLY ORGANIC MINERALS.** It is physiologically impossible for your body to use an inorganic mineral. It simply cannot and will not do it. Anyone who knows biochemistry and physiology knows this to be true. It is frustratingly ironic how many people who should know better fail to recognize this simple fact. Your body can no more use an inorganic mineral than your car can run on Coca-Cola.

It's true that *chemically* an organic mineral is the same as an inorganic one. But there the similarities cease. *The human body cannot use inorganic minerals*—that is, minerals that have not already been organically processed. Minerals are only usable as they are found in organic forms of life such as plants, which make up an amazing link between the soils of the earth and animal life. Would you go into a gravel pit and pick up a piece of gravel and try to chew it up? Would you go out and pick up a handful of soil and eat it? Obviously not. Well, let your common sense answer here. Would you eat that piece of gravel if it were pulverized into particles small enough to swallow? Would you eat the soil if it were ground into a fine powder? There is no difference except in particle sizes. We are not rock or soil eaters. Your body cannot incorporate rocks into its cell structure. When you drink water containing minerals, they are inorganic. They're finely ground rocks! They have no more virtue in the human body than if the soil or rock itself were eaten.

Your cells must be furnished the minerals they need in order to accomplish their work. The minerals a cell cannot use will, if absorbed, only interfere with the cell's function. Therefore, cells reject inorganic minerals. In due course, this rejection leaves a surprising accumulation of discarded minerals, harmful debris. These minerals are deposited by the body in various tissues—organs, joints, bones, and the circulatory system. They lead to kidney stones, gallstones, ossification of the brain, arthritis, and heart disease. Bound up by cholesterol and fats in the arteries, these inorganic minerals form a thick concretelike plaque that causes "hardening of the arteries." They literally clog up the body and vascular system. Precious few people are aware of the havoc wreaked by inorganic minerals. If the minerals you provide your body are not organic, your body will reject them at great expense to its vital powers.

So how do we get our organic minerals? Through plant life! Plants take minerals from the soil and transform them. The plant takes in carbon dioxide, water, and elements from the earth. It also takes in sunlight through its chlorophyll and, through the process of photosynthesis, forms carbohydrates. As the plant grows, minerals from the earth become *organically part of the plant itself*. Then, and only then, can the minerals be assimilated by the human body.

Which plants are these? All fruits, vegetables, whole grains, nuts, seeds, and sprouts. These are the foods that supply you with the finest minerals: *organic* minerals. *All* others, whether from water or supplements, are nothing more than rocks or pulverized metals. Anyone who tells you otherwise is either selling mineral supplements or should be wearing a dunce cap to give you fair warning of his or her lack of understanding of this vital issue.

As for distilled water leaching out minerals, this is one of the grossest misrepresentations of data in all the field of physiology. It reminds me of the story of the scientist running a study to note the effect of removing the legs from a flea. First he trained the flea to jump on command. He successively removed each leg, giving the command "Jump!" after each removal. The flea obeyed every time. Even down to its last leg, the flea feebly attempted to jump on command. The scientist removed the last leg and gave the command, "Jump." No movement. He loudly shouted the command—"JUMP!" Absolutely not a move out of the flea. In reporting his findings in the scientific journals, the scientist wrote, "It has been conclusively demonstrated that if all the legs of a flea are removed, it will go deaf."

It may *look* as if the flea went deaf, but that's not why it wouldn't jump. It may *look* as if the sun moves across the sky, but actually it's the earth turning. It may *look* as if distilled water is leaching out minerals, but it's *in*organic minerals and mineral wastes that the distilled water is removing.

Distilled water has an inherent quality. Acting almost like a magnet, it picks up rejected, discarded, and unusable minerals and, assisted by the blood and lymph, carries them to the lungs and kidneys for elimination from the body. Referring to the elimination of these damaging minerals as a leaching out of minerals is erroneous. The statement that distilled water leaches out minerals from the body has no basis in fact. It doesn't leach out minerals that have become part of the cell structure. It *can't* and it *won't*. It collects and removes only minerals that have already been rejected or excreted by the cells.

Water is not where you should be looking for nutrients. Water is needed in the body simply as water, not as a source of any incidental impurities it may have picked up from soil and rock. *You should never try to get anything from water but water.*

To state that water leaches or does anything in the body is to make a very fundamental mistake. Water doesn't *do* anything. It is the body and only the body that acts. The body directs and controls the chemical absorption and elimination processes that go on within itself. Water is a totally lifeless substance. To say that water leaches out minerals is to ascribe to water powers of action that are inherent only within the living body.

The body is master. The body is the actor. Water does not determine what it will or will not carry into the body. *The body uses water. Water doesn't use the body.* To suggest that distilled water takes up minerals from foods so that the body derives no benefit from them is absurd. This is not an issue to take lightly. There is no more reason to put other than distilled water in your body than there is to put kerosene in your gas tank.

Perhaps it *seems* like too much fuss to make over this matter, but it's altogether clear that *not one* function of your body can be performed without water. Why would you *not* want the purest possible? Remember, the body cannot use *in*organic minerals. They only contaminate water, placing a burden on the body, as it has to expend energy to eliminate them. Besides that, they clog up vital tissues and arteries. Consider iodine as an example of the superiority of organic minerals over inorganic. Iodine is a mineral the body vitally needs, but *only* in its *organic* state. In its inorganic state, it's deadly poison, sold in pharmacies with a skull and crossbones on it.

While on the subject of water, let's turn our attention to two common "purifying" treatments used for tap water. The first is chlorination. With few exceptions, chlorine is added to the water supply of every large city in the United States. It's supposed to *poison* and kill germs. And it is well equipped to do so, considering how chlorine was first used. It seems we gullible Americans have been lulled into a stupor by the commonness of poisons being routinely added to our foods *and* water.

Chlorine was used during World War I *to kill people*—our enemies, of course. It was pretty nasty, too. Burned up their innards, it did. In fact, quite a few soldiers and civilians who only got "a touch" of the chemical were permanent physical wrecks because of its damages to their bodies. Now we've progressed.

We *drink* it! Good grief! Naturally we'll be treated to another verse of, "You'd have to drink enough water to launch the *Queen Mary* just to get enough chlorine to burn out one cell." Yeah, yeah. Ever notice how many times we get that song sung to us? And it's always to convince us to swallow another poison served up by the chemical industry. Our bodies are practically a dumping ground, for God's sake.

Chlorine (as in chlorinated tap water) combined with animal fats in the diet (consumed by the ton in this country) results in a chemical union of the chlorine and fat into a sticky pastelike substance. This stuff adheres to arterial walls, thus causing atherosclerosis—heart disease, in plain English, the biggest killer in this country. Chlorination of water supplies is sufficient reason in itself to consume distilled water.

The second treatment of water represents the most flagrant kind of abuse against an innocent public by commercial big business interests. Fluoridation.

The argument used to convince people that fluoride in our drinking water is beneficial or that it has some positive effect on our health is ludicrous. I wonder how many people are even aware of what fluoride is. Considering the way that the entire subject has been clouded with everything but the truth, I doubt it. For starters, take out your dictionary and look up *sodium fluoride*. You will find that it is a *poisonous* substance, among other things used for treatment of teeth to prevent decay, which is in itself a doubtful application, considering that tooth decay is just as rampant today as it has ever been.

Using poisons on human beings has become so commonplace that any dictionary matter-of-factly lists them as standard items in our diet. There are other uses for sodium fluoride, too. They include rat poison, glass etching, cockroach powder, industrial products such as dyes and plastics, pharmaceuticals (of course), tanning agents, metalworking agents, fumigants, insecticides, fungicides, germicides, fire extinguishers, solvents, and fire-proofing compounds. Doesn't that sound like just the perfect thing to be put into your drinking water for your consumption or sprayed on your child's teeth every time he or she goes to the dentist?

In 1945 the sales engineer at the biggest aluminum manufacturing plant in the United States realized that millions of pounds of aluminum were going to waste during processing. This waste was in the form of aluminum filing tailings, an extremely fine dust separated from the body of the aluminum during processing. Company executives figured out that if they could sell this waste at even the minuscule price of one-and-a-half cents a pound, they would reap a handsome $15 million dividend each year.

The dust was so poisonous that it posed a problem just disposing of it. It was used primarily as a rat poison, because it ground the digestive organs to shreds just as ground glass would. So poisonous was it to the human system that aluminum cooking utensils had been under attack for nearly forty years because of harmful metallic matter being given off into the water and food, especially acidic foods, during cooking. Many countries, including Germany, France, Belgium, England, Switzerland, Hungary, and Brazil, prohibited the sale of aluminum cooking utensils. Moreover, there was a definite link apparent between aluminum and Alzheimer's disease.

It was discovered that the water in Hereford, Texas, had a high content of calcium fluoride in its *natural* state—produced by nature over thousands of years—which seemed to assist in making teeth strong. So the aluminum trust decided arbitrarily to call the tailings dust ''sodium fluoride'' and then to sell *all* the cities in the United States on adding it to their municipal water supplies. Public enthusiasm for a tooth decay preventative resulted in logic and reason being overshadowed by hasty, unsubstantiated tests and claims based on those inadequate tests. The powerful aluminum industry put its resources behind overriding opposition to their grand plan to make a profit on their problem child, highly toxic aluminum wastes.

The argument promoting fluoridation was based on tests conducted in two cities in New York State, Kingston and Newburgh. The tests conducted there in the 1940s are still used today to justify fluoridation. The results, *as reported by the aluminum trust*, were that 817 children tested and living in Newburgh, the fluoridated city, had 60 percent fewer cavities than the 711 children tested and living in Kingston, the unfluoridated city. That all sounds convincing, and who's going to New York to check the records for themselves?

The facts are these, however. What industry researchers did was take a fraction of the children from each city and check their teeth. They used children from Newburgh who did not have many dental problems and children from Kingston who did. That way it looked as if the fluoridated city had far superior results with fluoridated water. But the true numbers were not 817 and 711. *All* the water in Newburgh was fluoridated, and *all* the children drank it. There were considerably more than 817 children drinking water. I quote from *The New Drug Story:* "The water from Kingston was left pure. The water from Newburgh was fluoridated. The U.S.P.H.S. [United States Public Health Service] announced that in five years it would examine the teeth of school children of these two communities and the examination would show that fluoridation would reduce tooth decay fifty percent."*

This test backfired, and how! A preliminary survey by the U.S.P.H.S. showed that fluoridation was *causing* a lot more tooth decay than pure water. So they dropped the subject, hoping it would not come up again. The New York State Board of Education had other ideas. They had their school doctors examine the teeth of the children of both cities, and this is what they found:

"In Newburgh [the fluoridated city], 4,969 pupils were inspected and 3,139 found with tooth defects. In Kingston [the pure water city], 5,308 pupils were inspected and 2,209 found with tooth defects. The box score: Newburgh [fluoridated] found 63% of its pupils with bad teeth; Kingston [the pure water city] had only 41%. Thus, in four years, the record indicated that fluoridation *caused* 50% more tooth troubles than nonfluoridation."† Those are the facts. Unfortunately, commercial interests twisted them and changed them until it looked as if fluoridated water was the best thing since sliced bread.

It was for profits and profits only that the pushers of "sodium fluoride" wanted all water systems fluoridated. And consider this: only 5 percent of a city's water is used for drinking purposes. The other 95 percent goes for domestic uses, sanitation, lawn and garden sprinkling, industrial purposes, sewage dilution, street flushing, and fire fighting. Again from *The New Drug Story:* "Mayor John S. Johnson of Fulton, New York, announced that after three years of fluoridation, brass rods that supported gears in city water meters have been eaten away by fluoride. The City Council has removed fluorides from the city water.

"In Chicago, Illinois, when fluoride was being put into South Chicago reservoir, the community newspaper in that area published a picture of the proceedings. It showed workmen in asbestos cloth-

*Morris A. Bealle, *The New Drug Story* (Washington, D.C.: Columbia Publishing Company, 1958), page 127.
†Bealle, page 127.

ing and space helmets. The label on the fluoride shipment read thusly: 'WARNING: The standard label for this material reads ''corrosive liquid.'' This label really means what it says. The vapor or liquid material is very dangerous when it comes in contact with the eyes, skin or any part of the body, *or if taken internally* [my emphasis]. When in contact with the skin, it can cause painful and slow-healing burns. Exposure to more than fifty part fumes per million of air is known to be fatal in thirty to sixty minutes. You are dealing with a substance so corrosive that it will eat through a quarter inch steel plate in a few minutes.' ''*

That is taken directly from the label of the stuff to be put into your drinking water. So there you have it, a known poison winding up in our drinking water. Paying to have your water fluoridated with aluminum filings (sodium fluoride) and then drinking it makes as much sense as paying some thug fifty dollars to punch you in the mouth. Not only do you lose some teeth, it costs you money to do it. Again from *The New Drug Story:* ''The coup de grace to the illusion the U.S.P.H.S. has been spreading far and wide that 'fluoridation is harmless' or that it 'saves the kiddies' teeth' was administered in Worcester, Massachusetts, by a group of fifty-nine medical doctors and one hundred and fifty-one dentists in that city.

''They had been hoodwinked into endorsing fluoridation without knowing anything about it. Wiser heads prevailed and an investigation was made. The Worcester Dental Society repudiated its own endorsement with a frank and honest statement, admitting its endorsement had been given after hearing only one side, that of the sales engineers for the aluminum trust. The repudiation signed by a hundred and twenty-seven of the W.D.S.'s members reads: 'Having heard, since approval without discussion prior to approval, the other side of the fluoridation plan, and having learned of its dangerous and unscientific nature: that it is not essential to development of good teeth; that it does not prevent tooth decay; that there are better and less devious ways to control tooth decay without polluting our water supplies and compelling an entire nation to drink medicated water which is of no value to them, which is known to be harmful to all human beings as a slow and accumulative poison, that all benefits attributed to fluorides are not due to fluorides at all, but are due to better nutrition, better hygiene

*Bealle, pages 138–139.

and better supervision. All of the foregoing statements being supported by universities in many parts of the country, by eminent scientists, biochemists, physicians, and dentists, we demand that this hollow approval of the Worcester District Dental Society obtained by telling only one side of the fluoridation story, be rescinded.' ''*

The fluoride pushers are still managing to sell you their poison. When it comes to the business of taking in money, their repertoire of schemes is seemingly unlimited. Enough people were sufficiently aware of the dangers of fluoride not to allow it to be added to their water. So the producers of fluoride came up with a ''fluoride rinse'' they could sell to the schools in communities without fluoridated water. At least 20 million children in nonfluoridated communities could possibly use the rinse. It would be sold to the schools at fifty cents per student. That is at least $10 million more a year to be reaped by the fluoridators. Every little bit counts. How nice it is to know that they are looking out for you and your children's teeth with *rat poison*!

In case you're not convinced of fluoride's deadliness, consider this. If it takes you about half an hour to read this chapter, during the course of the reading, three people will have died from cancer caused by fluoride. According to Dr. Dean Burke, former chief biochemist at the National Cancer Institute, *more than 50,000 Americans a year are dying of cancer caused by fluoridated drinking water!* In his words: ''We've now had time to look at fluoridation and see its effects on human health and we know it's a killer. Any institution who supports fluoridation is guilty of mass murder.'' That's strong language! Dr. Burke used these words at an Environmental Protection Agency hearing on June 18, 1985. He was imploring the EPA to do whatever it could to end this horrific poisoning of our water. At the same hearing, Dr. John Lee, a physician from Mill Valley, California, testified that fluoride is also a major cause of birth defects. Dr. Burke cited a study of cancer death rates in Birmingham, England, and found that after only a few years of artificially fluoridating their water supplies, there was an extraordinary increase of cancer in that city as well.

The cancers that fluoride is primarily associated with are of the gastrointestinal tract, kidneys, bladder, breast, and ovaries. The dangers of fluoride have long been known.

*Bealle, page 144.

Dr. John Yiamouyannis, a biochemist and science director of the National Health Foundation, is considered one of the world's leading authorities on fluoride and its effect on health. In a study he conducted with Dr. Burke of the death rate among people age forty-five and over in the ten largest fluoridated American cities, they found the death rate among these people to be significantly higher since the start of fluoridation than in the largest nonfluoridated cities with similar cancer death rates from 1944 to 1950.

Even in the area in which fluoride is *supposed* to provide benefit, less dental cavities, there are serious doubts, considering the findings by dentists that it causes mottling of the teeth. Why not become educated on how to prevent tooth decay with diet instead of risking cancer with a virulent poison? In the words of consumer advocate Ralph Nader: "Fluoridation is a diversionary issue to a more basic problem. It's helping divert public awareness of the role of junk foods in helping to cause cavities. I've often wondered why all the people who are so gung-ho for fluoridation never say anything about how poor food choices cause so many dental cavities in our children."*

Don't think for one moment that the fluoride issue is not a financial-political one. Ever hear of AIDS? You can't pick up a newspaper or magazine or turn on the television without something about this dreadful situation being reported. Ever hear anything about how many people are dying from fluoride poisoning? In the same five years, from 1981 to 1986, that 10,000 people were succumbing to AIDS, a whopping *one quarter of a million* people died from fluoride poisoning. Twenty-five times more deaths and not a word. How come? I'm certainly not suggesting we ignore AIDS, but I'd sure as hell like to know why fluoride deaths *are* being ignored.

When you reflect on the spectacular, incomparable wisdom and functionability of the human body, you can't help but be in awe of its magnificence. Whatever each of us can physically do to *assist* rather than thwart the operations of the body, we must do. We have an obligation to do our best for ourselves. Now that you know the full extent of the important role water plays in *all* of the operations of your body, by all means make the smart choice in

*Edith K. Roosevelt, "Poison in Your Drinking Glass," *Nutrition Health Review*, Vol. 20, October 1981, page 23.

the type of water you drink. There should be only *one* choice—
PURE! And pure means distilled.

By the way, if you have the kind of clothes iron that you fill
with water for steam, you know what kind of water is *always*
recommended for use. Distilled. Know why? Because if you use
other than distilled water, the minerals in it will corrode and destroy
your iron. I know people who would no more fill their iron with
tap water than they would fill their shoes with glue, yet they drink
the very water they wouldn't put into their iron. If nondistilled
water will destroy the insides of an iron, what might it do to *your*
insides?

CHAPTER 8
Food

HARVEY:

Ahhh, yes, food . . . one of my *only* weaknesses. I love food. I really do. Always have. One of the reasons I am so happy to have learned how to eat and maintain a healthy body weight is that I get to eat, enjoy my food, and not gain weight. At the rate I was going, if I hadn't learned what to do, I might have become 600 pounds by now—if I had lived.

Here's an interesting piece of information for you. In an average lifetime, we each will eat somewhere between fifty and ninety tons of food. That's a lot of food for one little stomach to process, don't you think? Fifty to ninety tons! *All* of the elements of health are important. No doubt about that. And although air and water are by far the most vital in terms of what we must have to fulfill our most immediate needs, it is food that plays the most crucial role in terms of our *long-term* health and longevity. Of that there can be no doubt whatsoever.

What happens if you stop eating? You die. You may last a month, two months, or maybe more, but without food you're going to die. Every single day your body loses hundreds of billions of cells, and every day they are replaced with new ones. What are these new cells made from? The food you put into your body. It is only logical to conclude that **THE QUALITY OF THE FOOD THAT WINDS UP IN YOUR BODY IS GOING TO BE A *MAJOR* CONTRIBUTING FACTOR TO THE QUALITY OF YOUR HEALTH**.

The food you eat is going to become you. Quite literally, your very cells will be built from what you eat. There really is no escaping this conclusion. That is why this chapter is such a critical one, because food is the area where we have *most* flagrantly forsaken our biological needs, and we are paying a dear price for this fact—paying with our health.

I want you to think about something for a moment. Do you realize that we are the *only* species on this entire planet *not* eating our food in its natural state? Please don't say that our pets or animals in zoos don't either. When under the domain of humans, animals eat what we give them, and then they suffer the same health problems we do. Left to their own devices, animals in the wild *all* eat their food in its natural state. Humans do not and we are entirely alone in that respect. Also, do you realize that we are the *only* species that combines different foods together at one meal? Do you realize that we are the *only* species taking billions of dollars worth of drugs after we eat to deal with the discomfort *eating* has produced?

An odd thing has happened in this country when it comes to food. Even though **HAVING THE BEST, FRESHEST, MOST WHOLESOME FOOD POSSIBLE IS ONE OF THE MOST SIGNIFICANT CONSIDERATIONS OF DAILY LIFE**, frequently food does not receive the attention it deserves. Because of vested commercial interests, greed, convenience, apathy, and *gross* misinformation, far too many people have been lulled into believing that *anything* they can get down their throats is okay to put there. It's not.

You may be convinced to buy someone's product through advertising, false claims, promises of value, or what have you. But much of the food foisted on the American people is as worthless as eating crushed adobe bricks. There is a lot of ill health in this country, and *far* more of it can be traced to what people eat than you might expect. Let me tell you about the greatest threat to your health on this planet. No, it's not nuclear proliferation. **THE GREATEST THREAT TO YOUR HEALTH IS PROCESSED FOODS!**

There is more phony, adulterated, devitalized, worthless "food" offered up to the American people today than real, honest-to-goodness, authentic fare that is necessary for our sustenance. And we have the food processors to thank. As our waistlines (and arteries) get fatter, so do their wallets.

We use the term *processed food* so routinely that for many of us it has come to represent "just another kind of food." Understand what it *really* means.

Understand that when the word *processed* is used, it refers to procedures that ultimately undermine your health. It is a term that you can easily and accurately interchange with the word *destroyed*. Processing is the practice of taking a perfectly good food, one that contains the nutrients necessary to prolong life, and stripping it of everything and anything of value and then offering it up for sale. In other words, processing is making something to put into the human stomach that no longer resembles what nature produced and intended for consumption.

Let me describe for you a successful little scenario the food processors have devised.

First, as step one, a food that was once actually a food, created by nature and capable of supplying the needs of your body, is processed. In other words, it is denatured and devitalized—heated, reheated, adulterated, pulverized, fragmented, impaired, de-graded, and otherwise despoiled—until it bears absolutely no re-semblance whatsoever to the product of nature that was grown for your consumption.

Next is step two. Chemicals are added. More than *one billion pounds* of chemicals are routinely added to food Americans eat each year. There are chemicals for everything and anything you can think of: colorings to either intensify or modify existing colors; dyes to enhance the appearance; preservatives to prevent spoilage—so that three weeks after buying a loaf of white bread (what we like to call vitamin-enriched Styrofoam), it is still soft; conditioners; stabilizers; antifoaming agents; chemicals to prevent fermentation; chemicals for texture, firmness, thickening, and emulsifying; flavoring agents by the trainload, most of which are synthetic coal tar products produced in a laboratory; chemicals to either increase or decrease moisture content; and a host of artifi-cially produced nutrients to try and add back at the end some of what was destroyed.

The day science entered the food industry was a sad, sad day, indeed. Natural foods are routinely turned into a conglomeration of high-priced chemicals designed to *simulate* food. Once the food processors have these abominations produced by the miracle of modern food technology, it is time to get you to lay down your hard-earned money for them.

Step three is deviousness carried to new heights. The food processors hire lobbyists to get legislation passed allowing them to call these foods, of all things, *natural*. Ever wonder how a food that is over 50 percent *processed* white sugar and dripping with additives can be called natural? Legislation, m'boy, legislation!

Food processors have actually been successful in getting laws passed allowing the use of the word *natural* on a label as long as *some* percentage of the ingredients did indeed come *from* a natural product. Tricky, tricky. When you look at the ingredients of a packaged product labeled "All Natural" and see several words with more syllables than you can count on both hands, it's *not natural! Natural* means as occurring in nature—period. I don't know about you, but when I was a kid, I did not relax in the shade of the old hydrogenated methylchloride tree.

Such dubious claims are possible because there is no generally accepted definition of a natural food. So the FDA pretty much allows the manufacturers to define the word for themselves. How convenient. That would be like telling auto mechanics that they have to be honest when making out your bill for work rendered but what's honest is up to them. You could then "honestly" be charged $650 for changing your oil or $300 for fixing your windshield wiper.

Now comes step four, packaging. Very important. More money is spent on the package than the product itself: Four-color boxes scream out promises of value and taste, free coupons, "ALL NATURAL" in huge letters, and include perhaps a free whistle or some other gimmick to get you to buy. Lots of claims.

Finally, we have step five. A marketing/advertising firm is hired to convince you to buy the product. Enough advertising could get some people to buy and eat tar if it were presented in the right way. Don't laugh. People are already eating things as bad—or worse. The ads don't really sell you food. They sell you "fluff." Ads depict happy, healthy people enjoying the product to the tune of a snappy jingle; everything but the actual value of the food is advertised. Remember the ad for ketchup that, instead of talking about how that brand tastes more like tomatoes, sold you on the fact that this ketchup took more time to drip down a plate than a competing product?

This highly successful food processing scenario has quite the appropriate name. It's called a "cashectomy," and it is carried out with the precision of brain surgery. Your cash is expertly extracted from your wallet and in return you are given something not only worthless but *harmful*. That's a first-rate cashectomy.

What would you think if you found out there was a group called the National Water Contaminators Association (NWCA) whose job it was to make sure your water is contaminated? Or a National Air Polluters Association (NAPA) whose job it is to see to it that your air was polluted? Or a National Food Processors Association (NFPA) whose job it was to process your food? Would you be outraged, surprised, disappointed, or what? You're probably saying, "There are no such groups as those." Well, you're right . . . mostly. Two of these groups don't exist, but the NFPA does exist. It has conventions, sponsors conferences on food advertising and labeling, and its members are out there processing your food and performing "cashectomies."

Allow me to introduce you to Paul A. Stitt. Mr. Stitt is a biochemist dedicated to helping Americans get some *real* food and exposing the big food giants who have used fancy million-dollar advertising campaigns to convince people that nonfoods are the right things to eat. His outspoken opinions on the American food industry have gotten him written up in practically every major newspaper and magazine and interviewed on practically every major radio and television show in the country. He has written a book entitled *Fighting the Food Giants*. He wrote it because he was outraged. When I read it, I was outraged. And if you read it, you will be, too.

What makes Mr. Stitt's book so engrossing and meaningful is the fact that he didn't simply write the book as an outside antagonist. He was a professional food processor himself for four years, working for two of the larger food giants in the United States. He was fired when he protested against some of the underhanded, devious, and deceitful tactics used by the company he was working for. When he insisted that more nutritious foods be offered to the public, he was terminated. The fact that his book was written from the *inside* is what affected me so intensely. He *knows* what is going on. It's not speculation.

In the introduction of his book, Mr. Stitt states, "There is a force in this country that's out to poison your food, to make it addictive, to manipulate your very body chemistry. This conspiracy wants to keep you overfed but undernourished. Who's behind this conspiracy to take your life? The food giants.

"Without your knowledge or consent, they control what you eat, when you eat, how much you eat, even the way you think of food. The food giants have done everything they can to keep you from finding out. They've warped your food consciousness to make you a willing participant in your own demise."

Good grief! That's scary! Just read this quote over a few times to get the full import of what he is saying. You . . . your children . . . are being poisoned *on purpose*! It's one thing to make a buck selling a product that you think is beneficial even though it may not be, but to put something on the market with total knowledge of its inferiority and harmfulness is unconscionable.

Have you ever heard anyone say, "I don't understand it. I eat all the time but I'm always hungry." Or perhaps you have found yourself (or your child) prowling around the kitchen looking for something to eat only an hour after a meal, even though there is simply no reason you should be hungry. That seemingly baffling and frustrating situation is no accidental occurrence.

Ever hear of the appestat? The appestat is an organ located in the base of the brain. It is something like a thermostat. The appestat is responsible for your appetite. It constantly monitors the bloodstream for nutrients. When they are not present in the necessary amounts, you feel hungry. So what do you think happens when you eat food that has had its nutrient content destroyed? You fill up, but because the food is "empty" the appestat registers that you need still *more* food. You keep eating and eating but the appestat just doesn't turn off. The result is that familiar complaint, "I eat all the time but I'm still hungry." The body is tricked into thinking it needs more food when it's actually crying out for *nutrients*. Sadly, there is a beneficiary of this tragic situation— *the people making and selling you the empty foods!* Your apparently insatiable appetite is a result of the most detestable kind of manipulation of your body chemistry imaginable, and it's all done to increase profits while diminishing your health. This is what so incensed Mr. Stitt that he jeopardized his chosen career in an attempt to get the truth out.

He found out that the company employing him—and plenty of others—had people working on foods that would *bypass* the appestat. They intentionally created foods devoid of nutrients—processed the nutrients right out, then soaked the foods with chemicals to make them look and taste good. That way you eat and eat and eat and buy more and more and more of their product. They get rich. You get fat and your body suffers. And it is done by design! It's planned. It's calculated. It's being done this very second, as you are reading this!

In Mr. Stitt's words, "The food companies *know* that compulsive eating is caused, not cured, by filling you up on worthless nutrition-free diet snacks which are actually empty calories in disguise. They even know that some of the products they pass off as wholesome and nutritious actually *cause* harm and poor health, but they've kept the truth from you."

Here is just one example that is liable to make you livid with rage:

While doing some research for a project he was working on for a large food processing company, Mr. Stitt came across a report that the company printed in 1942. It detailed a study in which four sets of rats were fed special diets. Group 1 received plain whole wheat, water, vitamins, and minerals. Group 2 was given puffed wheat—a product that the company sold—water, and the same vitamins and minerals. Group 3 was given water and white sugar. And Group 4 was given nothing but water and the nutrients. The rats that received the whole wheat lived for more than a year. The rats who got nothing but water and vitamins lived about two months. Those fed white sugar and water lived one month. The rats given the puffed wheat died in two weeks! They didn't die from malnutrition. There is actually something toxic about puffed wheat itself. When the grain is subjected to 1500 pounds of pressure per square inch, evidently that produces chemical changes that turn a nutritious grain into a poisonous substance. The company had known about this toxicity for thirty-eight years!

Mr. Stitt, shocked, took the report to one of his colleagues, who was equally shocked and went to the president of the company to implore him to reconsider selling this "food" to the innocent public. Here is a *direct* quote of what the president said: "I know people should throw it on brides and grooms at weddings. But, if they insist on sticking it in their mouths, can I help it? Besides, we made nine million dollars on the stuff last year." Mr. Stitt was instructed to keep his nose in his own business and not to worry about what was going on in the rest of the company. Obviously, these people had figured out a way to get to sleep at night. Mr. Stitt couldn't and was fired when he pressed the issue.

In the context of this book, when we refer to a processed food, we refer to a food that is lifeless, therefore dead . . . therefore valueless. Under *no* circumstances will the vast intelligence of your body ever attempt to incorporate any dead matter into live cell structure. It can't and it won't. **YOUR BODY IS *ALIVE* AND CAN *ONLY* BE BUILT WITH LIVING MATERIALS.** How smart do you have to be to realize that if most of the fifty tons of food you eat is dead (processed), then that is what your body will become, *dead!* In other words, you have a degree of control over the length and the quality of your life. If dead food is what you *don't* want, then, obviously, its opposite is what you *do* want—living food! **IF YOU WANT TO BE ALIVE, EAT LIVING FOOD!** Do you need proof of that or does your common sense reverberate with the obviousness of it?

Allow me to explain to you what a living food is. A living food is *any* food that has not been altered in *any* way from the way it was created by nature. Another way of saying living food is *raw food*. Either term describes the same thing: food in its pristine state, the way it was produced by the Grand Provider.

Every animal on earth is biologically adapted to eat a certain type of food. A lion is biologically adapted to eat zebras and wildebeests. A horse is biologically adapted to eat grass. A koala bear is biologically adapted to eat eucalyptus leaves. An orangutan is biologically adapted to eat fruit. Etc. Etc.

Two things are true of all animals' dietary habits. First, they *never* cross over in terms of their biological adaptation—a lion does not eat grains; a horse does not eat zebras. Second, they *all* eat their foods *raw*, no exceptions, not one anywhere in nature.*
Barring being eaten, guess what the animals in the wild usually die of. *Natural causes*, that is, reaching the end of their natural life-span.

Now, let's take a look at the human animal—ourselves. Have we crossed over from our biological adaptation by eating foods not designed for us? Are you kidding? Name something we *won't* eat. We eat grains, fruit, vegetables, fungus, ants and other insects, fish eggs, other animals—including pigs' intestines, cows' livers, lambs' brains, frogs' legs, snails, baby cows, horses, dogs, rats, snakes, worms—rotten cheese, and a host of manufactured items that no other animal in its right mind would eat. Yes, we have

*Again, remember that I am referring exclusively to animals in their natural habitat, not to animals in zoos or kept as pets and forced from their natural biological inclination.

very definitely crossed over. Surely we have to be biologically adapted to *something*. Could we really be the only animal on earth created to eat absolutely anything we can get past our lips? Hardly.

THE HUMAN SPECIES IS BIOLOGICALLY ADAPTED TO EAT FOODS FROM THE PLANT KINGDOM. We may have learned to eat other foods and that's okay, but in terms of what we are *biologically* adapted to, the plant kingdom is it. Of course, there are going to be those who laugh this off while stating that we are designed to eat flesh as well as plant foods. Statements like that are not based on physiology. Those who insist that we are intended to eat flesh foods are either selling hamburgers for a living or they're on the payroll of companies making their living from the sale of animals for food. This is not speculation, guesswork, or wishful thinking.

The physiology of our bodies is what it is, and neither fancy talking nor credentialed "experts" can *ever* change that to fit their fallacious premises. All of the animals that are truly designed to eat the flesh of other animals have digestive tracts shorter than those of animals designed to eat from the plant kingdom. There are no exceptions to this. Match the digestive tracts of animals that are carnivorous or omnivorous against our digestive tracts and this becomes crystal clear. Our digestive tracts are very much longer than those of the flesh eaters. There is simply no getting around this.*

Not only have we crossed over, but we no longer eat our foods raw. Far from it. The greatest percentage of our food is either processed or cooked or both! And what do humans usually die from? *Disease!* In fact, the percentage of deaths due to natural causes is so small that it's not even listed in statistical charts. What do your instincts, common sense, and logic tell you about all of this? All animal groups on earth except one—us—eat food they are biologically adapted to, in its raw state, and they live out their lives with precious little pain or disease. The one species that does *not* stick to its biological adaptation and does *not* eat its foods raw suffers pain and dies more frequently of disease than anything else. These are the cold, hard facts, and all of the blathering and gibberish from an army of paid-off professionals will not alter these facts one iota.

*The effects of flesh eating on the human species are discussed more extensively in chapter 14.

Let me be explicitly understood here: *In no way* am I implying that to be healthy and live a full life you must eat *only* foods you are biologically adapted to in the raw state.

Inevitably, some dietitians, nutritionists, and pseudointellectuals somewhere will read only the table of contents, bibliography, and a few selected pages of this book, then dismiss it out of hand with a sneer about my suggesting that you can't eat anything but grass, uncooked. I do *not* mean to give the impression that you must eat exclusively uncooked food from the plant kingdom to experience health and longevity. However, I do *strongly* want to suggest that the more unprocessed, living plant foods you do eat, the better. Obviously! It's a simple matter of finding a happy balance that works in your life.

We must always consider what we call the real versus the ideal. It would be *ideal* to eat only totally pure, living food from the plant kingdom, but that is simply not a realistic expectation. The reality of it is that we like meat, pasta, bread, pizza, ice cream, and a host of other foods that may not be ideal but have played a role in our diet. It's best to get as close to ideal as we can while still enjoying ourselves. That there should be pleasure in eating is right and normal, but pleasure is not the only end for which we should eat.

When I am talking about living food, I am talking about fruits, vegetables, nuts, and seeds. If those foods predominate in your diet, then health will predominate in your life. A nice, simple equation. What we are suggesting is not that you try to turn your life around overnight with a total commitment to eating only living food, but that you increase the amount of living food according to your life-style and level of commitment. If that's a lot, great! If that's a little, great! Your improvement will match your level of commitment. These changes should never *ever* become an ordeal or a contest. Eating should remain a joy. As you feel better you will automatically become more enthused and you will naturally progress *at your own pace*.

There's a lot of talk about the prevention of disease these days. Ironically, as recently as ten years ago the relationship between diet and disease was all but denied by the "experts." As a matter of fact, when Dr. David Reuben first introduced the high-fiber diet, it was vociferously attacked (standard treatment for new information) by the American Association for the Advancement of Science, a group of top scientific authorities who are *supposed* to be on the cutting edge of what's best for the population. They actually maintained that a high-fiber diet would "shred the intestines and cause liver cancer." Are we on a high-fiber diet today? As recently as April 1986 the Memorial Sloan-Kettering Cancer Research Center put out a newsletter suggesting that those who propose a relationship between cancer treatment and diet are "quacks." Put a little new information in front of some "experts" and they turn into ducks—"Quack, quack, quack."

Notwithstanding the resistance of the "experts," the correlation between diet and disease *has* been made, but except for the most cursory advice (e.g., cut down on fat and cholesterol and increase fiber), we don't get a lot of direction in specifically what to do or how to do it. This is what Marilyn and I have endeavored to do with our combined total of twenty-nine years of study: give you *specific* tools to use. And these are our specific recommendations:

1. Eat high-water-content food.

2. Properly combine your food.

3. Eat fruit correctly.

4. Refrain from eating heavy food during your elimination and assimilation cycles.

5. Consider your biological adaptation and increase the amount of appropriate living food in your diet (fruits, vegetables, sprouts, nuts, and seeds).

When you start to eat less cooked food in favor of more living food, immediate positive changes take place, both physically and mentally. Because you are supplying your body with what it biologically craves, *all* your body functions improve: better digestion, better utilization of nutrients, better elimination, better cleansing of the system, better everything. Like any machine, the better the fuel, the better the performance. As usual, our wish is not that you take our word for it. Our wish is only that you try it and witness the results for yourself.

The reason that changing over to more living food has such a profound beneficial effect is because you reduce exposure to the unhealthy effects of cooked food in your body. Cooking creates the environment for disease. It is itself disease producing. This has been shown to be true in numerous studies. To anyone who has examined these studies the evidence is overwhelming. Cooking food destroys the potential benefits inherent in living food—it destroys or makes unavailable some 85 percent of the original nutrients. Almost all enzymes are killed off because they are sensitive to heat. Amino acids are destroyed or converted to forms that are either extremely difficult or impossible to digest. Under a microscope the etheric body of a living cell scintillates with sunlight. Dead cells do not polarize light; the color display is extinguished. If you take a seed from a plant or from a food and you heat it to the same degree of heat you cook food, *it will not germinate, it won't grow*.

Here is a little experiment you can perform for yourself. Buy two apples at the supermarket. Bake one, then put them both on your windowsill. You will witness the raw apple lasting for quite some time while the baked apple ferments and spoils very quickly.

In her book *Be Your Own Doctor*, Dr. Ann Wigmore states: "The most thrilling experience I can recall was to see cancer cells taken from a human body and *thriving* on cooked food but unable to survive on the *same* food that was uncooked."

One of the most impressive and impactful studies of cooked food versus live food was conducted by Dr. Francis M. Pottenger and published in the *American Journal of Orthodontics and Oral Surgery*. Dr. Pottenger carried out a meticulous, thorough ten-year experiment using 900 cats placed on controlled diets. Only two items of food were used and were given either in their raw state or cooked state. The results were so overwhelmingly conclusive and convincing that there can be no doubt whatsoever of living food's superiority over cooked. The cats fed only the living, raw food produced healthy kittens year after year. There was no disease, no ill health, no premature death. Death came only as the natural consequence of old age. However, cats fed the same food, *cooked*, developed every one of humanity's modern ailments: heart disease, cancer, kidney and thyroid disease, pneumonia, paralysis, loss of teeth, arthritis, difficulty in labor, diminished sexual interest, diarrhea, irritability so intense that the cats were dangerous to handle, liver impairment, and osteoporosis (resulting in bones and teeth becoming thin and brittle). The excrement from these cats was so toxic that weeds refused to grow in the soil fertilized with it, whereas weeds proliferated in the stools from the cats fed living food. Here is the clincher: The first generation of kittens born to the second group of cats were sick and abnormal. The second generation were often born diseased or dead. By the third generation, the mothers were *sterile*. Dr. Pottenger conducted similar tests on white mice, and the results coincided with those of the tests run on the cats.

Cooked food takes its toll! That's why anyone wishing to live a life as free of ill health and disease as possible *must* see the wisdom of at least somewhat increasing his or her intake of living food.

SICKNESS DOES NOT JUST HAPPEN. It is built just as surely as health is built, and we have a choice as to which we build. In the words of Dr. Robert S. Mendelsohn, "Health is a matter of choice, not a mystery of chance." If you are building a thirty-story building and you use worm-eaten wood for the frame, inferior structural supports, and other fourth-rate, low-grade materials, what kind of finished product do you think you will wind up with? No need to answer. So if you're building a human body and the material that will become your blood, bones, skin, organs—indeed, *every* cell of your body—is inferior and of poor quality, what kind of body do you think you will wind up with? No need to answer.

Considering the case I've presented against cooked food, you might assume that my next step will be to try to convince you to eat just living food or practically all living food. Don't panic. As I've already noted, while that would be *ideal*, it certainly is not very realistic. Let's face it, cooked food is an integral part of our lives. I know I consume my share, but I try to eat more living than cooked food, and the cooked food is as pure and unprocessed as possible. And that is all we would hope for anyone reading this book.

If you knew the home you had worked and scrimped for and cherished was directly in the path of raging floodwaters and all you had to do to save it was stack sandbags around it, would you make the effort? Why would you *not* make the effort? What force could prevent you from taking this protective measure? Surely your life is as important as your house. There are protective measures you can take to *prevent* ill health, and no measure is as effective as upgrading the quality of the food that you eat. There is just no getting around it.

Your food is the single most important factor in building and preserving your health. In the past, the failure to accord diet the importance that it warrants was a glaring oversight of monumental proportions. To think that at one time it was actually considered absurd to link diet to ill health! Today, of course, that would be like saying the ocean has nothing to do with the waves that lap up on the shore. Every day it becomes more and more apparent just how crucial food is to health, and someday people will look back on those who doubted this fact with the same incredulity we now express in looking back to the practice of bloodletting. Now is the time for you to recognize that you can dramatically affect the length and quality of your life and the lives of your loved ones. Don't wait until it is too late or until the evidence is so overwhelming that it is practically passé. Do it now!

The more living food you eat, the more alive and free of infirmities you will be. Even if the changes you make are almost imperceptible, you will *still* see improvement. The Two-Week **Living Health** menus in this book are designed to help you incorporate more living food into your diet while allowing the eating experience to remain a joyous one. Just give it a try. See for yourself the remarkable difference you can produce in *every* area of your life by rewarding your body with less processed dead food in favor of more natural, living food.

A NEW ATTACK ON YOUR HEALTH— FOOD IRRADIATION

Having made the case for how crucially important one's food is to overall health, indeed to our *lives*, I cannot conclude this chapter without bringing to your attention what is probably the most outrageous attempt to defile our food (and therefore our health) ever to be concocted in the history of this planet: food irradiation, the exposure of your food to radioactive material. That's right, the very same radioactive waste that people all over this country are up in arms about, marching in the streets to protest its being buried underground in their state, is now going to be used to bombard your *food!* Give me a break! And we're just supposed to go merrily along and say, "Golly gee, ain't life grand?"

Now, I know that a good many people reading this are saying, "What on earth are you talking about? I never heard anything about radiating my food." You bet you haven't. A mammoth effort is being made to keep it that way, too. The perpetrators of this bit of lunacy are using every means possible to get the laws passed and put into effect without your knowing a thing about it. And what else would you expect, considering what they are trying to pull off? If someone were trying to rob your home, do you think he would knock on your front door and ask to be shown to your jewelry box? No, he'd sneak in at night when no one was home. One day you'll be turning your head rapidly from left to right asking, "What happened?" If you do not voice your displeasure with this *right now*, by the end of this decade, *much* of the food you consume will be treated with radiation emitted by deadly nuclear material and waste.* It's "Stop it now, or eat it later!"

"Well, who's behind this evildoing? The Russians? We'll run 'em out of town." No, no. It's not the Russians. That would make too much sense. It's the Department of Energy (DOE) and the International Atomic Energy Administration (IAEA), and they have the support of the World Health Organization (WHO) and the United States Food and Drug Administration (FDA).

You can be certain that whatever possible benefits this misuse of "progress" provides will be glorified until they sound like the second coming, while whatever dangers there are—and there are plenty—will be minimized to appear no more bothersome than an itchy foot.

Irradiated food will receive very high doses of radiation—from several minutes to much longer, depending on the food. The dose is measured in RADs (roentgen absorbed doses). One RAD is more than the radiation emitted by an X ray. Three hundred RADs will kill half the people directly exposed to it and sterilize the rest. Guess how many RADs the FDA wants to allow on your food? *One hundred thousand* on fruits and vegetables and *3 million* on herbs and spices. And I thought all this time that the FDA was out there to protect us! The foods currently approved for irradiation in the United States include potatoes, wheat, wheat flour, pork, forty-seven herbs and spices, seeds, and tea. Did you know? Irradiation is touted as increasing shelf life. What's wrong with getting a *fresh* potato rather than one bombarded with nuclear waste so it can sit in a bin for two months and not go bad? *Let it go bad*. Nature intends food to go bad if not eaten, so that we will

---

*Two by-products from nuclear weapons production are cobalt 60 and cesium 137. These will be used on your food.

seek out the freshest food possible. Who benefits from longer shelf life? Not you!

The FDA is quick to point out that irradiating food does not make the food radioactive *unless there is an equipment malfunction or leakage*. That's the biggest "unless" in the history of human-kind. Now, if the equipment that makes washing machines mal-functions and you wind up with a defective machine and have to return it for a new one, that's very annoying—but at least your life is not jeopardized. When the equipment irradiating your food malfunctions, you and your children eat radioactive food. Is *any-thing* worth that risk? I mean *anything*. Do machines ever mal-function? Did the space shuttle blow up? Did Chernobyl happen? Of course, some "expert" will tell you that the chances of that happening are one in a million and that's very reassuring—until your child pays the price for that "one" with leukemia or who knows what. When it's your child, it doesn't matter if the chance is one in a million quadrillion.

The FDA maintains that radiated food is "safe and wholesome." But their newest proposal also states, "Destruction of nutrients, however, is not a concern." Marvelous. Not a concern. To whom? Destruction of nutrients is not a concern; other than that irradiation is wholesome. Want to buy this house? Other than the fact that the roof has no support and will collapse if you shut the door too hard, it is perfectly safe. Would you buy a car that is advertised as safe as long as you overlook the brakes not working on downhill slopes and the steering failing on sharp turns? No wonder the proponents of this atrocious innovation want to sneak it through before you find out what they are up to. Who would take seriously someone trying to sell you as "wholesome" food whose nutrients have been destroyed? And destroyed they are. Amino acid (protein) groups are broken down; fats and fatty acids, very sensitive to radiation, break down into toxic substances. Carbohydrates break down into substances that impair cell division. Some enzymes are destroyed, and vitamins are destroyed or depleted. This the FDA considers "safe and wholesome." The FDA's track record in being right on what it has declared safe has a few blemishes. Among other items given its stamp of approval are thalidomide, bendec-tine, sulfites, EDB, DES, asbestos, and the Dalkon Shield. Shall we now trust that irradiated food is just as safe?

Although the FDA states that food irradiation will be strictly regulated, these are empty words, dishonest because, as they admit, "the FDA has not compiled a list of radiation facilities or companies in the United States that treat foods. Companies treating food need not register with the FDA." How on earth will they closely regulate facilities if they don't know who or where they are, what they irradiate, and in what products it is going?

And just how "safe" is it?

German scientists have found that plastic containers and wrappers in which foods are irradiated impart toxic substances into the food during the process. An internal 1982 FDA audit showed that only 1 percent of 413 studies conducted over thirty years appeared to support safety. Two Russian studies of rats fed irradiated food showed kidney and testicular damage. Children in India fed irradiated wheat showed chromosome damage and blood abnormalities associated with leukemia. German scientists found so many ill effects that West Germany has forbidden food irradiation by law. These effects include mutations, reduced fertility, metabolic disturbances, decreased growth rate, reduced resistance to disease, changes in organ weight, tumors, and more. Great Britain has also banned the irradiation of food. A Japanese doctor, Takahashi Kosei, reviewed the studies upon which the World Health Organization based its approval of irradiation. He reanalyzed the data and found they did not prove safety. They showed rather that irradiated potatoes caused arterial problems, higher mortality, mutations, and increased organ weights; irradiated wheat caused white blood cell changes; irradiated onions caused higher death rate and ovarian and testicular changes; irradiated rice caused disturbances in the pituitary, thyroid, heart, and lungs as well as giving rise to tumors. One thousand two hundred and twenty-three Hungarian studies failed to support the safety of irradiated food.

And does it actually increase shelf life? There are many studies that question the effectiveness of irradiation in prolonging shelf life, one of its primary rationales. Dr. Noel Sommer at the University of California at Davis, paid by the Atomic Energy Commission from 1963 to 1973 to study the feasibility of irradiation as a preservative technique for fruits and vegetables, came to the following conclusions:

1. Irradiated strawberries weep from irradiation-caused injury when cut.

2. Citrus fruits are more sensitive to disease and chilling injury after being irradiated.

3. There are changes in the color, odor, flavor, and texture of irradiated produce that make the process questionable and may necessitate chemical additives.

4. Food irradiation is probably not a sufficient means of handling agricultural emergencies such as fruit fly infestation, one of its purported uses. It would be prohibitively expensive to build and maintain enough plants to be available when they might be needed.

5. It is doubtful that any fresh [living] commodity's shelf life would be increased by more than a few days by using irradiation to control rot organisms and there is utterly no possibility that gamma radiation could possibly replace fungicides.

Another claim is that irradiated food would be less expensive. Ha! There will be added costs to the consumer in spite of the Department of Energy's and the food industry's insistence that reduced spoilage would lower prices. These include estimated price increases of two to twelve cents per pound of irradiated food, depending on the food, millions of tax dollars already budgeted for financing the building and operation of the facilities, promotional expenses for winning public acceptance of irradiation, and the astronomical costs of "clean up" in the tragic event of an accidental leak of radioactive materials into the environment.

The FDA is trying everything it can to fool the public and protect itself from blame should something go wrong. They wanted to replace the existing labeling laws with a no-label requirement at the retail level. Fortunately, a consumer activist movement led by the NCSFI forced the FDA to adopt a label requirement. The FDA's position was that consumers lacked the background to understand the words "treated with gamma radiation" and might resist purchasing food that had been so labeled. Oh, brother! That takes some kind of nerve. They actually have to take measures to combat your natural instinct for survival, lest you might protect yourself unnecessarily from harm. Can't have that. That would be such an annoying delay in their plans. When cows are being led to slaughter, every once in a while one of them will bolt for freedom and will have to be rounded back up. That is also quite an annoyance to the herders leading them to slaughter.

On December 12, 1985, the FDA stated in a press release that irradiated food will be labeled "Pico-Waved." But there is no such term in physics. How clever. Such ingeniousness to get you to do what they want you to do. A word was simply made up and used so as to be less objectionable than the truth . . . plus they want to change food irradiation from an "additive" to a "process," which in FDA terms means that no longer will food irradiation automatically be subject to safety review or toxological testing. This, plus the establishment of the joint commission, takes the FDA out of the picture as an effective force for regulating the industry. The industry of food irradiation will be left to "regulate" itself—that is, to do anything, anytime, anywhere. No one will have any control whatsoever. How does that make you feel?

The purpose of irradiating food is to rid the Department of Energy of its nuclear waste problem and to make a profit for the food industry at the same time. It authorizes the leasing of radioactive material by the United States to private industry for the purpose of food irradiation. The same nuclear waste that is presenting such a problem to so many people and has created fear and apprehension among the public will now take on an aura of respectability. Rather than government agencies figuring out how they can possibly contain it safely, it is now going to be leased and distributed to companies to make money on it. And how are they going to make that money? They are going to *treat your food* with this waste.

Guess how you'll know if you are buying an irradiated food? There will be a *flower* on the food—not a skull and crossbones, *a flower!* They could at least make it a *dead* flower.

The Health and Energy Institute, a nonprofit watchdog group concerned with the dangers of radiation, summed it up best: "The DOE is not trying to find the best way to preserve food or protect human health, it's trying to find a convenient way to get rid of some of its nuclear garbage created by building nuclear weapons." *We must not allow them to get away with it.*

If the Department of Energy has its way, there will be a thousand food irradiation facilities across the country within ten years. The truth is that these food irradiation facilities are nothing more than nuclear waste dumps with a fancy name. Think about that. That's an average of twenty irradiation facilities or nuclear waste dumps in every single state in this country. This brings up grave questions regarding the hazards of transporting, handling, and using radioactive materials. The Nuclear Regulatory Commission does not have a good track record of monitoring safety violations and preventing accidents at the present ninety-eight nuclear power plants. Pay attention! *Ninety-eight* nuclear power plants! They want to have a *thousand* food irradiation facilities. The amount of radioactive material that would move in and out of one facility in five years would equal five times the total of *all* sources of low-level radioactive waste produced in the United States in 1981. Currently, it is estimated that there are 400 million pounds of high-level radioactive waste buried in temporary storage sites all around the United States—perhaps in *your* neighborhood. The life span of this radioactive waste is *250,000 years*. When you consider that there will be an average of twenty of these sites in every state in this country, it's very likely there will be some sites around where you are living—if not you, then someone you know. Do you want to have one of these sites in your neighborhood? Do you want to run the risk of your child's being poisoned by nuclear waste? Do you want to stand idly by and allow for a *thousand* sites to be put all over this country?

On October 17, 1986, President Ronald Reagan stated, "The danger of toxic wastes is perhaps the most pressing environmental problem facing our country."* It is beyond human comprehension that while the president is being wildly cheered by the public for earmarking $9 billion to create a Superfund to clean up these toxic waste sites, the Department of Energy is planning *behind your back*, to create *a thousand* nuclear waste sites all over the country—not merely toxic waste sites but *nuclear* waste sites, the ultimate toxic substance.

Then to rub in our faces how gullible and stupid they think we are, we're told that they're *not* waste sites, they're food irradiation sites. Despite the fact that it is the *very same nuclear waste* most of the people in this country are deathly afraid of, we're supposed to take a sigh of relief simply because those standing to rake in some big profits from this most outrageous assault against our health have come up with a less objectionable name for it.

Be very clear on one thing. Notwithstanding the attempts to justify this abuse and defilement of our food as a beneficial treatment, it really has very little to do with protecting food. The truth is that the entire food irradiation controversy is a slick coverup and a smokescreen designed to divert attention away from the real issue: plutonium and nuclear warheads.

*Los Angeles Times, October 18, 1986.

There are currently 1,800 nuclear warheads produced in the U.S. every year. This calls for a considerable amount of plutonium. America's aging military reactors, which now produce the plutonium for warheads, can barely keep pace with the present nuclear buildup. And at ten billion dollars per new reactor, constructing new reactors is not affordable. Guess where else plutonium can be found. *It can be extracted from commercial nuclear waste*. But . . . in 1982 there was a congressional ban on reprocessing commercial wastes which virtually prohibits the military from crossing over and using civilian-generated wastes.

Here the plot thickens. A byproduct of plutonium extraction, which is one of the waste's most radioactive components, is Cesium-137. If the DOE could just figure out a use for Cesium-137 they could then go after all that swell plutonium sitting fallow in dump sites across this country. Well, they have figured it out; we get to *eat* it!

Knowing how important it is to build five new nuclear warheads *every single day*, no sacrifice is too great so long as we get that precious plutonium. So thinks the DOE. In a statement to the House Armed Services Subcommittee in 1983, the DOE stated, "The measure of success (in the program) will be the degree to which this technology is implemented industrially and the subsequent demand created for Cesium-137."* CREATED! The demand had to be *created*. Food irradiation has *nothing* to do with shelflife and killing bacteria. It has to do with plutonium and nuclear warheads.

Mark Twain once said that there were two things that were infinite: space and man's stupidity. And his statement was made without even the benefit of this particular example of madness to reflect on.

Dr. Donald B. Louria, professor and chairman of the Department of Preventive Medicine and Community Health at the University of Medicine and Dentistry at New Jersey Medical School and author of several health books, has written a letter expressing his views on food irradiation to a colleague. With his permission we have taken some excerpts from that letter:

> I am enormously concerned about food irradiation. By
> 1990, a lot of the food we eat and our children eat may

*THE NATION, "Why Is D.O.E. for Food Irradiation?" February 7, 1987

have first been irradiated by Cobalt 60 (half life five years), or Cesium 137 (half life thirty years). The proponents tell us such treatment is absolutely safe, that such irradiation can reduce use of potentially dangerous pesticides and that the longer shelf life of irradiated foods will help us to feed the poverty stricken parts of the world.

Is it really safe? The answer seems to be that no one knows. There have been many hundreds of studies over the last decade, but only a handful (69), have been thought to be sound enough to provide truly useful data. Of these, roughly half conclude that irradiation is safe, half that it is not. That is hardly a ringing endorsement. There are valid concerns that the radiolitic products in food are not safe and these concerns include the potential for genetic damage. There are other safety issues. The amount of Cobalt 60 or Cesium 137 used in irradiation plants is enormous. These plants show little evidence of adequate security. An accident or terrorist attack could spew enormous amounts of radiation into the neighborhood. A plant with a few million curies of radiation with the potential for major environmental contamination is not a good neighbor. Additionally, an enormous amount of Cesium 137 or Cobalt 60 will have to be transported long distances on a continuing basis. Accidents with inadvertent release of radiation are inevitable.

Is it effective? There is a continuing debate whether irradiation will significantly increase shelf life. At 100,000 RAD irradiation, it will be effective against certain pests, but will not prevent spoilage. Thus, a major argument of the food radiation proponents, its use to feed the impoverished of the world, is probably invalid. To achieve significantly longer shelf life would require a much greater amount of irradiation; that in turn would mean more radioactive substances in the food and a great likelihood that the nutritional value of the food would be significantly reduced. Even at the lower radiation dosage, the issue of loss of nutrient value is not at all settled. So the pest control effected by radiation may be offset by lesser nutrient value. The notion of using irradiated food to feed the world is wishful thinking without substance.

Are there subsidiary issues of importance? There is one of immense potential implications. There is a drive by the United States to replace Cobalt 60, largely enriched in Canada, with Cesium 137, that is available from our own nuclear waste cesspool. We wish to make use of the approximately eighty million curies we have stockpiled. But that will not last long. A small number of plants will use that up quickly. Much, much more would be needed and there is only one possible source. Our spent fuel rods in nuclear reactors, both civilian and military. To get the needed Cesium 137, nuclear waste would have to be reprocessed and the reprocessing that provides Cesium 137 will also make available the plutonium our military wants for Star Wars and other military endeavors. There is a strong suspicion that the food irradiation drive doesn't reflect a determination to feed the world, but rather it is a ploy by the Department of Energy and the Department of Defense to get rid of some of our nuclear waste and simultaneously fuel our war machine. We could soon be in the disquieting situation of contributing to the arms race by turning on our lights at home. Since the arms race is increasingly likely to kill our children, we could be, in essence, contributing on a daily basis to the death of our own children. It would be interesting to see what happens to the food irradiation industry if Cesium 137 were prohibited as the radiation source.

When asked by an officer of Radiation Technology, Inc. (one of the companies that stand to get rich on this scheme) why he was supporting the anti-food irradiation side, a New Jersey parent replied, ''If I follow their path and they are wrong, my children won't get hurt. If I follow your path and you are wrong, my children might die.''

Is there anything you can do about this? You'd better believe there is. First of all, be prepared to hear this and many other writings against food irradiation attacked and ridiculed. There is big money and power pushing it. They want what they want and these powers will use any means necessary to *get* what they want. So the biggest effort will be to discredit anyone they see attempting to prevent them from achieving their goal. More importantly, when you go shopping for food, ask the manager of the store if they plan to sell irradiated food. Tell him or her that you will buy your food elsewhere if they do. The most cherished commodity of a retail market is a satisfied customer. If enough people express displeasure over irradiated food, believe me they won't want it any more than you do.

This is not something to be lazy or noncommittal about. If you don't tell them you don't want it, you soon will have no choice. The most important thing you can do is to contact the National Coalition to Stop Food Irradiation (NCSFI), Post Office Box 59-0488, San Francisco, California 94159-0488; telephone: (415) 566-2734. They can give you a great deal more information and tell you exactly how you can help prevent this monstrous assault upon your well-being.

CHAPTER 9
Rest and Sleep

HARVEY:

We spend about one third of our lives in sleep. Its remarkably recuperative effects are well known. This is one area where evidence is not demanded to prove it works. The greatest remedy for being tired is . . . sleeping. Without this natural restorative, true health is an impossibility. Healthful, soothing slumber that rests muscles, nerves, and brain is one of nature's greatest rejuvenators. It is during periods of rest and sleep that the body repairs itself, reenergizes itself, and prepares itself for renewed activity. It is every bit as essential to life as air, water, and food.

We generally accept sleep as commonplace, but when we can't sleep we crave it more intensely than the most precious gem. People rarely give much thought to sleeping, viewing it merely as a time of inactivity for the body.

You would be making a huge mistake to think that your nights are any less significant or complex than your days. During the hours of sleep, when we appear to be most passive, something within us is intensely active, recharging us for the next day. When we are active, we are expending energy; when we are seemingly inactive, we are building it. It's interesting that energy is always noted in its expenditures, never in its accumulation. The brain and nervous system operate on nerve energy in the form of electricity. The body, like an electric car, needs to be recharged at night. Sleep is a partial shutdown for recharging.

The primary purpose of sleep is the regeneration of nerve energy. The vitality of the body is restored. During sleep the body is bustling with activity—repair of tissue, healing, restocking of organs and cells with fuel, replacement of old cells that have lost their vitality with new ones (cell reproduction occurs at more than twice the rate at which it occurs during waking hours). The heart pumps blood through the body to pick up wastes and debris une-liminated from the previous day and take them to the channels of elimination. Muscles tense; pulse rate, temperature, and blood pressure rise and fall; we are sexually aroused; our senses evoke a world of sights and sounds. Only part of the brain is asleep, for the nervous system continues to conduct billions of processes while we are sleeping.

The brain is the most marvelous, complex, and astonishing organ known to science. During fetal development the brain grows by about 360 million new nerve cells a day, ultimately totaling about 100 *billion* of the most highly developed, sophisticated cells any-where in the universe. Over the last few decades, a great deal has been learned about the brain. However, despite advances in com-prehending this awe-inspiring organ, we have only the barest un-derstanding of the intricacy and wonder of this marvel of Creation. Many doubt that we will ever be able to fathom the true extent of the intelligence necessary for the mind and body to interact the way they do. Truly it is biology's ultimate challenge. There are some who believe that the entire purpose of our bodies is simply to supply food and oxygen to sustain the brain.

All body processes and functions are under the overall control of the brain. Everything that concerns the interactions of cells, tissues, and organs is under its control. The brain is the supreme judge of the body's best welfare. And marvelous beyond imagi-nation, almost all brain functions and their results occur beneath the level of awareness. Brain functions at the subconscious level are unimaginably more diverse, extensive, wise, and precise than at the level of consciousness. In fact, at the level of consciousness we are simpletons compared to the seemingly infinite intelligence of our brain's subconscious. Even the most sophisticated computer that we can envision is crude compared to the apparently limitless complexity of the human brain. When one reflects on the brain's astronomical number of tasks simultaneously performed with pin-point perfection twenty-four hours a day for decades, one has to stand humbly in awe. Remember, the body has some 75 to 100 *trillion* cells, a number we can't comprehend. If you had to spend $75 trillion, you would have to spend a $1 billion a day every day for over 200 years. We're talking big numbers here. Consider that all of those 75 trillion cells are alive and sending out messages that they need responses to. Your brain at *any* given moment is literally receiving, analyzing, and sending messages to *all* 75 trillion. That's why the brain is the biggest enigma in our universe.

The billions of signals flashing through your brain incessantly carry a mind-boggling load of information, monitoring not only the status of your body's inner environment but your outer environment as well. You can't swallow or breathe or sing or sharpen a pencil or think about last night or tomorrow or *anything* without your brain's involvement. At the same time that your brain might register that you have an itch on your neck, you smell a fresh-cut piece of watermelon and hear a friend's funny story. Signals are processed, analyzed, cross-checked, and categorized so that you can immediately respond—scratch your neck, pick up a piece of melon, and giggle at the joke. Meanwhile, your brain is also monitoring your blood chemistry, temperature, breathing, and all of the other essential processes that keep you alive—all this beneath your awareness. In recognizing that consciousness, or awareness, is but a fractional function of our brain and is but one of its *lesser* activities in view of the magnitude of its role in administering the entire body, we can begin to appreciate the need for rest and sleep and their role in enabling the brain to recharge itself with nerve energy.

No doubt about it, rest and sleep are two essentials of life important beyond description, but the full import is unrecognized by most people. They just "hit the sack," wake up when it's over, and go about their business. Sleep is *so* critical that it simply overtakes us when it's needed by the body. It can be put off for a while or deferred in an emergency, but put it off long enough and you just conk out. The body must have it, for it perishes without sleep, so it just *takes* it.

Many people are apt to confuse the words *rest* and *sleep* as being synonymous. Not so. Though both are vitally important, they definitely are not the same. The condition of sleep exists only when consciousness has ceased. Not too many people need convincing that sleep is important. That would seem as necessary as trying to convince someone that water is wet or fire is hot. However, when it comes to the importance of rest, people don't seem to have a sense of how essential it is in preserving health.

What is rest? It is a period of inactivity during which the body can restore expended energy. When we've depleted our energies faster than they can be restored, a period of inactivity enables the body to catch up. You've experienced this. You're tired, fatigued, so you sit down and close your eyes for a moment or two; your head nods a few times, then all of a sudden you "come to," and in those few seconds you feel refreshed and invigorated.

There are four kinds of rest that can be used to replenish and refresh oneself.

1. *Physical rest* may be obtained by discontinuing physical activity—sitting or lying down and relaxing.

2. *Sensory rest* is secured by quiet and by refraining from using the eyes, which curtails a great drain of energy.

3. *Emotional rest* is achieved by withdrawing from involvement in the ups and downs caused by personal interaction.

4. *Mental rest* is obtained by detaching the mind from any and all intellectual demands or activity.

Essentially, rest is the curtailment of energy expenditures, which permits the body to redirect energies to restoration. It can be used very effectively to rejuvenate yourself and improve your outlook.

For various reasons, sometimes a night's sleep may be inadequate, perhaps due to a particularly stressful day, some disturbing toxic crisis your body is undergoing, or arousing thoughts of a momentous situation in your life. When your sleep is inadequate due to any of these conditions and you become drowsy, sleepy, listless, or down during the day, you need rest. To some people suggesting they take a nap in the middle of the day is akin to suggesting they poke themselves in the eye with a sharp stick. *Nap* is virtually a bad word. In today's hustle and bustle atmosphere of workaholism and efforts to succeed and get ahead, the body's biological needs are sometimes sacrificed in favor of productivity at any cost.

Much of the stress that so many working people struggle under can be traced to forcing the body to go beyond its capabilities and thereby pushing it to the brink. I think our "succeed at any cost" culture has some people thinking they would rather be caught stealing than caught taking a nap. So they push themselves though feeling in need of a rest and resort to stimulants (coffee, tea, soft drinks, "uppers," etc.) to perk themselves up. This practice takes its toll. The problem is aggravated rather than solved. People who take this route further drain nerve energy, even though the drain may not be evident at the time. In many countries around the world a siesta is the *normal* practice. Animals in nature also rest during the heat of the day. Napping contributes to health and well-being.

It is far better to take some time to rest quietly, with eyes closed and body still, so as to perform more efficiently in the afternoon and evening hours than to forgo a needed nap and drag through the whole afternoon performing at a greatly reduced productivity level—the impaired efficiency more than offsets the extra time you work when not alert or not feeling well. Napping is also important in that it improves body functions, including digestion, thereby promoting better health through better nutrition. Resting prevents excessive fatigue, promotes better and more efficient work, and increases productivity. When you are fatigued, mental sharpness and physical powers are greatly diminished. Resting sharpens the mind and prevents the fatigue that otherwise makes you nervous and irritable at night. It also allows you to fall asleep more quickly and sleep more soundly.

Try this: Instead of gulping down two cups of coffee at your next coffee break, which will catch up to you later with the demand for more coffee, find a quiet place, still your mind, close your eyes, and take a few deep breaths and relax your muscles. Turn your coffee break, your stimulation break, into a rest break and see for yourself what a positive difference this will have on your day. Just try it!

The healthful custom of taking a short noontime nap has been largely destroyed by the needs of an industrial society. This loss has, to a great extent, contributed to our ill health and stimulated habits that make industrial nations so highly stressed and diseased. Our parents knew what they were doing when they called us in during our childhood for our afternoon "snooze." **RESTING AND NAPPING IS NOT A SIGN OF LAZINESS. IT IS AN** *INTELLIGENT AND PRODUCTIVE* **USE OF YOUR TIME.**

Some 50 million people in this country suffer from sleeplessness or insomnia. Obviously this interferes with the body's ability to recoup the nerve energy needed for the next day, so it is a very serious problem for people.

There is a line about a friend telling his neighbor that he knows just the thing for insomnia: Get lots of sleep. This may be funny but it is no joke for the individual who either can't get to sleep or has a very broken, fitful sleep. Sadly, many of these individuals resort to drugs (sleeping pills, tranquilizers, alcohol), which ultimately makes the problem worse, because this approach only deals with the symptoms, not the cause. A far wiser thing would be to look for the cause rather than look for methods to induce sleep. Sleeplessness is not an uncaused phenomenon and it will speedily end when its cause is removed.

There are several reasons that contribute to the inability to sleep. Caffeine, for instance. It takes twenty-four hours for *one* cup of coffee to pass through the kidneys and urinary tract. People who have several cups of coffee, chocolate, and sodas have lots of caffeine in their bloodstream. The distress and stimulation from caffeine can inhibit sleep, especially sound sleep. The body must expend energy in expelling the caffeine, plus it generates less energy at the same time because of lack of sleep, a terrible cycle. Those supposedly innocent cups of coffee during the day take their toll during the night. Fresh air is another factor that affects sleep, as we noted in the chapter on air. Those who sleep in fresh rather than stale air invariably report better sleep. Exercise (covered in the next chapter) also helps to oxygenate the blood and facilitates the removal of toxins from the body, giving the system less to do in terms of removal of waste at night, so better sleep is enjoyed.

By far, the factor that most affects one's sleep is food. Nothing can disturb sleep more than eating at bedtime. The primary reason for sleep is to regenerate nerve energy. Eating before sleeping redirects much of the energy to the digestion of the food. Since the brain is involved in digestion, less sleep will result. You simply should not expect to sleep well while the body is conducting digestive tasks. At least two hours should elapse between eating and going to bed.*

The more toxic you are, the more difficult it will be to sleep through the night. An eating life-style that is based on more wholesome food requires less digestive energy. Wholesome food lessens sleep needs and increases sleep efficiency. This is why diet and eating practices weigh so heavily on how much sleep we need and how well we sleep. **THE BIGGEST SINGLE FACTOR CON-**

---

*The only exception is if fruit is eaten on an empty stomach.

TRIBUTING TO SOUND SLEEP, WHICH IN TURN SOUND SLEEP CONTRIBUTES TO, IS GENERAL HEALTH.

Since the quality of our food so dramatically affects our health, it is easy to see why it's such an important factor in the quality of our sleep. Over the past seventeen years in which I have been studying the field of health, I have been told by many hundreds of people that their sleep improved dramatically immediately upon upgrading their diet. Some people who had consistent difficulty sleeping for over *twenty* years were able to sleep through the night without any drugs whatsoever. If you are one of the 50 million Americans who can't sleep well, we want you to know there *is* hope. In fact, there is a lot more than hope; there is reason for jubilation. The simple fact is that sleep is just too important to your overall well-being for it not to occur spontaneously when needed. By improving your eating habits and employing some of the tips you'll find in chapter 19, "Two Weeks of Living Health," you can look forward to some sound, peaceful, restful slumber.

How much sleep does one need? Let's put it this way. You should go to sleep when you're sleepy, and you've had enough when you wake up. Actually, enough is what is required to re-cuperate nerve energy, build up reserves, replace and cast out spent cells, and eliminate the by-products of metabolism. There is no single set amount for everyone. Different conditions require different lengths of sleep. Some people do fine with four hours, some need ten. If you supply the best conditions in terms of air, water, food, sunshine, exercise, and positive influences, you will stay asleep as long as your system needs you to, then you will wake up. As long as the purposes of sleep are fulfilled, it doesn't really matter how long you are asleep.

There really is no such thing as oversleeping. The body will not sleep beyond need. Consciousness returns when needs have been met. However, there certainly is such a thing as undersleep-ing, and it is an affliction of our times. It is a transgression that far too many people commit against themselves. Talk about sab-otaging one's well-being. It would never occur to you to deprive yourself intentionally of the air, water, or food necessary to carry out the functions of life. But for some reason, sleep gets sacrificed. *Big mistake!* When we undersleep, not enough nerve energy is generated to meet needs. The longer we are awake, the more energy we use. The less we sleep, the less energy we generate. That's not a good combination. When energy is squandered unnecessarily, all body activities are seriously lessened. *This means poor digestion and impaired elimination*—a surefire way to put on weight, feel tired and stressed, be lacking in energy, invite disease, and just feel generally lousy.

I don't know exactly when this happened, but somehow it has become almost chic not to sleep many hours during the night. You will hear people saying, "Boy, I worked until two A.M. and was up at seven!" And someone will answer, "Wow! That's great!" Or people will be bragging about how much sleep they get, and the one who gets *the least* seems to be the winner! That's just not how it's supposed to be. Sleep is a vital commodity, like good, wholesome food or a walk in the fresh mountain air. It is not something to be done *without*. Quality and quantity are *both* important.

Use your common sense for a moment. Are we as a species really designed to "burn the midnight oil" the way we do? We turn nights into day in modern times and yet, our ancestors, more in tune with Nature and their biological needs, could *not* have done what we do. In more natural times, the hours for sleep began as the light of day ebbed. Without electricity, people had no way to prolong the daylight hours. They went to bed at dark and woke with the light which, except in the "land of the midnight sun," is at least an eight-hour stretch. To this day the health philosophy of the yogis includes going to sleep by nine and arising with the sun. In terms of quality sleep, *the hours you get before midnight are most valuable and most restful*. This is something that you can verify for yourself. Try going to sleep early as often as possible. It is no accident that the old adage "Early to bed, early to rise makes a man healthy, wealthy, and wise" is so often repeated. Or that an early night is called "a beauty sleep." Sleep as much as you need to and, for heaven's sake, don't be ashamed to do so.

Sometimes we tend to do things without considering the consequences simply because we weren't aware that there might be negative ones. If you have, for whatever reason, jeopardized your sleep for other activities, be it work, play, or whatever, you are undermining your health. Turn that around and start to allow your body the rest and sleep it requires as a *biological necessity of life*, and you are in store for a most rewarding change in your life.

CHAPTER 10
Exercise

HARVEY:

Life is motion and the less we move the less alive we become. We have bodies exquisitely designed for motion. In order for health to be achieved and maintained, we must establish a proper balance between rest and activity. If we rest too much and do not balance our rest with sufficient physical activity, fulfilling our true health potential becomes quite a task. There is certainly no need to spend several pages trying to prove that exercise is an important ingredient in a healthy life-style. Anyone who thinks that this is *not* the case is past praying for. I think you will be better served by an overview that shows you some benefits of exercise you may not be aware of, simplifying the entire subject and creating in you a desire to exercise regularly.

There is an exercise routine for everyone. These routines may vary enormously from person to person, as well they should. Different people need different routines, and you should not try to do more than your body type and life-style demand just to be "in." Some people exercise vigorously every day for three hours or more. Others look upon physical activity with the same enthusiasm as facing the Sahara Desert. Physical activity should be a joy that you look forward to and participate in out of eagerness, not out of guilt. The benefits from even seemingly negligible amounts of regular exercise are so extensive and so profound that anyone who merely begins to exercise even on a very small scale will soon become aware of its value and genuinely *want* to participate in some sort of vigorous activity daily. There is nothing like results to spur on interest.

The musculoskeletal system of the human body is yet another example of the magnificence of our bodies. Some six hundred and fifty muscles interact with over 200 bones and are responsible for *every* movement of the body. The mass of skeletal muscles in the body can be viewed as one large organ of movement. Practically every activity, and especially athletics, is the result of the integrated action of nearly all the muscles in the body. It takes over 200 muscles to take just one step. It takes 40 just to lift a leg.

Bones are usually pictured as a solid mass. They're not. Bones are living, breathing, *porous* structures. Very fine blood vessels keep blood flowing through the bone. In fact, blood is manufactured in the marrow of bones and at a phenomenal pace. In the second it takes you to turn this page, about 3 million red blood cells will be lost from your body, and during the same second, 3 million new ones will be produced. And this happens *every second of your life!* If all the red blood cells in your body were stacked on top of one another, they would reach 31,000 miles into space.

Bones are alive and just like every other part of the body, they benefit greatly from exercise. The more activity one engages in, the stronger and more durable both the muscles and bones become. Perhaps you have seen the results of someone breaking a bone or tearing a muscle and having to wear a cast for several weeks. The muscles and bones in the cast begin to atrophy, to shrink in size and strength. If the cast is left on long enough, the area may become completely useless. But once the cast is removed and motion is again possible, the muscle and bone respond by regaining their normal size and strength.

Every part of your body depends on regular physical activity. When a specific part of the body is put into action, the body responds by sending more blood, nutrients, and energy to that area. This response leads to an overall improvement in the health and vitality of the particular part involved. If exercise is neglected, the body will become weak and all its physical powers will be diminished, but with regular exercise the *entire* system will be strengthened and invigorated.

Life depends on the flow of blood in our bodies. Every drop of blood circulates through the entire body, every minute! Exercise greatly increases the effectiveness with which the heart delivers blood and with it oxygen and other vital nutrients to all areas and tissues of the body. With this increase in efficiency, vital blood pathways are cleaned out and overall circulation is enhanced. This, in turn, serves to ensure optimum performance of all the organs and keeps them functioning properly.

Probably the strongest muscle in your body for its size is your heart. Held in awe by anyone who has ever studied its operations, this fist-sized masterpiece is a tireless organ of incalculable functionability. It beats 2.5 billion times in an average lifetime, driving five quarts of blood every minute to every cell in the body to cleanse and nourish the entire system. That's 220 million quarts over a lifetime. It has valves as thin as tissue paper, ten-millionths of an inch, which are *sturdier* than iron. When surgeons replace heart valves with silicone parts, the hard man-made materials become battered and out of shape after only a few years, but the delicate durable tissues of a healthy heart exert their force and withstand the beating for a *lifetime*. So powerful and enduring is the normal heart that it is almost impossible to work the rest of the body hard enough to injure this marvelous organ. This exquisitely designed, incredibly durable, magnificently proficient study in perfection is in constant and absolute control of the river of life that is our bloodstream. Can you think of a more worthy undertaking than to ensure your precious heart is in its best possible condition? Do birds fly? Do flowers grow?

Possibly the greatest virtue of regular exercise is that it makes the heart a stronger, more efficient, and *larger* organ. That's right. You can actually increase the size of your heart muscles, thereby increasing its capacity to perform. Like any muscle, if not sufficiently used the heart will become small, weak, and even atrophy if neglected long enough. Or this same muscle can be exercised vigorously and regularly to be made large and strong.

A larger heart is a healthier and stronger heart. It has a slower and stronger beat. The blood load is greater and the heart contraction is stronger, sending a greater volume of blood through the arteries at each beat and providing for a longer rest period between beats. The fact is that the heart is not nearly as delicate as sometimes imagined. It is much stronger for its size than any other muscle in the body.

Any good exercise routine should address basically three areas of fitness: (1) cardiovascular, or aerobic, (2) strength, and (3) flexibility. Aerobic exercise is the form that strengthens the heart.

Aerobic exercise gets you panting and perspiring and doubles your resting pulse rate for twenty to thirty minutes. This oxygenates the blood. The word *aerobic* literally means "with oxygen."

An individual's capacity for muscular work is dependent upon the supply of oxygen to the working muscles. Swimming, bike riding, jogging, rope jumping, handball, tennis, basketball—all are aerobic exercises. And although walking has to be of somewhat longer duration, it is also highly effective and certainly an aerobic activity.

Aerobics classes are very much in vogue today, and this is a very positive trend. However, one word of caution: You need to work up to the demands of some of these classes, and it is a mistake to attempt to force your body to a level of performance that it may not be ready for. Trying to keep up with the instructor (who does this all day for a living) may *not* be in your best interest. For many, a more natural aerobic exercise like walking or swimming may be more beneficial in the long run.

Whatever aerobic exercise you do activates many wonderful changes in the body, and you should engage in it regularly. If you see a wild cat—a lion or tiger—you will see it running, leaping, stretching every day. It is trim, fit, and vital and has a tremendous endurance level. Put that animal in a zoo, and even though it will continue to stretch, its physique deteriorates and the animal becomes lazy. Why? Because its aerobic exercise has been discontinued.

RESISTIVE REBOUNDING

A unique exercise that we enthusiastically recommend for both cardiovascular fitness and strength is called Resistive Rebounding. Rebound exercise has been available since the trampoline was first invented in 1936. However, for the most part the only people to take advantage of it have been gymnastics students. Trampolining was introduced to the armed services prior to World War II and used to develop balance, dexterity, coordination, rhythm, and timing. It also produced strong, well-developed physiques. Resistive Rebounding was developed several years ago by Dr. Harry Sneider, an athletics and fitness coach for thirty years. Resistive Rebounding requires only a mini-trampoline and one-, two-, or three-pound weights. It is so simple and convenient a means of exercising the entire body that many people tend to think, "How could something so easy and fun be so good for you?" If it were a bit more complicated, more costly, or caused greater discomfort, it would probably be more popular. The fact is that Resistive Rebounding will probably revolutionize the fitness movement in the next decade, not only for world class athletes but for *everyone* interested in fitness, from the weakest to the strongest, from the clumsiest to the most fleet of foot.

Resistive Rebounding is probably the best home aerobics training program in existence today. Surprisingly, rebounders are quite reasonably priced. Equally appealing is the convenience. You can use your rebounder anywhere—in your bedroom, your den, even in your backyard. And you can rebound no matter what the weather. This is a cardiovascular and strengthening exercise that cannot be "rained out." Anyone, from the youngest toddlers to oldsters, can benefit from simply bouncing on a rebounder, even if only doing the "health bounce," a rhythmic up-and-down movement. People who are bedridden or in wheelchairs can also benefit simply by placing their feet on the rebounder while someone else jumps. Here's why!

Muscle movement is a *cellular* function. Each muscle is a community of cells that band together to perform a function that cannot be performed by any single cell—that is, the movement of part of the skeletal system. We have already mentioned that there are around 650 muscles in the body. They are really highly organized communities of cells, individual cells actually in communication with each other through an intricate system of nerve cells or neurons to get their work done. Without these nerve cells, the muscle cells would be unable to function.

Rebound exercise provides a stimulation for the neuromuscular system that can be achieved with no other exercise. It does so by combining three forces—gravity (an ever-present, never-changing downward pull), acceleration, and deceleration (the two opposite forces of movement). In the words of Albert E. Carter, president of the National Institute of Rebounding and Health, "The neural muscular stimulation of rebound exercise is close to phenomenal. Rebound exercise also provides a refreshing aerobic activity void of the joint jarring shock of hitting a hard surface." We personally know many joggers who have switched to rebounding. You can get just as much aerobic benefit as you would receive from jogging, but without the injuries frequently suffered by runners: knee injuries, Achilles tendon injuries, shin splints, ankle strain, and foot fractures. The *true* test is in the doing.

The Resistive Rebounding routine that follows, a product of extensive rebounding research by Harry and Sarah Sneider, has a multitude of benefits. It is virtually a scientific breakthrough in fitness and athletic training. The alternating weightlessness and increased gravitational pull (called G forces) produced in rebounding, combined with a sequence of exercises that work each muscle group through its full range of movement, result in total body fitness and tone. *Every single cell, organ, and muscle is exercised.* Resistive rebounding additionally stimulates the activities of the lymph system, helps circulate more oxygen to the tissues, strengthens the heart, aids metabolism, enhances digestion and elimination, builds muscles, corrects poor eyesight, improves overall coordination, improves posture and body alignment, strengthens joints, and brings flexibility to the neck, hips, knees, ankles, and back. This may sound like hyperbole, but you'll see—it is *all* true!

Rebounding is probably the best all-around exercise you can get. We have been rebounding for over six years. We own three rebounders, which everyone in the family uses, and we would feel lost without them. In fact, we like to give rebounders as gifts to people we love. We are presenting this exercise program to you because we believe in it. Even if you are already actively involved in some sort of exercise, we hope you will investigate rebounding. It will serve to support whatever other exercise you are doing. If you have not yet found your "perfect workout," this may be it! We hope you will try it and discover what a boon it will be in your life.*

On the following pages you will find the **FIT FOR LIFE "PERFECT WORKOUT"** of Resistive Rebounding developed by Sarah and Harry Sneider. Dr. Sneider is this country's leading rebounding authority and trainer. Having used the rebounder to overcome the loss of his hip joint during World War II, he has worked successfully in developing a rebounding program for all types of

---

*If you have difficulty finding a rebounder and the weights for your "Perfect Workout," write to us at 2210 Wilshire Boulevard, Suite 118, Santa Monica, California 90403.

bodies. Additional workouts for people of all ages or those with specific goals and much more information on rebounding can be found in his excellent book *The Olympic Trainer*, which can be ordered from: Sneider's Family Fitness, P.O. Box 3374, Arcadia, California 91006.

The Perfect Workout for Every Body*

NOTE: Some exercises may not be suitable for your particular body condition. Do not do any exercise that causes pain to your body. If you are uncertain about which exercises are appropriate for you, consult a physical therapist or exercise specialist. Use your common sense. Do what makes sense to *you*!

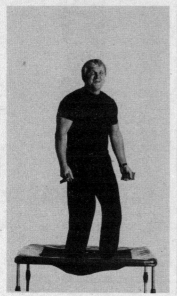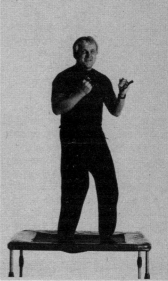

1. CURL: Firms upper arms and forearms and strengthens grip.

Directions: Grip sandbag weights. Jog or shuffle in the center of the rebounder with palms up and your elbows close to your sides. Raise both weights together to your shoulders, then bring weights back to original position. Do 12 reps.

*All repetitions are merely suggestions. Do what is comfortable for you.

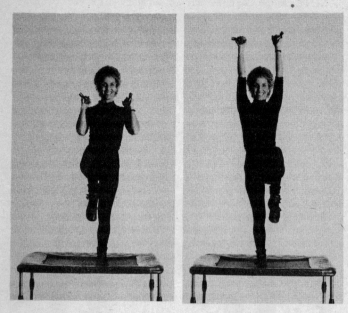

2. PRESS: Firms and works upper back, shoulders, arms, and grip. Presses provide excellent overall toning for the arms.

Directions: Grip sandbag weights. Jog or shuffle in center of the rebounder. Bring weights to your shoulders, push both arms together overhead, then bring back to shoulders after each repetition. Do 12 reps.

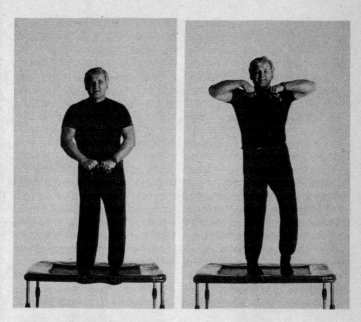

3. UPRIGHT ROW: Excellent for posture, upper back, chest, and forearms.

Directions: Grip sandbag weights. Jog or shuffle in the center of the rebounder. Hold hands close together in front of lower body. Pull both hands up to your chin with elbows out in a straight line from the chin. Lower hands to original position after each repetition. Do 12 reps.

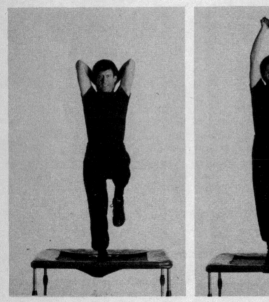

4. TRICEPS PRESS: Works back of upper arms and shoulders and strengthens grip.

Directions: Grip sandbag weights. Jog, shuffle, or bounce in center of rebounder. Place hands behind head, holding weights together. Press weights up over head, arms extended, and then bring back down to original position.

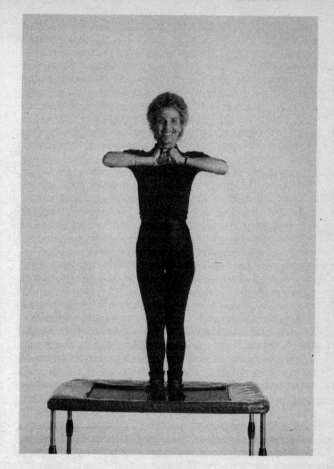

5. SQUEEZE: Strengthens grip, forearms, and chest muscles.

Directions: Hold weights with elbows bent four to six inches from chest as you shuffle or bounce in the center of the rebounder. Squeeze firmly and release. Do 12 reps.

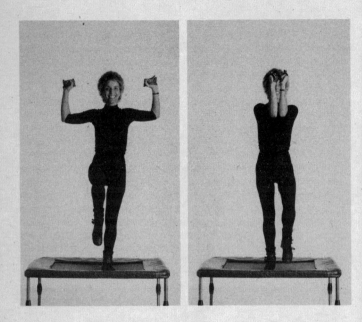

6. HIGH BENT ELBOW TOUCH: Works chest, shapes and firms upper back, shoulders, and arms.

Directions: Grip sandbag weights. Jog, shuffle, or bounce in the center of the rebounder. With elbows bent at chest level and parallel to the ground, bring forearms together in front of you. Extend back to open position. Do 12 reps.

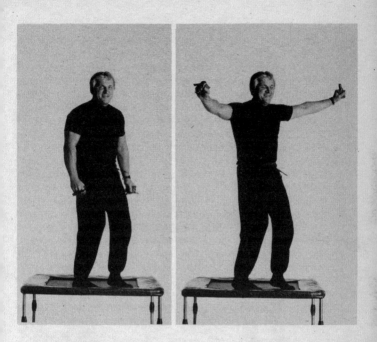

7. SIDE RAISE: Works shoulders, arms, and upper back.

Directions: Grip sandbag weights. Jog, shuffle, or bounce in the center of the rebounder. Keeping arms straight, raise the weights to at least shoulder level—do not bend elbows. Slowly lower extended arms to your sides. Do 12 reps.

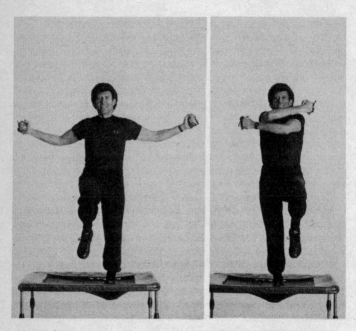

8. CROSSOVERS: Firms upper chest, shapes arms and shoulders, and strengthens upper back.

Directions: Grip sandbag weights. Jog, shuffle, or bounce in the center of the rebounder. Extend arms out to the side at shoulder height. Bring hands around in front of your chest and cross over in a ''hug yourself'' motion. Return arms to original extended position. Do 12 reps.

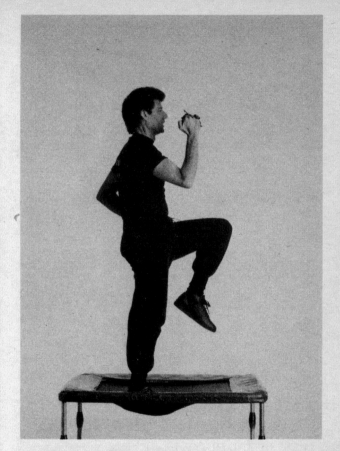

9. SPRINT KNEE-HIGH: Conditions all muscles, particularly waist, hips, thighs, calves, and upper body.

Directions: Grip sandbag weights. Run in place in the center of the rebounder, raising knees as high as possible. Do for 30 seconds to 1 minute.

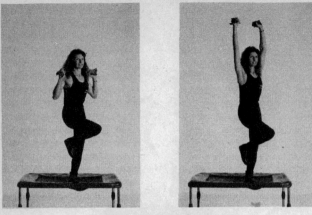

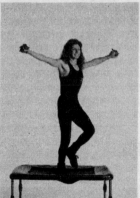

10. PRESS UP AND OUT: Firms upper back, shoulders, arms, and chest.

Directions: Grip sandbag weights. Jog, shuffle, or bounce in the center of the rebounder. Pull weights to shoulders, push overhead together with palms facing each other, then bring back to shoulders. Now push weights out to side, extending arms straight out from shoulders, and returning back to shoulders. Alternate pressing overhead and pressing to the side. Do 12 reps.

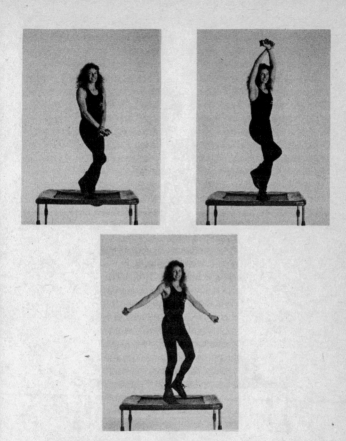

11. WINDMILLS: Works chest, shoulders, arms, upper back, hips, and thighs, and aids posture.

Directions: Grip sandbag weights. Jog, shuffle, or bounce in the center of the rebounder. Holding your arms straight, make large circles with your arms, rotating them in an upward motion. Reverse direction for second set. Do 6 reps in each direction.

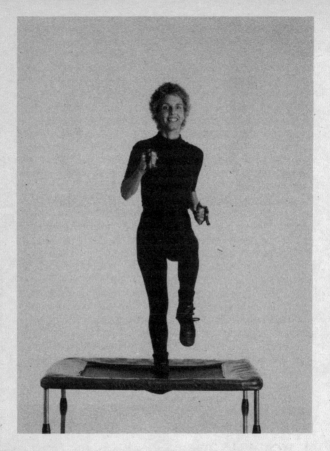

12. JOG EASY: An overall good body conditioner.

Directions: Grip sandbag weights. Jog easy in the center of the rebounder, elbows and knees moving together in easy cadence. Do for 30 seconds to 1 minute.

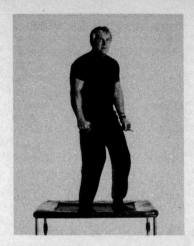

SPECIAL EXERCISE FOR THE ELDERLY OR WHEN HEALTH IS IMPAIRED

LYMPHATIC BOUNCE: Works to pump and cleanse the lymph system, your body's in-house "vacuum cleaner."

Directions: Bounce lightly in the middle of the mat without feet leaving mat. Keep hands at sides; hold sandbag weights if you desire. Maintain erect posture.

> *Beginner:* 1 to 2 minutes
> *Intermediate:* 3 minutes
> *Advanced:* 5 minutes

NOTE: Some rebounders are constructed with a hand support for elderly or infirm people. This is the exercise which can be adapted to benefit people who are in wheelchairs or who are bedridden. Simply place their feet on the rebounder while they remain seated in a chair and have someone else bounce gently.

WEIGHT-LIFTING

Unlike the cardiovascular and strengthening exercises and unlike stretching for flexibility, which we will soon discuss, weight-lifting serves primarily to develop muscular strength and endurance. The most common form of weight-lifting involves using Nautilus-type exercise equipment or free weights. But it also includes sit-ups, push-ups, pull-ups, etc. Although professional bodybuilders work to develop every muscle they can work with weights, each weight-lifting exercise concentrates on a specific muscle or group of muscles, unlike the whole body workout provided by an aerobic routine.

While weight-lifting exercises can be extremely beneficial for muscle building and endurance, they do very little for the development of the rest of the body. In fact, if not balanced with aerobics and stretching, weight-lifting exercises can sometimes prove detrimental. Keep in mind that strong muscles and a weak heart do not make for a good combination. Ideally, one should utilize weight-training one day and aerobics/stretching the next. This way you will be concentrating on different body areas daily while allowing other areas a chance to recover.

The proper use of weight-lifting, coupled with good eating, is the best way to increase your body weight and size. Considering that 90 percent of the population wants to *lose* weight, a lot of people might respond, "So who cares?"

You would be surprised at how many letters we receive from people wanting to increase their size and weight. For those of you who fall into this category, the combination of fresh, wholesome, *unprocessed* food and weight-training is your best bet for putting on *healthy* weight. The weight-lifting does not have to be a full-on, superstrenuous routine. Even the use of light weights will create a demand in your muscles to increase in size, which they will do as long as your diet is supplying the best possible building blocks available.

Since muscle weighs more than fat, you will fill out and put on weight as you start to build up even a little. It does not take long for someone who is very thin and has that hollow look to fill out just enough to improve his or her appearance considerably. It is certainly not difficult these days to locate a health club or gymnasium with professional trainers who can put you on the right track and set you up with a nice comfortable routine designed to fit *your* life-style and *your* wants and needs.

A young man once called us and complained that although he was eating good food according to our principles (including enough pasta to feed a family of four) and working out with weights regularly, he could *not* gain an ounce. He said he had been trying for several months. This was hard to believe, because ordinarily that kind of discipline over an extended length of time brings results. Not until I spoke with him on another occasion did he happen to mention that he was a marathon runner, competing in two or three marathons a year in addition to running hundreds of miles a month.

There seems to be a real honest to goodness shortage of fat marathon runners. I have yet to meet a marathoner who has successfully built up his or her body with weight-lifting. Perhaps it can be done, but *I've* never seen it. Of all forms of exercise, marathon running is the exception in terms of ''norms'' in diet and weight-training. Marathoning requires special diet and training.

STRETCHING

Regardless of how superb and strong a physique may appear, without proper extension and stretching of muscles the body cannot reach its highest potential. A thorough stretching program exercises every muscle, nerve, organ, and gland in the body. It promotes a fine build, one that is strong and elastic without being muscle-bound.

MARILYN:

There are many approaches to stretching. Some can be helpful. Others can be harmful because they are done without an understanding of how the body works. Of the many philosophies regarding stretching that we have explored one that yields great benefits is Hatha Yoga.

In chapter 6, in the discussion on breathing, I talked about the autonomic nervous system, which regulates all involuntary body processes—breathing, blinking of the eyes, in fact, all the workings of all the organs of the body. This autonomic nervous system has two sides: the sympathetic side, which responds to all our immediate needs, and the parasympathetic side, which calms us down after each response. In other words, whenever you are challenged or threatened, the sympathetic nervous system kicks in. Your heart beats faster, your glands produce more adrenaline, the sweat glands open, your hair follicles stand up. All of this takes place as your body becomes alert to protect itself—to either flee or fight. Even if the situation is imaginary, even if the threat is not real—for example, a scary moment in a movie—the response is still the same. The brain has no screening device. In a movie you can know totally that all that is really there is a screen full of images, but you can go through the same physical shock as if everything were really happening to you. Your body has no way of knowing. It reaps the results of what you pass through your mind. A constant barrage of stressful situations, real or unreal, forces your nervous system to lock tension into all your organs and muscles. This tightens you up, constricts the organs and the blood supply to them, and creates the stress that so many people experience.

If the sympathetic side is too dominant, you will be overreactive, nervous, and full of stress. If not relieved, this stress leads to disease.

The function of the parasympathetic side of the nervous system is to calm us and quiet us down after a strong response so that we don't keep on buzzing. After bouts of great laughter, anger, or fear, the parasympathetic nervous system comes into play to restore our equilibrium. However, if the parasympathetic is *too* dominant, we become *too* laid-back or depressed or lazy. A perfect balance between the sympathetic and the parasympathetic is what is needed and this is what Hatha Yoga provides us.

Hatha Yoga is the science of balancing your body. *Ha* means "sun" and refers to your sympathetic nervous system, your activating state. *Tha* means "moon" and refers to your parasympathetic or resting and healing state. *Yoga* means "union." So *Hatha Yoga* signifies the union between the active and passive—the union of sun and moon, the oneness of being in balance in the most productive state of existence. This is what Yoga poses are all about. They stretch us, teaching us how to release the tension and stress locked in our muscles and organs, in the very depth of our being. They strengthen us, giving us balance, determination, and the willpower to deal with life.

We move from this understanding to a series of Yoga postures developed for **Fit for Life** readers by Alan Finger, a second-generation yoga master whose *YOGAWORKS* studios are presently located in Los Angeles and New York. When Alan teaches, he introduces Yoga in the following way.

The ancient Yogis studied how animals release stress, how cats, dogs, and various other animals stretch and balance themselves. Then they studied the human being and noted how when humans became tired they would yawn as they stretched their arms or when they had been working in the fields they would try to stretch their spines out. Thousands of years ago, the Yogis began from their observations to develop a philosophy of stretching. They noticed that breathing was always interrelated with this process.

Whenever humans stretch there is a release, a sigh. In the process of Yoga, when you exhale you release the tightness in your body. When you inhale, you strengthen and develop your body. The therapy in Yoga takes place as you breathe during a pose. If you hold your breath, you are resisting the release of tensions. If you breathe *with* the pose and *through* the pose, in and out, smoothly and evenly, your body will, little by little, begin to let go. *In Yoga, you only go as far as you can, never overdoing. Enough is enough, but enough is necessary. There is no competition with yourself nor with others.*

Yoga is about opening up your own being. Whenever you do a pose, do it the best you can, breathing smoothly through, and the therapy will take place in the doing. The sequence that I have formulated for you is a minimal but highly effective sequence that you can do every day to work every part of your being.

If you are inerested in learning more about how to make yoga part of your lifestyle, Alan's video and audio tapes are available through:

YOGAWORKS
146 E. 56th St.
New York, N.Y. 10022

Daily Yoga Set

CAUTION: Some yoga postures may not be suitable for people with lower back problems. If a posture causes you any discomfort in the lower back area, do not do it. Consult a physical therapist or exercise therapist if you are in question as to whether certain exercises are appropriate for your body.

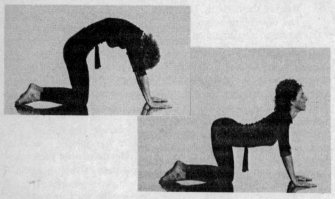

1. THE CAT POSE: Teaches you how to keep suppleness in the hip structure, which is the foundation of your spine. The condition of your hips determines what kind of agility you will have in your spine. Your spine is the central part of your nervous system and hence the highway of your life. By learning to move the hip structure, the spine moves to its extremes each way. In this fashion you keep the spine healthy and the hips mobile. In old people the hips become frozen. Keeping your hips loose and supple keeps the life flowing in your nervous system and spinal column.

Directions: Kneel on all fours with your knees and feet hip distance apart and your hands lined up with your shoulders. Exhale, humping your back upward, chin into chest. Tuck seatbone in. Inhale, arch back *down*, and lift face up, turning seatbone up in the air at the same time. Initiate spinal movement from the hips. Repeat 5 times, inhaling as you lower your spine, exhaling as you arch your spine.

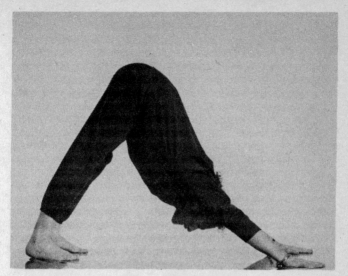

2. THE TENT POSE: Works to release pressure from the back of the legs. This is where unconscious suppressions are locked, where things not even in your awareness are taxing you. Little fears, shocks, even shame or discomforts that you never think about are locked into the back of the legs. The sounds of cars blowing their horns, brakes screeching, and all the little disturbances that register unconsciously lock in behind your legs, and that is why your legs get so tired and stiff.

In the Tent Pose you lengthen your spine and stretch out the back of your legs by rotating the hip structure. You are releasing all the tension that locks behind the legs, tension that actually pulls the hip structure down and out and thereby creates so many back disorders. This pose releases pressure on the spine by loosening the hip structure.

Directions: Kneel with feet and knees six inches apart and parallel. Place your palms, fingers spread, on the floor where it meets a wall. Align the thumb and first finger against the wall. Keep your feet flat and your legs apart and straight. Work your abdomen and thighs toward each other, and raise seatbone up in the air. Hold for 6 even breaths. Keep inhalation and exhalation smooth.

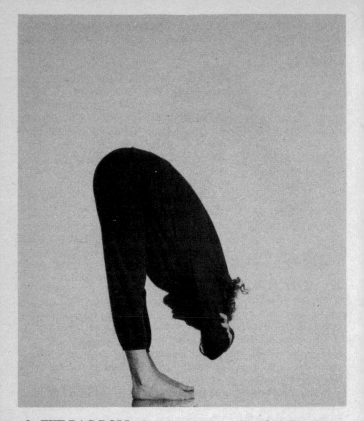

3. THE RAG DOLL: A more extreme version of the Tent Pose. The same benefits are provided, with the difference that you get a lot of extra blood pouring into the brain from bending forward and hanging down. It's like turning halfway upside down.

Directions: Assume the Tent Pose and walk hands toward feet. Fold your arms, letting your elbows hang toward the floor. Turn your seatbone up in the air. Keep the front of your thighs tight and concentrate on keeping your seatbone up in the air. Hold for 6 even breaths.

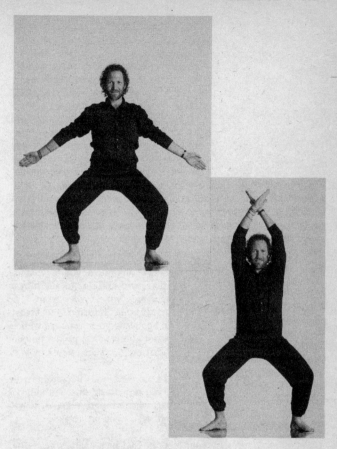

4. ARM ROTATION: Helps release subconscious suppressions, those that you can't deal with but that remain on your mind nonetheless. They lock in from your shoulders to the hips.

Directions: Stand with your feet three feet apart and turned out 45 degrees. Bend knees slightly in line with your feet. Rotate arms 10 times in each direction, forward and back.

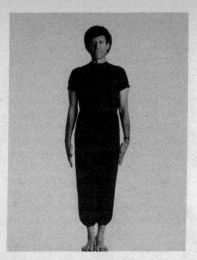

5. THE POSTURE POSE: An exercise of stance. It teaches you how to correct your posture. When you slump, you compress all your organs; you force your spine out of alignment; you set yourself up for bad posture, spinal disorders, and disease. In addition to bad posture, you also create great pressure on your heart. The heart is situated between the lungs. If you slump and your breastbone sinks in, you're actually strangulating your heart, as well as all your internal organs. You are not allowing the proper amount of blood to flow through your heart or the other organs of your body.

It is important to stand tall and keep the blood circulating in the heart. The Posture Pose teaches you how to do this. Although it is not how you are going to stand when you are relaxed, it will teach you to stand straight and tall when you are relaxed.

Directions: Stand with your feet one-half inch apart, spread your big toes to touch, and distribute your weight in the area of each foot between the big toes, two little toes, and your heels. Tighten your front thighs, forcing the arch in your feet to rise. "Pinch in" the seat and pubic areas tightly, lifting your spine upward. (Be sure your seat is tucked under, not arched out!) Relax your shoulders and imagine that you have lead weights in your fingertips. Feel yourself being pulled *up* from your breastbone and the crown of your head. Hold for 15 seconds.

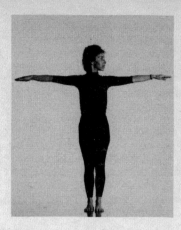

6. THE NECK RELEASE: Conscious suppressions are locked into the neck. When you get tense and busy, your neck tightens and becomes stiff.

Directions: Stand in the Posture Pose, raising arms out to the sides until they are parallel to the floor. Point your chin over each shoulder, twice to each side. Rotate your head to four points—chest, side, back, side. As you press your head back, project your chin up into the air. Do 2 rotations clockwise and 2 rotations counterclockwise.

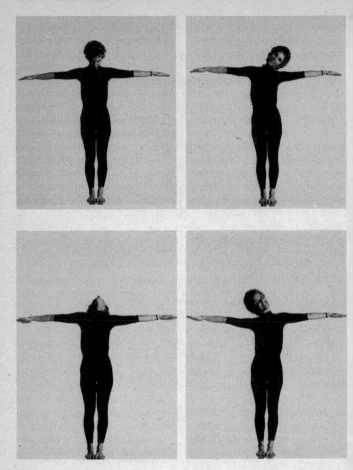

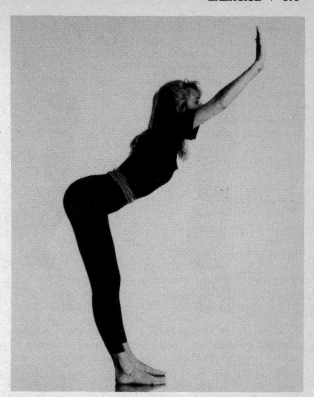

7. ARM EXTENSION AT THE WALL: This posture will release tension in your shoulders and open your chest cavity, taking pressure off your heart and lungs. It allows the blood to flow freely to these major organs. It also eliminates hunchback and round shoulders.

Directions: Stand at arm's distance from the wall, with your feet shoulder distance apart. Place your palms on the wall well above your head. Press your seatbone back as you arch your upper back, pulling your chin, neck, and chest forward toward the wall. Breathe through 6 breaths with slow, even breathing.

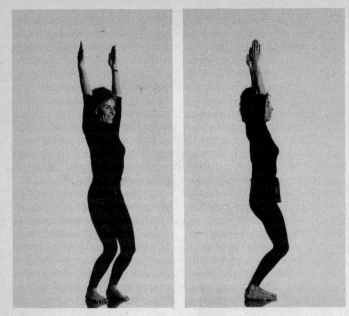

8. THE CHAIR POSE: Helps to build strength in the thighs, the seat, and the abdomen. These muscles must be strong to hold your spine in alignment. They are the seat of determination and will-power.

Directions: Stand in Posture Pose. Separate feet six inches apart, keeping them parallel. Raise your arms above your head, so that your biceps line up next to your ears. Keeping your feet flat, back straight, and seat tucked under, bend your knees and hold at the point where you can be comfortable without straining. Hold for 6 even breaths. With arms still held above your head, come up, go up on your toes, then bend your knees again, this time remaining on your toes. Hold for 6 even breaths. Come up, lower your arms to be parallel to the floor in front of you, then come up on your toes again, bring your knees together, and lower all the way down to sit on your heels, keeping your back straight and seat tucked under. Hold for 6 even breaths and return to standing position.

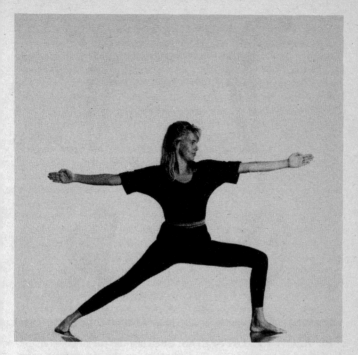

9. WARRIOR: This is a dynamic posture to develop strength in your seat, thighs, and abdomen. It opens your hip structure and corrects posture problems.

Directions: Stand with your legs spread wide apart, at least four feet. Turn your feet to the left, your left foot 90 degrees and your right foot 10 degrees. Bend your left knee to a right angle, so that your thigh is parallel to the ground. Keep your right leg straight, extended behind you. Stretch your arms out to the sides and parallel to the floor. Keep all your joints on the same plane. Hold for 6 even breaths. Alternate sides, reversing left and right in instructions here.

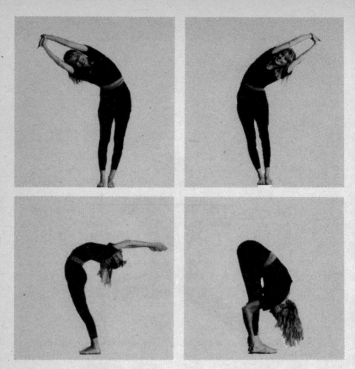

10. BLOWN PALM SERIES: Stretches the spinal column and all the major organs in all directions—to the sides, back, and forward.

Directions: For *side bends*, stand with legs together. Take hold of one wrist with the opposite hand, then stretch up and over to one side, keeping your biceps beside your ears. Your hips should project to the opposite side. Hold for 6 even breaths on each side. For the *back bend*, extend arms straight up in the air; look up between your fingertips. "Pinch in" your seat, and stretch up and back, lengthening your lumbar spine. Go only as far back as is comfortable, and hold the pose by squeezing the seat. Hold for 6 even breaths. For the *forward bend*, bend forward and take hold of your ankles, thumbs tipping the floor and elbows kept behind your calves. Press your seatbone up in the air as you straighten your legs. Hold for 8 even breaths.

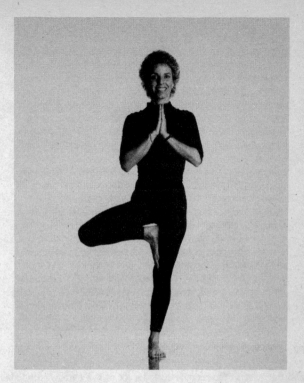

11. THE STORK: This pose balances left and right brain. Besides aiding physical balance, it opens the hip structure and the knee joints.

Directions: Standing in the Posture Pose, take your left foot and place it on the inner, upper thigh of the right leg, working the foot as high up as possible. Try to keep your knees and hips in the same plane. (Focus your eyes on one point for balance.) Bring your hands up into a prayer position in front of the chest. All your exerted strength should be in your thighs, seat, and abdominal muscle. Your shoulders and chest should be completely relaxed. Hold for 4 even breaths. Then separate hands to six inches apart, palms facing forward, and extend your arms straight up into the air. Hold for 4 breaths. Release slowly. Repeat on other side.

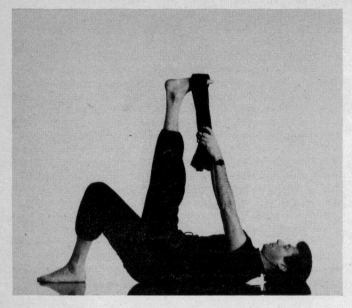

12. LYING LEG EXTENSION: Releases stress from the legs. The leg muscles are where unconscious suppressions are locked, and they act as the receptacle for a lot of the narrow-mindedness of life. Ridding oneself of that stress enlightens and freshens you. This posture also releases pressure from the hip structure as it releases the tightness of the hamstrings, which are attached to the bottom of the seatbone.

Directions: Use a folded towel for this posture. Lie comfortably on your back on the floor, with neck and shoulders flat. Roll the towel lengthwise, bring your left leg up so that your foot is flat on floor against your seat, with your knee bent. Raise your right leg perpendicular to the floor, loop the towel around the ball of the right foot, and gently pull down on either side of towel, keeping your shoulders and neck flat on floor. Climb your hands upward on the towel while slowly releasing the back of the leg, keeping leg as straight as possible. Hold for 15 seconds to 1 minute on each side, breathing evenly.

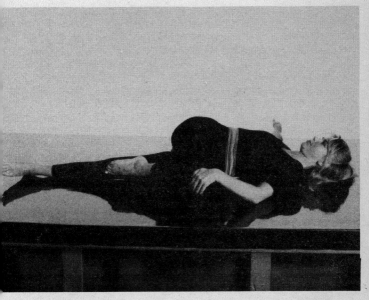

13. MALTESE TWIST: This pose releases tension from along the entire length of your spine. It massages the gangliated nerve trunk that extends down either side of your spine. It also massages your digestive system. This will give a tremendous sense of relaxation.

Directions: Lie on your back with arms out to your sides at right angles to your body. Raise your right leg to a bent-knee position and place your right foot on your left thigh just above the knee. Place your left hand on your right knee and *gently* pull the knee down toward the floor as far as it will go, keeping your right arm and shoulder flat on the floor. Hold for 6 breaths. Return the right leg to a straight position on the floor. Repeat with your left leg.

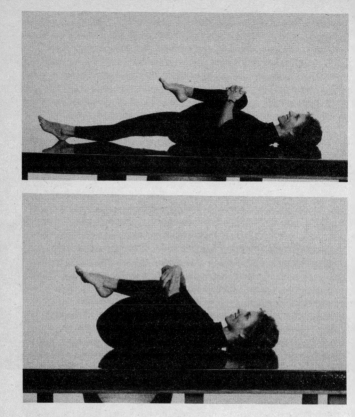

14. WIND EXPELLER: Massages the digestive system. It releases gases from the system, massages and loosens the hips, and positions the spine.

Directions: First, while lying on your back, bring your right thigh up to your abdomen. Interlace your fingers and clasp both hands two inches below the right knee. Keep your neck and back as flat to the floor as possible. Hold for 6 even breaths. Repeat with the left leg. Second, bend both legs up, holding your thighs against your abdomen with your arms. Hold for 6 even breaths.

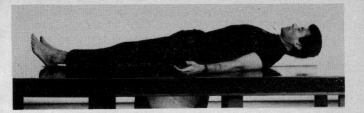

15. RELAX ON BACK

Directions: Place a rolled towel under your spine from the top of your head to your hips. As you relax on the towel feel yourself breathing from the abdomen—as you breathe in, your abdomen rises; as you breathe out, your abdomen lowers. Do for 2 to 5 minutes.

Try to practice these Yoga postures every day to keep your body strong and supple. It is good to do them after a walk and a warm shower in the morning when your body is warmed up. When you live in a society such as ours, stress tends to make you crumple into yourself and stifle all your organs. The result, in the words of Alan Finger, "is like throwing a blanket over a fire—you stifle it." You block the blood supply to and from all your organs. The postures teach you to stand tall, to keep upright, and to allow the blood to circulate correctly. As people get older they shrink into themselves; the muscles become weak, stress pulls them down; the aging process sets in, diseases come, and they accept it all, saying, "Oh well, we're getting on; we're aging." That's not necessary. You can keep the muscles strong and stretch the tension out of them. You can keep the correct alignment. You will lead a fit and healthy life. *Yoga will not only add years to your life but will add life to your years*.

BACK PAIN

Afflicting millions of people in this country, back pain is second only to headache pain in the numbers of people it affects. Sufferers can be in a particular quandary about how to exercise without aggravating their problem. A great deal of back pain can be traced to poor posture. Most people do not stand, sit, lie down or walk correctly. A method for improving body movement and posture which well deserves the greater acceptance it is recently gaining is called the Alexander Technique. Originated over half a century ago in England and taught by certified Alexander teachers throughout this country, it combines a gentle hands-on system of adjustment with unique verbal direction to the subconscious to forget old postures and begin holding the head, neck, shoulders and spine in the biologically correct way. The result is pain-relief and an amazing sense of lightness as the body naturally realigns itself. As an additional measure to quality chiropractic care, the technique is a logical first step in fighting back pain since it deals with the *cause* of the problem, rather than fighting the effect.

HOW MUCH EXERCISE?

HARVEY:

Exercise is not in itself some sort of panacea. Some hold the notion that exercise by itself will protect us from disease. Supposedly, if we run every day we can eat all kinds of fatty foods and still ward off plaquing of the arteries, blood cholesterol, and arterial sclerosis. The death at age fifty-two of Jim Fixx, the father of running, laid that particular bit of nonsense to rest. Although he ran every day, the three main arteries from his heart were severely blocked.

The point must be made loud and clear: Exercise does *not* insure us against disease, nor does it remedy disease. That it helps the body by making it stronger and more capable of dealing with ill health is certain, but exercise has no magical ability to correct the results of an unhealthy life-style. Of course, there will always be those who point to some isolated case of a person exercising rigorously but eating abysmally and faring better than someone who neither exercises nor eats properly. The difference can be explained by the fact that the latter ignored *two* elements of health while the former ignored only one. Exercise will *not* undo the effects of dietary abuses, but a lack of exercise can certainly compound their effects.

How much exercise should one engage in? This is determined

by several factors of an individual's life-style. You surely do not have to become an outstanding athlete or become a marathoner to supply your body with its physiological need for exercise, which is not as great as some people believe. Rather than trying to meet the requirements on an arbitrarily formulated chart some "expert" devised, it is far more useful to do as much as *you* are comfortable with. We have one strict rule: **DO MORE THAN NONE!** As long as you are doing *some* exercise, you will gravitate toward what is the best type and amount for you.

All too frequently people get hyped up about exercising, go on an all-out program of much more exercise than they are comfortable with, then become frustrated and wind up cursing exercise and doing none. Guilt sets in and the entire issue of exercise becomes a sore spot. Try not to be influenced by what others are doing or to keep up with them. Be influenced by your own desire to experience a long, robust, and fulfilling life. *Some* form of exercise is simply one of the ingredients of realizing that goal.

Of considerable importance is *when* to exercise. From my own experience and that of numerous people I have questioned—and in the opinion of quite a few authors writing on exercise—the best time appears to be in the morning hours. However, this is definitely a generality. I know people who exercise vigorously every day for two or three hours in the late afternoon or early evening. Follow your personal preference. But keep in mind that when you awaken in the morning you have a full complement of energy stored from the night's sleep. So morning is when your body is physiologically best equipped to engage in and reap the benefits of exercise—in my opinion. By all means, try exercising at different times of day and settle upon what is best for you.

Of more crucial importance is when to exercise in relationship to when you eat. *Ideally*, any exercise, no matter of what type, will be most beneficial when your stomach is empty of all food. Except for fruit or fruit juice, you are best served by not eating before exercising. It's obvious why.

Our lives are based on energy. Everything you do requires some expenditure of energy, from reading to running. Exercise takes a considerable amount, and we know that eating takes more than anything. If you have food being digested in your stomach, thereby using a good portion of your available energy, exercising at the same time will only put too much of a burden on your system. Your body has to divide its energy between these two activities, therefore neither is well served. If you eat and then exercise, the food will stay in your stomach much longer than necessary, more energy than normal will be expended, and the overall effect will be to leave you feeling depleted. Exercising *before* eating allows your body to *fully* involve itself in that activity without also having to meet the demands of the stomach. Fruit or fruit juices are the only exceptions, because as we indicated earlier, they are the only foods that do *not* demand digestive energy in the stomach.

This is all very easy to verify for yourself. Whatever your particular form of exercise is, do it for one week at the same time of day, exercising *after* eating. Then do it for one week at the same time of day, exercising *before* eating. You'll have as much difficulty discerning which is more desirable as you would have deciding which would be more comfortable, lying on a down quilt or falling down a flight of stairs.

If you are partial to some form of activity after eating, then take a light stroll, which many people find actually helps them digest their meal. More activity than that will only prove counterproductive. The only other activity that we might recommend is very, very light stretching. I can't think of a time when *light* stretching would not be helpful.

Exercise is a basic biological need. There is *no* way to achieve **living health** without it. Remember to walk whenever you can. Walking is a "dying art" in our country; there is a direct correlation between the automobile and large, "unused" thighs. The "Perfect Workout" and the "Daily Yoga Set" are suggested to help you get into some regular, enjoyable exercise pattern. But realize that every time you become aware of your body, you are in fact exercising it. When you suddenly realize you are sitting in a slumped and twisted posture and you straighten out and pull yourself up nice and tall, *that* is a form of exercise—you are *using your muscles* to support your body. When you are walking, straighten your body. Take long-legged strides (for the long-legged look)! Swing your arms! When you bend over to pick something up, *be aware* of how you do it; use your legs, not just your back.

All body movement and the awareness of that movement is exercise. Cleaning your house and garden are exercise. Exercise is part of life, ingrained in human existence, not something you have to view as an alien discipline. Feel good about moving your body. You will gravitate toward moving it more and more.

CHAPTER 11
Sunshine

HARVEY:

Picture the planet Earth without the sun. Not an easy task, since there would be very little to picture. First of all, it would be pitch black, so you couldn't see anything anyway. Moreover, there would be no life—no plants, no animals, no humans, *nothing*. Picture a large, dark, cold, barren, ice cold rock and you have our planet without the sun.

Throughout history the sun has been worshiped and revered by those aware of its health-enhancing properties. Planning activities in the beneficial rays of the sun is as much a part of natural living as the procuring of food or water or any of the other elements of health. Ancient civilizations such as the Babylonians, Egyptians, Assyrians, Greeks, and Romans were all aware of the hygienic use of the sun and equipped their cities with sun gardens for this purpose. One of the Egyptians' first temple complexes was erected in honor of their sun god. It was named Heliopolis, or City of the Sun.

The extraordinary, magnificent creation that is the sun is the source of *all* life as we know it. It is your friend, *not* your enemy. It is not possible for us to attain and sustain a full degree of health unless we establish and maintain an intelligent relationship with the sun. We are constituted for life in the sunshine, and we need the benefit of regular contact with its rays, not only for its warmth but also for its light.

Light is necessary for vision and for warmth, but it is also a vital nutrient required by the body, although few people realize that. Sunlight is essential for plants and animals. So important is sunshine to life that denying ourselves its life-giving rays directly contributes to our own undoing.

Both animals and plants make use of the powers of sunlight. Vegetation is at its most luxuriant and at its highest form of development in the tropical regions near the Equator, where the sun's rays are most consistently abundant. In the higher latitudes we find the near sterility of the frigid zones, where the sun's rays are less powerful—indeed absent for an extended period of each year. Deprive plants of sunlight, and the result is an inferior plant that is pale or colorless.

Earlier, in chapter 6, we pointed out our dependence on plants to transform carbon dioxide into usable oxygen for breathing. This is accomplished by the process of photosynthesis, which is *not possible without sunshine*. Were it not for the sun we couldn't breathe!

A number of people in northern latitudes suffer from what is called "severe winter depression." People who otherwise live normal, happy lives experience an abysmal depression come winter that deprives them of practically any pleasure. They are sad, lethargic, unable to perform simple tasks, and tend to cry for no apparent reason. Researchers at the National Institute of Mental Health have been able to eliminate this malady in people merely by subjecting them to a couple of hours daily of *full spectrum* fluorescent light, which simulates sunlight. The decrease in sunlight in the winter months occasions this severe depression.

Tadpoles that are deprived of sunlight fail to turn into frogs. They just continue to grow as tadpoles. Animals who live out their lives in a complete absence of light are commonly blind, even eyeless. Chickens raised in sunlight produce eggs with harder and thicker shells than those not so exposed. Studies by some of the early Natural Hygienists, notably Russell Trall, confirm that hospital patients lucky enough to be in rooms on the sunny side of the hospital make quicker recoveries than those on the shady side.

There have been numerous studies verifying the extreme importance of sunlight in nurturing healthy plants and animals. One of the most well-known and respected researchers is a gentleman named John Ott. Mr. Ott, author of three books on the subject, founded the Environmental Health and Light Research Institute to coordinate his ongoing studies into the ways in which light can enhance the health of plants, animals, and humans.

In Mr. Ott's words, "My studies have indicated that light is a nutrient similar to all the other nutrients we take in through food and that we *need* the full spectrum range of natural sunlight. This is a fact long since proven by science."*

Mr. Ott has coined the term *malillumination*, a lack of the necessary amount of sunlight (just as *malnutrition* is a lack of the proper nutrients in our diet). One of the tests he conducted was with rats and mice bred in captivity for laboratory experiments. Usually the males have to be removed from cages before a litter arrives or they'll eat the young, but Mr. Ott found that when the cages are placed in natural daylight, that does not happen. In fact, males displayed normal parental instincts and helped take care of the young. He moved the cages back and forth from natural to artificial light. Under natural light males are calm and manageable. Moved to artificial light for the next litter, those same males will start attacking their young again.

Mr. Ott also ran studies on humans. In 1973 he ran a five-month study in the Sarasota County School System. He equipped two classrooms with full-spectrum light that simulated natural light. Two other classrooms, the control group, were left with their regular fluorescent light. In the classrooms under the full-spectrum light, several extremely hyperactive children calmed down completely and were able to overcome their learning disabilities. Time-lapse cameras were used in each classroom to record incidences of disruptive behavior, and the fluorescent classrooms always had more.

Of the many experiments that have been conducted so far to demonstrate the beneficial effects of sunlight, one is particularly remarkable and significant. That test was conducted with twelve bean plants in order to determine whether indirect or diffused daylight had the same effect on plants as direct sunlight. The bean plants were of the same variety and in the same stage of development. They were planted near one another in such a way that six always had full direct sunlight while the other six received only the diffused daylight. When the pods were harvested and the weight compared, the beans grown in full sunlight were three times larger than the beans grown in indirect light. This result was expected. What followed the next year was totally *un*expected.

*John Ott, "The Light Side of Health," *Mother Earth News*, January/February 1986, page 17.

When all the plants grown from the harvested seeds received the full amount of direct sunlight, those whose parents had been raised in the shade yielded only one-half the amount of the previous year's harvest, while the fourth-generation descendants of those plants blossomed but did not mature. The deprivation of direct sunlight during *one* summer weakened the plant genetically to such a degree that the *species became extinct after four years!*

In humans it is common knowledge that the problem of rickets is a condition caused by vitamin D deficiency. Rickets usually affects children. It is a terribly sad affliction characterized by an abnormally low concentration of calcium in the bones, resulting in severe skeletal distortion and muscle pain. The problem is *not* an insufficient amount of calcium in the body. It is a shortage of *vitamin D*, which assists in regulating the transport of calcium to the bones. Guess what the absolute *best* source of vitamin D is? That's right. Sunshine.

Vitamin D is unique in that it can be formed in the body. There is a fluid right under the skin called ergosterol, and when it comes into contact with the ultraviolet rays of the sun, it is converted into vitamin D and absorbed into the bloodstream. **THERE IS NO BETTER SOURCE OF VITAMIN D THAN SUNSHINE,** and those who tell you that the artificial vitamin D added to foods is just as good are doing you a grave disservice. The sad truth is that all too frequently the people telling you that vitamin D supplements do the same job as sunshine just happen to sell them. For example, you have the dairy industry telling you that the little squirt of artificial, inorganic vitamin D added to their products somehow meets the requirements of the body. Rubbish! That's merely another instance of cashectomy.

Vitamin D is instrumental in a host of other bodily functions, not the least of which is its role in preventing osteoporosis by ensuring a proper calcium balance. The reason you should depend upon sunlight for the proper amount of vitamin D is that *too much* artificial vitamin D (supplements) will *interfere* with calcium absorption, which is as harmful as too little. Our natural inclination to be in the light of day provides us just the right amount of the vitamin D we need. When industry and pseudoscience start to meddle in the natural relationship between our bodies and our environment, *look out!*

Unfortunately, the fear of overexposure to ultraviolet light is causing many people to overprotect themselves from sunlight to the point that they're creating a vitamin D deficiency. Because of the fear of skin cancer, many people never let the sun reach their skin. This is an outrageous overreaction, a most ignorant bit of reasoning. There is a marked difference between sun*bathing* and sun*burn*. No one is suggesting you lie in the sun until damage is done.

You can intelligently use or ignorantly abuse *any* of the elements of health. You can overeat valueless food until you become fat and sick. Does that mean you should not eat food? Or does it mean you should eat food properly? You can very rapidly push all air from your lungs, then hyperventilate until you pass out. Does that mean you should not breathe at all? Or does it mean you should breathe properly? You can exercise aggressively and violently and push yourself until you collapse in pain and depletion. Does that mean you should not exercise at all? Or does it mean you should exercise properly? You can hold your head under water until you drown. Does that mean you should not use water? Or does it mean you should use water properly? Similarly, you can be in the sun until your skin resembles a potato chip. But that doesn't mean you should not use the sun. Rather, you should use the sun properly.

We must not consider the sun, the provider of life for our planet, as our enemy. Sunbathing is every bit as essential and beneficial as any of the other elements of health, but sunbathe properly! The best time to lie in the sun is during the early morning hours or the late afternoon hours, when it is least strong. You should expose as much skin as possible and refrain from using suntan lotions, oil, or sunscreens. These will prevent the ultraviolet rays from being absorbed and will inhibit the oil-secreting glands of the body from working properly. Remember, it is not mere tanning that you are after but a general revitalizing of your entire body that is not confined to the skin alone.

Now for those harbingers of doom who have managed to scare people half to death with threats of cancer if they so much as step into the morning sun, unless they are swathed in clothes or caked in chicken fat, let me make our position quite clear so we are not accused of trying to promote skin cancer. **SUNSCREENS ARE ONLY NECESSARY WHEN YOU ARE IN THE SUN FOR A PROLONGED PERIOD OF TIME DURING THE MOST INTENSE HOURS.** I don't think that sunbathing in extreme heat for hours on end is a very good idea, sunscreens or not. People who like to spend long hours in the hot sun should indeed take precautions to protect their skin. To do otherwise is foolhardy and invites trouble. When we say, "Don't use sunscreens," that is for the *least intense time of day* (early morning or late afternoon, when ultraviolet rays are at their lowest) and for exposures of only about half an hour at a time. That is the *proper* use of sun. To suggest that any sun under any circumstances is harmful is dumb—and I mean rock dumb!

For those of you who have an absolute aversion to sitting in the sun or who redden and blister easily, be aware that just being outdoors in sunlight, even though it is not directly on the skin, is also extremely beneficial. We take in the light through our eyes, and it is extremely valuable to do so. So spend at least some time in the sunny outdoors, even if you just sit in shade. If you wear sunglasses, make sure they are *full-spectrum* glasses that do not keep out any of the rays that you need and are outdoors to get. According to Mr. John Ott, the best sunglasses are full-spectrum neutral gray, which can be ordered from your local optometrist.

The knowledge of sunlight's importance is no new discovery, although, typically, the people who control health care in this country have attempted to perpetuate the notion that only when *they* discover something should any credit be given. A case in point is an article in the *New York Times* (November 13, 1984) entitled "Surprising Health Impact Discovered for Light." The writer states, "Light can have health benefits far beyond those imagined by science even as recently as four years ago." Golly gee! Four *whole* years ago! The article gives the false impression that this "discovery" is new. It is not. The sun bath has been employed in this country for more than a hundred years, especially among pioneer Natural Hygienists who have never received their due recognition. In 1843 Sylvester Graham wrote *Lectures on the Science of Human Life*, stressing the benefits of sunshine for bone growth and development. In 1850 Russell Trall, M.D., pointed out the importance of sunlight in speeding the recovery of hospital patients. In 1855 Arnold Rikli established a healing institution on an island in the Adriatic Sea and prescribed sun baths for all of his patients. He wrote seven books describing his methods. In 1875, Earnest Wellman, M.D., writing in *The Science of Health*, pointed out that sunshine is an indispensable necessity for *all* forms of life, animal and vegetable. An extraordinarily enlightening book on the importance of sunshine is *Sunlight* by Zane R. Kime, M.D.

To deny yourself the life-supporting, health-enhancing rays of the sun is tantamount to refusing yourself water when thirsty, food when hungry, or sleep when tired. When done *intelligently* in concert with the other elements of health, by taking in the sun you are taking a measure necessary to ensure yourself the highest level of health possible.

CHAPTER 12
Loving Relationships

MARILYN:

Love. Is there a sweeter word in the English language? Is there anything nicer you can say to someone than "I love you"? Coming from the lips of your own true love or from your dearest child, are not these three words life's greatest reward? In times of need, hearing "I love you" spoken in sincerity by a friend can turn your blues into joy. Love is a force so great that in its name the greatest of feats can be accomplished.

Could it have been anything but love that inspired Michelangelo to paint the Sistine Chapel? Could it have been anything in the Universe other than love that inflamed the desire to build the Taj Mahal? And what else but love would give a frail woman the strength to lift the family car off the legs of her son after it had fallen from a jack?

When you think about it, is there anything that you value more than the love in your life? In our experience, we have noticed over and over again that it is the love that flows in our lives that makes everything work. Interactions devoid of love never bring satisfaction and rarely lead to a successful outcome. As an element of health, love affects *every* aspect of human existence. It particularly affects your well-being and happiness. No matter how much you amass materially or how much prestige you gain in climbing the occupational or social ladder, without love you are not complete. And yet people put so much time and effort into material acquisitions. They value themselves by how much they have or how successful they are and spend a minimal amount of their energy working at full, rich relationships that would nourish their lives.

Without the basic fulfillment of loving relationships we never really get any lasting satisfaction from our possessions or our positions. We can be powerful and successful in our work but lonely and alienated in our homes. Individuals and couples strive inexplicably to acquire more and more, yet their relationships are so empty and superficial that they are not happy, no matter how much they have. But they keep striving for more and more, not realizing that their energy is being wasted on "toys" in which they will quickly lose interest. If they would only put some of that energy into making their relationships work, their lives would become immeasurably more pleasant. The examples are there for us to see: tycoons who die lonely and abandoned; fur-clad, jewel-bedecked women who seem miserable; children or teenagers upon whom toys or cars have been lavished but who have been deprived of tender communication and as a result are unhealthy and un-balanced. It is so sad to see so many people running around ac-cumulating what they think will make them happy or devoting all of their energy to success without realizing the value of putting a matching effort toward working out their relationships along the way.

What is love after all? When we talk of love, we are certainly not only talking about relationships between men and women. There is a place for love in *every* human interaction. A sincere smile connotes love, whether you are talking to a stranger or to your mate. In short, *there is a way to be loving in all your inter-actions!*

"Yeah, sure!" you may be saying. "My interactions can *all* be loving? Most of my interactions are a pain in the neck! They are anything but loving!" That may be so. But that is, in fact, *your* choice. To realize the truth in this, one need only understand the nature of love.

In human experience, certain elements are clearly visible; others are abstract. The clearly visible elements are all that we see around us, all that we can touch and verify through our senses. Your car, your food, your possessions—all of these are clearly visible. Those things that take no definite form, however, are abstract. Those are health, beauty, hatred, peace, virtue, generosity, jealousy, envy, loneliness, gratitude, anger, and . . . *love*. The list goes on and on.

The most important aspect of the abstract elements is that they are all around us *all* the time. They are part of our lives at any given moment. We only have to tap into them. You can verify this for yourself. You can be relaxing, feeling wonderful, at peace with everything. Someone will put on the news on television, and at the very moment of feeling great, you become incensed about an injustice that is being reported; you instantly become angry. You have tapped into that emotion, and it has been your choice to do so. In the same manner, you can be out walking and see the beauty in your surroundings *or* the ugliness. *Both are there*. You make the choice of which you wish to perceive. Loneliness is there for you to feel *if you choose*. **LOVE IS THERE FOR YOU TO FEEL IF YOU CHOOSE.** You only need to tap into it. You can feel love in a crowd. You can feel it when you are all alone. Your thoughts can be loving whenever you choose for them to be so. If you choose to feel hatred or jealousy or envy, you can do that. You just tap into them in the same way. Want to live your life in disappointment or frustration? Just tap into those feelings. Want to be lonely? Tap into loneliness. Want to feel love? It's up to you.

You may know people whose relationships are all very full and rewarding. You say, "Boy, are they lucky. I wish I had that many good friends." Understand that it has nothing to do with luck. Somehow these people have learned how and chosen to tap into love. **LOVE IS AN ATTITUDE.** Just as the sun shines equally on everyone—it doesn't shine warmer, longer, or brighter on one individual in a crowd than another—love is there equally for everyone, too. Somehow some choose it and others do not. That is the only difference. But the choice is always yours to make.

Once you make the choice to be loving and interact in a loving way, you begin to experience what we call the "boomerang effect." This is a very positive aspect of love and always comes as a result of choosing love. The "effect" is simply this: As much love as you put into your interactions, that is how much love comes directly back to you. This can be verified. It might not happen immediately, but lovingness can overcome even the sourest or most petulant disposition, if the love that is given is sincere and consistent.

Once we knew *instinctively* how to be loving, but that knowledge is just another piece of information that we have learned to forget. Could our species have survived if in the beginning we were always alienated and at one another's throats? We would have done ourselves in long ago! And look at the innocent children, those of our species who are closest to their instincts. They only love. They do it unconditionally. Unless they have been abused and are full of fear, they dwell in a place of love. How have we come so far from knowing what we mean to each other? How have we lost our identity? Many people are disconnected from their ability to love to such an extreme that they are even at odds with themselves. The truth is that **UNTIL YOU LOVE YOURSELF, IT'S VERY HARD TO REALLY LOVE ANYONE ELSE.**

Do you love yourself? In your life, are you valuable? Do people take out their frustrations and complexes and disappointments on you? Do you dump on yourself? If you are treated unlovingly by those around you, perhaps one of the reasons is that *you do not treat yourself lovingly*. You actually set the stage for abuse by abusing yourself. You set the example, and everyone else follows. "How?" you ask. To start, look at your thoughts. What are they like? Are they pleasant, optimistic, uplifting, loving? Or are they sad, full of self-criticism and abuse, depressing, self-defeating? *You become what you think about most*. If your thoughts are mostly negative, there is no way you can be a positive person.

Notice how unstable your thought pattern actually is. It is so unstable that it demands that you take control of it. (A daily quiet moment when you sit in silence with yourself will help you be aware of this.) Your thoughts flit from one subject to the next, pulling your emotions along as if you were on a roller coaster. You can go from happiness to despair in a moment, from crying to laughter. You do this. We all do, and we do it while nothing around us changes. *Only we change as our thoughts change*. **BY CONTROLLING OUR THOUGHTS WE CAN FEEL HAPPY ALL THE TIME.**

On the other hand, if you are constantly in a state of self-abuse, what sort of treatment can you possibly attract to yourself? If you look in the mirror and consistently criticize yourself, do you expect others *not* to criticize you? If you become angry with yourself for misplacing your keys, do you expect others *not* to get down on you for something equally trivial?

TAKE THE INITIATIVE TO BE LOVED

A major tool in being fit for love is to **LOVE YOURSELF FIRST, BELIEVE IN YOURSELF FIRST, ACCEPT YOURSELF**

FIRST. For *you are who you are*. You are a creation of the Almighty. You are *not* accidental. Many of our scientists may deny that there is a God who created all of us, but that is like saying that a painting can happen without an artist. Someone painted the painting and some force created us. You have been created in your specialness, just as the rose has been. Would you fault the rose because it is not an orchid? Do you hate the petunia for not being a peony? Are trees unworthy compared to birds because birds can fly and trees cannot? Is rain inferior to wind? Wood less valuable than stone? From whose viewpoint? By what value system? What crazy questions! And yet we use the same kind of comparative thinking when we judge ourselves.

If you think you are not wonderful, it is because you are comparing yourself to someone else. If you decide you are not good or worthy or intelligent or talented, it is because there is some standard somewhere against which you are measuring yourself. Can't you see the folly in it? *You are you*, created to be who you are. **ACCEPT YOURSELF!** That is the first step. *Be who you are, not what others expect you to be. Love who you are, and love will begin to flow in your relationships,* because when you have finally made the commitment to love and accept yourself, you will then be able to love and accept others. Once you are comfortable with who you are, you will be comfortable with who other people are. Most important, because you see them *as they are* and not as you want them to be, you can accept them unconditionally and, in the most good-natured way, allow them to be themselves. This nonjudgmental attitude manifests in the relationship as love.

So it's a simple message. If you can love yourself and allow yourself to be who you are, you have taken quantum leaps toward healing. In allowing yourself to be who you are, you are able to allow others to be who they are and can begin to recognize the sublime existence that comes from living in *unconditional* love with your fellow beings.

We people tend to be hard on each other in this age. The crowded cities are a living death for the individual spirit—everywhere around you people are demanding that you be what they expect you to be. In nature there are no demands. Only we make demands on each other. The time has come for us to love who we are. In this era it is sometimes easier to learn how to do that away from the crowded cities. In nature you can hear the beat of your own heart and the sound of your own footsteps. Take yourself there as often as you can—to the sea, to the mountains, to the forests and meadows. In nature you can learn that you are part of a grand and beautiful scheme and that you are as valid a part of life's masterpiece as is everything that you see around you. We lose our sense of self in the rush of the cities. If you must stay in the city for long periods of time, balance that out with strolls through the park or visits to museums.

Why a park or a museum? Impressions. Everything you see has an impression upon you. Some are uplifting and can energize you, while others are depressing and can enervate you. If you witness an auto accident and see someone lying in the street horribly injured, that is a terrible, unnerving sight. It can drain and depress you. But if you are strolling through a park and come upon a nest in a tree with little baby birds chirping away in it, that sight can gladden your heart and brighten your entire day. Hours later you may excitedly describe what you saw to a friend.

Whenever you can create a more pleasant impression for yourself, you should do so, even in such apparently insignificant acts as driving home from work or shopping. Perhaps you can just as easily take a more scenic route through the park or by a lake or the seashore instead of one more ride on a freeway. Do that for yourself. It may seem like a small thing, but lots of small things add up. Besides, it sets an extremely positive psychological precedent in your life. When you go out of your way to create a nice impression for yourself, on a subtle level you are telling yourself, "I'm a nice person; I deserve to be treated nicely." And that's true! Similarly, consciously creating finer impressions for your loved ones makes for a more harmonious relationship. It shows you care and produces a more loving and joyous atmosphere. This is one of those simple little suggestions that is easily put to the test and verified. When you make an effort, even a small one, to improve the impressions you take in, you will be amazed at the positive results that seep into all aspects of your life thereafter.

Here's something to be aware of in your relationships. Some people who are unhealthy will try to gain energy from whomever they can. They will maintain their survival by drawing the energy out of others. Since their energy is low and they don't know how to regenerate it on their own, they will try to take it from those around them. These people are "energy thieves." What they steal from you is more valuable than your money. It is your life!

You know who they are. They are the nags, the critics, the people who are always telling you how much you have "messed up." They keep you abreast of your inadequacies. They are always ready to dwell on others' shortcomings rather than work on their own. They always remind you of how much you "owe" them. They *never* let you forget your trespasses, let alone forgive you. When they go into their song and dance, turn a politely deaf ear. Put yourself out of their reach whenever they begin to drain you. That is the best thing you can do for them.

Energy thieves are to be recognized for what they are and controlled in order to remedy the unhealthy relationship. No matter how close they are to you in your life, you must fortify yourself when they are around. Do not allow them to usurp your energy. They will soon realize that a source of life energy for them has been cut off. They will be forced to look elsewhere for a new supplier. When you no longer willingly feed their energy-draining detractions, the energy thieves will realize they have to figure out a new way to relate to you, or they will simply leave you alone. If they matter to you, you can teach them that the only basis for a relationship with you is positive interaction. If they don't matter, it is so much better that they move on.

A second tool to being fit for love is to **TAKE THE INITIATIVE IN MAKING YOUR RELATIONSHIPS WORK FOR YOU.** Granted, that is a little complicated in modern society. So many people seem very confused about how to relate to each other. Fortunately, today more people are trying to figure out for themselves what works for them. Rather than do everything the way their fathers and mothers did, they want to know who *they* are and what *they* need in the context of their relationships. This structuring of relationships along more personal, individual lines is a positive trend. We are no longer going through the motions of what has traditionally been acceptable, whether it seems to fit our needs and hopes or not.

New levels of consciousness resulting from self-awareness movements and the great reforms of the Women's Movement have led to our rejecting traditional and unworkable ways of relating, but they have not always supplied us with clear new models. In our opinion, certain traditional concepts probably should not be lost. Although male and female are intrinsically *equal*, they are also intrinsically *different*. Biologically, that is something that cannot be denied. Biologically, men are more muscular. Biologically, women are softer. Even when women take up bodybuilding, they cannot build the amount of muscle men can. Women are, however, uniquely capable of bearing offspring and giving sustenance from their bodies. Men are not. Thus there is in the female disposition, naturally, a quiet strength and a more nourishing, sustaining quality. Men are outwardly constructed physically. Woman are inwardly constructed. Sexually, the male gives and the woman receives. In the past these differences defined our roles in life. Man worked out in the world and supported the woman in the home; she cared for the home and offspring. Now in some cases men are home and women are out in the world. In some cases, men and women work equally together at home and in the world on a common project. In some cases they share equally the responsibility for their offspring. In other cases they avoid offspring because they are confused about *who* would do *what*. We are, in fact, in the middle of a great social revolution!

While all this is being worked out, respecting the differences between the sexes will keep us from going overboard. These differences are to be valued because they complement each other *naturally*. The sexes deserve equal treatment, equal compensation, and equal benefits, but it does not make sense for them to try to compete to the point that their inherent natural qualities are lost. There is a natural balance of masculine and feminine that must be maintained in the world, just as there is a balance of dark and light. If women abandon their feminine qualities rather than prize them, femininity will still have to occur somewhere in order for the natural balance to be maintained—less femininity in women, more femininity in men and vice versa with masculinity. Is that necessarily what we want to happen?

I don't think that the point of the Women's Movement was for women to take on the inherent qualities of the opposite sex and abandon their own feminine qualities. Its leaders have never advocated that. Far better than abandonment is a readjustment from traditional constraints to make relationships fit the reality of modern living.

One excellent "new" model that appears more and more frequently, the husband-wife team, is actually a return to a simpler structure from the past, when husband and wife worked together on the farm or at a trade. With both partners equally talented and strong in complementing areas, husband-wife teams are reaping success and a lot of fulfillment in their work *and* in their relationships. Couples frequently tell us that they are leaving their present positions in order to work together. There are the advantages of not having to be apart, of being able to work at home in some cases, of being able to work on a more personal schedule. Pursuit of a common goal brings additional opportunities to share. If children are part of the relationship, they are also made part of the team effort and the responsibilities for their care are also shared. Team relationships afford ample opportunity for getting to know each other better and, because you are frequently interacting with others in pursuit of your common goal, you get the opportunity to support each other's strengths and offset each other's weaknesses. This creates a very strong bond of love and respect. Best of all, work is no longer separate and routine. It becomes more challenging, more exciting in its ups and downs, and more intimate, because every aspect of it is shared.

LOVE AND COMMUNICATION

One of the reasons that relationships of all kinds seem to break down and become unloving is lack of communication. Communication takes dedication. It takes time and effort. You have to *want* the relationship to work and be willing to do *whatever* is necessary to maintain an open line of communication.

There are three highly effective tools that can be used to facilitate communication. During the first few years of our marriage, Harvey and I used these tools very extensively to make sure that we were continuously and consciously working on breaking down the obstacles that come up in many relationships. When you put these tools to work, especially if you agree to do this in the context of a relationship *with* someone, a new element of willing effort is injected and helps carry you to higher levels of mutual understanding.

1. *Giving space*. Giving space is a real test of one's ability to be alert and conscious of personal interactions. Ever notice that in practically every conversation between two or more people, more often than not before one person has finished a thought the other person is already starting to speak? Have you ever noticed its being done to you or your doing it to someone else? It happens *all the time*. But people rarely are aware of it, because it is so common.

If you don't think this is so, go, *right now*, to where two or more people are having a conversation and listen. You will be stunned at the regularity with which people talk while someone else is talking. In fact, once you start paying attention to this phenomenon you'll hardly be able to find a conversation where this does not take place.

This is why we all have little mechanisms to help us keep the floor without being interrupted. When talking you often need to take a breath, but you can see the person you're talking with ready to pounce on that pause and start talking. So you say something like "So, listen, here's what I did." This gives you the moment you need to breathe and then continue with what you were saying. Or you use a big obvious "And . . ." This lets the other person know that you're not through yet. However, frequently even ploys such as these don't work and people adept at pouncing on a pause will start talking anyway.

"So what?" you may ask. "Everyone does it." That's just my point. If everyone is talking over another's words or seizing on pauses to interject his or her point, there's not enough real listening going on. Most of us are so busy formulating what we're going to say that we're not listening to what is *being* said. And *not* listening does not make for effective communication. Moreover, on a subtle level, people who are interrupted feel a certain disappointment at the end of a conversation rather than satisfaction. When someone has to fight constantly to keep the floor or make what he or she feels is an important comment, it leaves that individual feeling frustrated.

Giving space remedies this situation and forces people to listen to one another. *It requires that a person be allowed to speak without interruption.* When someone is talking, you listen until they have finished. This allows them to complete their thought unpressured; it gives you the chance to really pay attention to what is being said and in turn provides you with an opportunity to speak without having to pry your way into the conversation like an unwanted salesman trying to get into someone's living room to sell something that is not needed. More importantly, the person with whom you are speaking feels less threatened and therefore becomes more open and relaxed.

Start to observe other people's conversations and you will see how infrequently, if at all, people give space. Observe *your* conversations and see if *you* can give space. I say "see if you can" because this seemingly simple practice is one of the most difficult things to do. You will see what I mean when you try it. However, once you become successful at it, you will start to see how much more satisfying and effective your conversations with others can be. As an added bonus, you'll become known as a great conversationalist because the people you talk with, even if they don't realize you are giving them the space to finish what they are saying, will find it so refreshing to be listened to without interruption and without being forced to fight to complete a thought. They will go away from a conversation with you feeling validated, important, and complete. And you will get the credit. This will help all of your relationships—in business, with friends, and with mates. Practicing giving space *with* someone is the most rewarding of all. When both parties are aware of giving space and consciously strive to do so in their conversations with one another, some of the most satisfying, loving interactions imaginable come to pass. Then communication truly becomes a most important part of your life.

Harvey and I actually have a hand signal we give to each other when we are in a conversation with a group of people and one of us forgets to give space and interrupts someone else. Have fun with this tool. It will not only make your conversations more rewarding, it will also benefit your relationships enormously.

2. *Avoiding the negative.* Ever notice how habitually we allow ourselves to express negative sentiments? In the most routine manner, we will start off an interaction with a negative emotion. Example: You're just getting home from work and your mate or a friend is waiting for you. The first thing you say is, ''I had such lousy traffic and this abysmal weather didn't make it any easier. Boy, I can't stand commuting in this city!'' Now, is that any way to set the tone for a pleasant interaction? Even if you are really fed up and must express it, how about *starting with something positive* that will assuage your irritability—''Am I glad to see you! Let's really relax for a while. I'm so happy to be out of that car and into this cozy house!'' The same phenomenon holds true for all the routine negativity we allow to creep into our casual communications. ''Isn't this weather awful?'' instead of ''Well, we sure do need all this rain.'' Or ''This darn elevator takes forever'' instead of ''This elevator gives me a chance to stand and stretch a little before I sit at my desk for the rest of the day.''

Do you see the difference? All the petty little negativities that we are in the habit of voicing unconsciously set a negative tone for conversation. We have a choice as to what tone we wish to set. If we consciously try to express ourselves more positively, people will find interaction with us more pleasant. Negative beginnings tend to make the other person want to get away from us as quickly as possible. Pleasant beginnings in communication lead to more fulfilling discussions.

3. *Body postures*. Your body speaks as loudly as your mouth. The position you assume with your body in a discussion can either thwart or facilitate communication. Realize that as you speak silent energy flows from you, and the same thing happens when you listen. If you speak or listen with your arms crossed in front of you, what you are portraying is that you are guarding yourself or placing an obstacle to frank openness between you and the person you are trying to communicate with. If you speak or listen with hands on your hips, you are silently expressing an authoritarian position. You are unconsciously overpowering the person you are supposedly communicating with. Remember that energy flows off your body and has an impact on whomever you are addressing. You want that energy to be as positive and direct as possible. If you are sitting or standing all twisted or slumped when you try to communicate, your energy flows in an erratic fashion and doesn't support your communication.

The most even flow of energy occurs when you have both feet planted firmly on the ground and your arms are at your sides, your hands are clasped in front of you, or your hands are clasped behind you. Any other position distracts and detracts. If you are sitting, cross your ankles and fold your hands in your lap. This consciousness about your body posture brings consciousness to your communication. The more conscious the communication, the more meaningful.

These three communication tools work, of that you can be certain. But once again, *don't take our word for it!* Try them and see for yourself the transformation that they can bring about. With something as important as having a loving relationship, every potentially useful tool is worth trying. All we ask is that you try.

Take the energy necessary to give space to the people you talk to so that they can feel relaxed and *listened to*. Meanwhile, hold your body in a position that promotes a smooth flow of energy, and when you speak do so with a positive attitude. You will see and feel things happen. Good things.

LIVE IN THE PRESENT

There is one more aspect that stands in the way of loving relationships: the "Past-Present-Future Syndrome." Unfortunately, most of us carry around a lot of attitudinal baggage as a result of our past experiences. We have either been burned in a relationship—rejected or mistreated in one way or another—or we have done that to someone else. We move on, but we hold on to all the negative feelings resulting from unsuccessful interactions and we load ourselves down with them and carry them wherever we go, including whenever we have a fresh opportunity to relate. We are like people who decide to go shopping but carry with them all the purchases they have ever made. That doesn't allow much of a free hand to assess new merchandise, let alone carry it home.

Here's what is important to know about the past: **IT IS OVER!** The past cannot touch you. You can let go of it. You can forgive yourself for whatever you have done, you can forgive others for whatever *they* have done, and you can start fresh *every day*. Doesn't that make sense? Doing anything else is *so* encumbering! If you carry all your past hurts with you, they inevitably color your present, and you perpetuate them right into the future. If you carry them with you, they never go away. Learn from them and let go of them.

If you see no prospects for a bright future, it is usually because you are holding on to your past. When you base your projections on a past that has not been good, you are holding on to that, fearing that it will recur in the future—and of course *it will*, because you are carrying it along with you. **THE ONLY WAY TO ENSURE A GOOD FUTURE IS TO MAXIMIZE THE PRESENT. FOCUS ON THE PRESENT. MAKE THE PRESENT GOOD!** If you are always nurturing the present, making it as positive and pleasant as possible, the future will be pleasant and positive because **THE FUTURE IS ONLY REAL WHEN IT BECOMES THE PRESENT.**

Lighten your load. Try to let go of your emotional baggage. There is no time to waste in the present. *It is all we have.*

Remember, *love is in the air!* It's another of those elements that is totally yours for the taking. Open yourself up to it. Go for it. You don't have to feel that it is not meant for you to experience. Starting right now you can weave love into every interaction of your day. Smile, breathe, communicate from your heart. See the other person as someone with whom you can share a pleasant interaction. It is such a relief when you do. Love is one of the easiest elements to incorporate into your life! We know you can do it from this moment on. Just start today! And remember, *we love you!*

SEX

Not hard to get your attention with that word is it? Madison Avenue knows that. Advertisers use it everywhere to sell us alcohol, deodorant, after-shave lotion, jeans, dandruff treatments, cigarettes, mouthwash, iron supplements, bathroom deodorizers, face creams, airline tickets, vacations, etc. I'm sure you could add scores more items to my list. In modern times, it almost seems that we have lost the conception of what sex really is and what its purpose is —we connect it with so much to which it has no relationship whatsoever.

If you have any questions about your sexuality, perhaps you will gain some new insights from this section, because Natural Hygiene very definitely *does* affect one's sex life. In the ten years during which we have been counseling people, we have *never* had any negative input from anyone concerning the effect of this lifestyle on sexual relations and sexual activity. We have, however, received much positive feedback about "improved relationships." The Natural Hygiene life-style has had a truly positive impact on our own relationship as well.

Sex has always been a motivating force in human life. The urge to perpetuate the species has driven us through the ages to become heroes, heroines, and great achievers. This vital act of species perpetuation has gone through some amazing transformations, considering that it is as basic to the species biologically as eating and sleeping. It is almost impossible to understand how something so much a part of our natural makeup could become so confused. The urge to perpetuate the species, which we have in common with all the other animals on the planet, has become an obsession in our time. What all the other animals do with complete naturalness has become a total "hangup" for many people. Abnormal sex practices have been called "bestial," attributed to "animal instincts," which is a real mislabeling. No student of nature would *ever* make that connection, inasmuch as the sex practices of the lower animal kingdom are *instinctively* well ordered and controlled, as are their eating, sleeping, and exercising.

Not too long ago, sex was an "unmentionable." It was *never* openly discussed. It was considered impolite to do so. It bore the stigma of something unclean and sinful! Our own grandparents and their grandparents lived through the end of that era. Our generation has forced rejection of that mentality. But even when sex was a repressed subject, early Natural Hygienists included in their writings for the lay population a treatment of sexual function that brushed away the cobwebs of ignorance and prejudice and stressed a reverence and respect for the human body *in its entirety*, no parts ignored. They treated sex just like eating, as a habit that *served the body* and therefore required a certain understanding, discipline, and restraint in order to help make it pleasurable and the body beautiful.

What has happened today? Sex has become an overindulgence, just as has eating. Now, don't get all flustered here. The intention is not to limit you, but only to point out ways to help you improve upon and enhance the quality of something that you value.

In our times, sex has become totally unrestrained. It has become allowable even in the lives of young teenagers, more and more of whom are now conceiving offspring at younger and younger ages. It is in no way disciplined. Instead of viewing it as a *normal* biological function designed for procreation and the expression of conjugal love, it has become permissible, even popular, to commercialize its sensuality and mass market it luridly as pornography. Objections to this are squelched as attacks on "personal freedoms."

Don't you think we've gone a bit too far? Instead of explaining, protecting, and respecting the normal function of sex in society, trying to put sex into healthy perspective in the wake of a puritanical background, our sex educators, including many psychologists and psychiatrists, seem to have accepted the other extreme; they are reluctant to take a constructive stand on promiscuity and adultery.

Here's the issue: If you criticize the "new sexual freedom," you're stamped as a prude or reactionary. From the biological point of view, however, **WHAT IS NORMAL PHYSIOLOG-ICALLY DOES NOT CHANGE.** The requirements and limitations that are biologically determined in the human body existed tens of thousands of years ago, are the same today, and will be the same in another 10,000 years. Sexually, in spite of our "new sexual freedom," we are today what we have always been as a species.

Ideally, sex serves two important purposes in normal human existence:

1. It allows the perpetuation of the species through the cellular union of two people of the opposite sex, who then have the obligation of providing adequate care for the helpless offspring that result from their union.

2. It provides a means of expressing the love between two people who have merged their destinies. This expression serves as spiritual food for these two people and helps to bind them in a special way that does not occur between them as individuals and *any* other person in their lives.

In our confusion over these two purposes, we have allowed sex to become a *sport*. Just as we often no longer "eat to live" but rather live to eat, frequently we indulge in sex for other than the ideal reasons. This is not to say that we expect all sexual activity immediately to become purely a function of love and procreation. That would be the *ideal*, but it is certainly not a realistic expectation.

This information is offered to allow you to view sex from a slightly different perspective than that being sold to you by Madison Avenue and the proponents of the "sexual revolution." In our times, to endorse anything other than "any sex, all sex, more and more sex, in more and different ways" is to incur a backlash reaction from those who seem to have pushed the pendulum to the extreme. I suspect a lot of people agree that society today has gone overboard in demanding unlimited sexual freedom, but they are afraid to say so for fear of incurring that backlash.

I'm not! I think we have gone overboard. Sex is not an appropriate pastime for fourteen- and fifteen-year-olds or teenagers in general. Those are not to me the ideal years for mating or parenting.

In my opinion, the atmosphere of sexual freedom we have demanded has created a lamentable situation. Our children should be taught not so much how to avoid conception, but that sex is a serious responsibility of *adult* relationships that is beyond their realm of capability. As Jo Ann Gasper, deputy assistant secretary to population affairs and head of the federal Office of Adolescent Pregnancy, said in November 1986, "Sexual abstinence is the only foolproof way of not getting pregnant. The message to convey is you do not engage in sex until marriage." This is a very encouraging trend in teenage sex education policy, after so many years of emphasis on supplying teenagers with contraceptives. In my own experience with teenagers, I have found that once they are supported *not* to engage in sex, they seem more carefree and sure of themselves. Sexual relationships are far too draining for them during the years when they are also dealing with finding out who they are.

The "acceptable" sexual expression on television and in widely distributed movies, books, and magazines promulgates images and attitudes that foster confusion and corruption in the undiscriminating mind and lead many people to believe that some very unhealthy and perverted practices may actually be considered "normal sexual behavior." Certainly we are being taught that infidelity and lust are a normal part of life—it's all over our television screens. And those who feel instinctively inhibited sexually are encouraged to "release those inhibitions" through the use of drugs and alcohol—"loosen up," in other words. All this right on prime-time television! As a parent, I'm not really interested in having my children exposed to what is so prevalent in the media concerning sex today. I personally find the general treatment of sex on many popular television programs to be infuriatingly inappropriate. A great deal of it is *very* harmful to the impressionable young in our population.

The fact is, when anything is overdone, it suffers in quality. A trip to Disneyland once in a while is enjoyable. Go every day and you're going to get sick of it. Thanksgiving dinner is enjoyable, too, but not as a routine event. Christmas every day loses its luster. With sex, when we go for quantity and frequency, there is a direct diminution of quality. In making frequency the driving force, as we do in our society, people have actually turned a beautiful, exciting, fulfilling experience into something routine, unsatisfying, and dull. In looking for a remedy for the routineness, the lack of satisfaction, and the dullness, they have sought to devise new titillations instead of understanding that frequency is the cause of the problem.

For health to be durable and a sex life to be vital, moderation is demanded. That shouldn't be a surprise! It's the same for all physiological functions. In order to be healthy and not to hurt yourself, you must be moderate in eating, sleeping, exercise, play, work, *and* sex! When you indulge in anything to excess, you pay with a deterioration in your health.

Unfortunately, you have been advised by numerous "authorities" that regular and *frequent* sex will "relieve tension," and movies and books continually tout frequency as the macho norm. Frequency, however, is *not* where it's at. Frequency brings the boredom, frustration, and enervation that should *not* be associated with healthful sex. Sexual activity and orgasm *deplete* rather than build energy, and energy, remember, is life's essence. You can relate to how much energy sex takes if you realize that after sex it's rarely "tennis anyone?" There is only one body function that rivals the energy use of digestion, and that is sexual activity. Overexpenditure in this area will leave you depleted and without sufficient energy to deal with toxic overload. Overindulging in sex will, in fact, bring on a toxic state.

Sex energy is valuable. It should not be wasted indiscriminately but should be stored and cherished for the perfect moment with the perfect person. *That energy is a gift!* It is powerful enough to make a baby, a precious baby. I don't think we were provided with this for the purpose of frittering it away much in the same way we would flick on the television set.

My own experience of Natural Hygiene has greatly changed my sexual life. First of all, before I began to recognize that my life-style determined my health, I thought infrequent sex was a curse, a real negative. I remember friends back in the early 1970s: educated, "sophisticated," affluent, married couples comparing notes on how often they had sex and actually *competing* with each other on a subtle level to be the couple that "did it the most." Those were the "Bob and Carol and Ted and Alice" years! However unfulfilling it seemed to be, frequency won the gold in the suburban Sexual Olympics that we were living through. When I changed my life-style it made an enormous difference in my sexual experience (of course, finding Harvey definitely made a difference, too, but Harvey would have been wasted on me sexually had I not also made the life-style change when I met him). When I began to cleanse my body of the waste that had been clogging it and allowed myself to rest and heal and *abstain*, something miraculous happened. I began to experience sex in a way that I had never before experienced it. One reason was the love Harvey and I shared, which provided the most appropriate background for meaningful and fulfilling sexual communication. The second reason was that I had become cleaner inside, and **WHEN YOU ARE CLEAN INSIDE, ALL PHYSICAL EXPERIENCES ARE HEIGHTENED, MORE VIVID, AND MORE INTENSE—INCLUDING SEX!** In fact, Harvey and I have both been quite surprised that so many people have been willing to talk about the increased sexual enjoyment they have experienced since embracing this life-style. Much of this feedback has come from people in their *senior years* who had thought the sensual pleasures they had lost years ago would never return. But they did!

It makes sense, doesn't it? Nerve impulses can register your pleasurable reaction better if you are *clean* inside. Furthermore, when you are in a healthy state, you are better at *everything* you do. If you play tennis, you are better at it. If you write, you're more creative. At work, you are more effective. Why would this not also be true of sex? The better the condition of your body, as a result of proper nutrition, rest, and exercise, the better your sexual experience will be. So restraint and discipline become very much a part of a fulfilling sex life, and discrimination also plays an important role. Whenever you involve yourself with someone sexually, you consent to mix your energy with theirs. Since sex can make a child, be sure your partner is a worthy choice, for the potential is always there for a child to result. Holding yourself in high regard and loving and respecting your body will help you attract the appropriate sexual partner. The cleaner and healthier you are, the cleaner and healthier the people you attract will be. The more restrained and disciplined you are, the more enjoyable the sexual experience will be. Before sex should ever enter into a relationship, the two people should know each other very well, trust each other implicitly, and care very much for each other. That may sound old-fashioned, but actually it is good, sound advice on how to stay healthy and happy.

According to Dr. William L. Esser, a leading authority on living healthfully, the "excessive use of sex generally results in an early reduction in vitality and function. When this occurs, medical help is usually sought. Hormones are frequently suggested but fail to correct causes. Changes in diet to include large amounts of protein, the use of aphrodisiacs, as well as mechanical stimulations are tried but invariably fail as long as causes are ignored. The psychiatrist is kept busy with cases of this kind. Failure to remove excessive practices as well as other enervating causes, plus errors in diet, lack of rest and sleep, which prompt an elevating toxemia, will also fail to restore sexual functions to normal.''*

Now, that's a pretty steep price to pay for overindulgence, if you ask me.

Here's another idea to consider. Perhaps an obsession with sex is an indication of a low level of health. As any farmer can tell you, "A plant in need is quick to seed." The unhealthy of the species, instinctively sensing their ill health, turn to sex as a means of ensuring perpetuation of their genetic line. Unfortunately, the less vitality in the parents, the less vitality in the offspring, and the species as a whole becomes progressively weaker and weaker. Is an obsession with sex a manifestation of diminished health? That is something we may do well to consider.

The case histories of Natural Hygiene are replete with stories of infertile couples who successfully conceived after adopting a more healthful life-style. Look at this from the point of view of common sense. The union of sperm and ovum is a delicate process. The environment of that union is significant. The minuscule sperm must travel a great distance before penetrating and uniting with the egg. If the environment of that union is clean and shiny and unpolluted by waste and food by-products, the process can more easily take place. If the female reproductive organs are cleansed rather than clogged, conception is easier. By the same token, if the sperm comes from a healthy body rather than a devitalized one, it will have the vitality to "carry out its mission." What is so lamentable is to see so many couples going through so much artificial medical manipulation in order to have a child without realizing that they are not conceiving for a very good reason: Something about their bodies' condition is preventing the conception of the child. It may be that one of them smokes. Or perhaps they are using coffee, alcohol or other drugs which inhibit conception. It has been shown in case after case that a few months

*William L. Esser, *The Greatest Health Discovery*, Chicago: Natural Hygiene Press, 1972.

of proper nutrition (plenty of fresh fruits, vegetables, whole grains, raw nuts and a minimum of meat, dairy, and processed foods), ample rest, exercise, sunshine, fresh air, and loving support will usually remedy the infertility, and the resulting offspring is also much healthier for the change.

Another aspect of sex that deserves attention here is the question of contraception. Many people find this issue to be perplexing. They are trying to treat their bodies more naturally and the idea of "the Pill," with all of its negative side-effects, makes them very uncomfortable. Justifiably so.

The IUD can also cause serious physical problems. Just consider it from a commonsense angle. If there is a foreign body placed inside your body, will your body just tolerate it? Or given the available energy, will it try to eliminate it? In past workshops and private practice, we frequently worked with women who were trying to detoxify their bodies and lose weight. Although they were following our program religiously, they did not have the expected results. And then we noticed that this was a predictable pattern in women who had IUDs. All the energy they were freeing up in their bodies by living more healthfully was being diverted *by the body* in an attempt to eliminate the IUD. Once the IUD was removed, the results were significant—weight loss, radiant skin, newfound energy, and lighter and more comfortable menstruation.

There *is* a nonchemical, noninvasive, *natural* form of contraception that you can use to prevent pregnancy. It is called the Ovulation Method of birth control and is based on the work of two Australian medical researchers, Drs. Evelyn and John Billings. When used properly it can achieve a 98.5 percent success rate. An international study, recently carried out by the World Health Organization, showed this simple method to be highly successful in five different areas of the world, three of which were developing nations, where the tests were run on illiterate women.

The Ovulation Method falls right in line with natural self-care, because it simply teaches you more about your body and how to read its signs. It shows you how to identify those days on which you have the best chances of conceiving. You learn to observe the clear signs of fertility that the female body manifests during each monthly cycle. In just a few months you can become familiar with those signs and begin to recognize when the safe and unsafe days for sexual relations occur. The Ovulation Method can thus be used to prevent pregnancy *or* as an aid for couples who wish to conceive.*

A second natural method of contraception and a highly effective one is the Sympto-Thermal method, which teaches a woman to recognize the three signs her body gives her that she's fertile. For information contact the Couple to Couple League, P.O. Box 111184, Cincinnati, Ohio 45211.

As you become more in tune with your biological needs and more capable of fulfilling them, expect your sexual experiences to become far more heightened and pleasurable. As we as a species become healthier, we will see future generations of healthier and healthier offspring. It's an idea whose time has come!

*There are many books available on the Ovulation Method and natural family planning. One excellent explanation of the method comes directly from its originator, John J. Billings, M.D.: *The Ovulation Method* (Collegeville, Minnesota: Liturgical Press). A second book explaining the method is Mercedes Argu Wilson's *The Ovulation Method of Birth Regulation: The Latest Advances for Achieving or Postponing Pregnancy—Naturally''* (New York: Van Nostrand Reinhold Company). Also very helpful are the explanations in *How to Choose the Sex of Your Baby* by Landrum B. Shettles, M.D., Ph.D., and David M. Rorvik (Garden City, New York: Doubleday and Company).

CHAPTER 13

Cleanliness, Pleasant Surroundings, and Quiet Moments

MARILYN:

Cleanliness, pleasant surroundings, and quiet moments are three additional elements of health that must be provided in order for us to thrive. Each is important and should not be minimized.

CLEANLINESS

"Cleanliness is next to godliness." We all know that! But listen to this: "In our opinion, once a week is often enough to bathe the whole body for purposes of luxury and cleanliness. Beyond this we consider bathing to be injurious." Now, where do you suppose a piece of backward thinking like that would appear? *The National Lampoon*? Close! It comes from an article entitled "The Abuses of Bathing" and appeared in the *Boston Medical and Surgical Journal* in 1850. Only 136 years ago, we were being told *not* to bathe more than once a week.

We've come a long way! It took the hygienic reforms of the Popular Health Movement of the last century and the concurrent education of the public to finally convince the medical profession of that era that frequent bathing was indeed an important factor in health. Health reformers who campaigned for frequent bathing were for decades attacked by the profession as "quacks."

Today's Hygienists are, in spite of similar disparaging attacks against them, campaigning for the cleanliness of the inside of the body. Millions of people have now experienced firsthand the validity of food combining, which cleans us on the inside. How long before we finally overcome the blind and stubborn resistance to it that some medical professionals vociferously exhibit? Hygienic reforms, in spite of great odds against them, have a habit of prevailing, which is so much the better for all of us.

We now know that **A CLEAN BODY INSIDE AND OUT IS A MAJOR PREREQUISITE FOR HEALTH.** Unfortunately, trying to compensate for the effects of a dirty inner body, many people just plain ''overdo it'' in maintaining a clean outer body. The chemicals and detergents that they use in the name of cleanliness are toxic and many contribute to disease. Shampoos, hair sprays, mouthwashes, toothpaste, breath sprays, scrubs and astringents, face lotions. powders, creams of every imaginable form, underarm deodorants and antiperspirants, feminine hygiene sprays, and foot deodorizers are used in unbelievable amounts in our culture. It's overkill. A lot of the television commercials for personal hygiene products are downright embarrassing; they really attest to our hangup about being dirty.

The irony of it is that we are not dirty on the outside, we're dirty on the inside, and no amount of perfumed sprays and creams can mask that. Even worse, they create problems. These sprays and creams are for the most part caustic chemicals that have no place on or near our bodies. They block the cleansing process by forcing the body to close the pores through which it releases toxins. Furthermore, since we obsessively demand the manufacture of these products, we can hardly fault the chemical companies for dumping the by-products of their manufacture into our waters. We asked for it, didn't we?

Are all these products harmful? You bet they are! Feminine hygiene sprays are irritants, often containing talc, which is a known carcinogen. Antiperspirants actually clog the sweat glands with aluminum chloride, and aluminum has been directly linked to Alzheimer's disease. The mouth sprays we use to kill odor-causing bacteria also kill beneficial bacteria. Toothpastes contain abrasives that take the enamel off our teeth, plus dyes and flouride, which are poisonous. A study by DuPont Labs revealed the freon content of propellants for hair sprays and spray deodorants to be dangerously high, and the particles in these sprays are often so small that they can penetrate the lung tissue and be absorbed directly into the bloodstream. In studies done on heavy spray users, all those tested had precancerous lung cell changes.

Why are we such a self-conscious society? Why do we feel that it's necessary to treat our bodies with all these anti-odor chemical agents? It's only because we have not cleansed the *insides* of our bodies. Therefore toxic material is coming out, causing us to smell bad. No amount of chemical agents will help the problem. They will only *compound* it. It is a case of fighting symptoms rather than going for the cause. The thing to do is *cleanse the inside of the body*. This will take care of the problem. The way to accomplish that is to follow the **Fit for Life** principles reviewed in chapter 5. When the inside of your body is clean you will not feel the need for all of these chemical deodorizers. **A CLEAN BODY HAS NO OFFENSIVE ODOR.**

For those who wish to use a safe deodorant in the interim, try the deodorant stone called "Le Crystal Naturelle." It is a body deodorant in the form of a fist-sized opalescent crystal stone made of natural mineral salts. It effectively eliminates body odor from the underarm area or feet without any harmful chemicals or perfumes, and it still allows you to perspire, which is one of the ways your body maintains its health. "Le Crystal Naturelle" is recommended for all types of skin; it doesn't clog pores or stain clothing. It lasts for a very long time, and you will find it to be extremely effective, safe, and economical.

Since most commercial body products and soaps are just full of chemicals, why not investigate some of the natural alternatives? There are many now available which contain all-natural ingredients. Look for them in natural food stores. There are other *truly* natural alternatives. The pulp that remains when you strain almond milk is an excellent body scrub and contains natural almond oil, so it moisturizes at the same time. Mint tea makes a good facial astringent. Instead of using a feminine hygiene spray, douche with two quarts of warm water in which you've mixed two tablespoons of lemon juice or apple cider vinegar. Substitute non-aerosol gels and mousses for hair sprays containing chemical propellants.

The best way to keep clean on the outside is with a warm, *not hot*, bath or shower every day—and a minimum of "products." Brush your teeth and gums with a soft brush and water only, and use dental floss regularly to remove plaque. Massage your gums to keep them healthy. Sweet breath comes from the inside, *not* from toothpaste. Instead of lathering your skin with creams for softness, drink plenty of water and eat plenty of fruits and vegetables. In addition, before bathing, dry-brush your skin with a medium-soft skin brush made of natural bristles. This will remove the dead skin cells that otherwise build up and roughen the skin. What's worse, these dead skin cells hamper elimination, much of which takes place through the skin. After dry-brushing, soak in a bath or shower and then thoroughly scrub your entire body with a loofah sponge—a natural sea sponge. This will really leave your skin soft and fresh. If you wish then to use oil, a little pure coconut oil is the best.

Avoid using talcum on babies. Just feed them properly with breast milk and nut and seed milk, fruit juices, and fruit. Wash them in warm water with a mild coconut oil soap if you feel you must use soap. Change them frequently. They will be sweet and rash free. (Jae Duckhorn of Pasadena, California, wrote to inform me that whenever she gave her baby dairy products, the baby had a diaper rash the next morning. I have heard the same from many other mothers.)

In keeping your body clean, the simplest, most natural solutions are the most intelligent. All those chemical body products are doing a lot more for the "big board on Wall Street" than they are for your health. Eliminate them! You'll save a lot of money, and you'll feel better without them.

PLEASANT SURROUNDINGS

The human species is a nesting species. We do not by nature thrive without some form of shelter. It is a great tragedy of our era and a symptom of the confused values of our times that so many of our fellow beings are forced to live without homes of their own.

Next to our bodies, the most chemically overtreated places in our lives may be our homes. Our homes have literally become chemical dumping grounds, and we who as a species require fresh air are paying the price with our health.

THE ONLY SAFE AND RECOMMENDED AIR FRESHENER IS AN OPEN WINDOW. The variables that contribute most to foul air are cigarette, pipe, and cigar smoke and greasy odors from the frying of meats and other foods. A healthy household where there is no smoking and where fresh fruits and vegetables play a big part in the diet will not experience most of the household odors that plague many American homes. A well-ventilated house will bring an end to stuffy odors. Even in winter, the house should be open briefly to allow a change of air between the inside and the outside. If there are smokers in your house, perhaps you can limit smoking to an area of one room. In many cases, people are successful in having smoking members of the family do so outside.

What are you using to keep your house "clean"? Do you know what is in the products you buy routinely? Do you realize what some of these products are doing to you? Many of the household cleaning products being used are not necessary; for many there are safe substitutes. Unfortunately, most people use toxic household chemicals regularly simply because they are not aware that these chemicals are injurious.

One of the best expenditures of time in your home when you are serious about living healthfully is to clean out and throw away anything that is no longer going to be useful. This effort to detoxify your surroundings will support and reinforce your goal to become healthier.

Go through your kitchen and throw out cleaning agents that are poisonous and polluting. Clean out from your kitchen cabinets and refrigerator the food products that contain chemicals. In your laundry room, eliminate all of the caustic agents you've been using to treat your clothes. When you do this, you'll find to your delight that you can replace all these toxic and costly products with fewer, more effective, harmless products at a *very* great savings. Moreover, the physical act of detoxifying your home will give you a greater sense of dedication to the detoxification of your body (and this planet!)

Kitchen cleaners in particular can be very dangerous. On the label of Easy-Off Oven Cleaner,* we read: "Danger: May cause burns to skin and eyes. Irritant to mucous membranes. Danger—contains lye. Keep out of reach of children. Do not get on exterior surfaces. Keep away from electrical connections. If taken internally or sprayed into eyes, call physician." Now why would anyone want to keep something as gruesome as that around? What is even worse, many poisonous chemical compounds like this are masked by "fragrances" so that they can be breathed in with less discomfort. How gallant of the manufacturers to do that for us! How thoughtful! Actually, oven cleaners are not necessary. First

---

*As of this writing.

of all, if you cut down on meats, your oven will not get as dirty. Secondly, the only reason ovens get caked with grime and require extensive cleaning is because stains and drippings from one day are baked on the next. The thing to do is clean up any spatterings that do occur *as soon as* your oven cools. That way you will be able to *avoid* the need for strong cleaning agents.

Drain cleaners are much like oven cleaners. They, too, contain a high percentage of lye. Along with toilet cleaners, they account for about 10,000 injuries a year. Worse yet, if a drain remains clogged after the cleaner is used, a dangerous caustic solution that gives off toxic fumes develops.

Sometimes the combination of two dangerous substances can be lethal. In November 1975 a sixty-eight-year-old Maine woman used bleach mixed with ammonia to remove egg stains from a window. When she brought the pail of mixed bleach and ammonia into the house, the fumes killed her. A niece who discovered her was killed by the fumes as she tried to give mouth to mouth resuscitation.

The cleaning agents that we use in our homes should help us clean without toxifying us. You just can't go on exposing yourself day after day to all this toxic material. Its effect is cumulative— a little bit from here, a little bit from there—and it severely interferes with your attempts to *de*-toxify. Furthermore, we routinely dump all this stuff down the drain—into our water sources—and then we wonder why we don't have any pure water to drink!

Most people are unaware of the many less toxic, less expensive, and *far* more effective alternatives to the household cleaners they are using. Here are some useful hints for substitution.

● *For general surface cleaning*, use several tablespoons of vinegar dissolved in a bucket of water. This solution is a *wonder cleaner* for windows and floors. Use baking soda to scour surfaces.

● *For bleaching*, use borax. It whitens without harm to the fabric, color, weave, or the water supply.

● *When cleaning utensils and greasy pots and pans* (which you will soon have fewer and fewer of since vegetables and grains rarely create grease), use a diluted solution for soaking or purchase baking soda or an Amway or Shaklee biodegradable liquid soap.

● *If you need to clean your oven*, scour with baking soda.

● *For unblocking drains*, put hot water down them and then flush with one-half cup borax. Unclog with a small plunger.

● *For washing dishes*, use Amway or Shaklee biodegradable dish-washing soaps. They are the *best!* (See page 204.)

Did you know that in this country we buy more detergent than any other product in the grocery store? More than bread, milk, or any other food! Detergents also cause more poisoning than any other household product. And if you have ever taken a walk along the coastline and seen all the foamy bubbles washing up with the waves, you know that all the detergents we dump in the water are ending up in our oceans. The problem with today's detergents is that many people do not understand that *they are no longer just soap*. Ordinary soap is relatively harmless and has been used for thousands of years. Today's detergents, however, are *chemical* products that include foam boosters, perfumes, enzymes, cleaning agents, fillers, and brighteners. If a little gets in your eye, you can experience severe corneal burns and eye damage. Ingestion causes serious harm to the upper digestive tract. You should be very careful to avoid using detergent the way you would use ordinary soap. Clothes washed in these detergents become permeated with artificial perfumes and other residues that are irritating to both the skin and the lungs. Enzyme detergents are often blamed for dermatitis, attacks of asthma, and flulike symptoms.

When Kathy Atwood, who was typing our preliminary manuscript, read this detergent section, she mentioned the experience she and her daughter had with terrible skin allergies as a result of using commercial detergents. She switched to Amway biodegradable laundry detergent. For the first several washings, the clothes actually appeared *dirtier* as the Amway product began to pull the chemical residues of commercial detergents from the fabric. After a few washings, the clothes were clean and bright. Even more important, now Kathy and her daughter no longer suffer from detergent-caused skin allergies.

There are several remedies to the harmful synthetic detergents that we now all use so unconsciously. First of all, you can cut way down on your usage. A Consumers Union survey says, ''Most people use twice as much detergent as is necessary.'' Secondly, you can cut down on all the other laundry-related sprays and additives—fabric softeners, antistatic preparations, stain remover sprays. The first two leave harmful residues in the clothes, and these irritate the skin. The last are particularly offensive because you breathe them in as you use them. (Believe me, none of the chemicals in any of these products is doing you any good.) Thirdly, you can use the biodegradable products that are now available, like those put out by Shaklee and Amway. These products can be purchased from your local Shaklee and Amway distributor, whose name you can find in your phone book.

The best solution to static problems is not chemical sprays. It is to buy more *real*, natural fabrics like cotton instead of all the synthetic ones. Real fabrics are much better for your skin, because they allow it to breathe.

Most people routinely spray their homes for insects. The fumes from these sprays linger for months and *you* get to breathe them! If they can kill bugs, how can they be good for you? The solution to insects in the home is a frequent "spring cleaning" during which you do away with all the clutter and dirt that may be attracting them. If you are living in an old place that had its insect inhabitants long before you got there, you may have to come to terms with the idea of settling for *control* rather than total eradication. After all, no matter how many poisons we use, the insects somehow seem to survive, don't they? As a matter of fact, while they survive our poisons, we succumb to them. Ever wonder why? Perhaps *they* are in harmony with nature while *we* are at war with it.

There are several ways to control insect pests. For roaches and like pests, remove all "gathering places" in and around the home. Eliminate any existing mosquito breeding grounds on your property. Use citronella oil as a natural mosquito repellant. A dab on the skin—better yet, on your clothing—will make you less attractive to mosquitoes. This works! Install screens on your doors and windows. If you *do* use pesticides, use the dry powdered variety that release no fumes.

Keep radiation out of your home, too. One of the questions we are most frequently asked is why we took a position *against microwave ovens* in **Fit for Life**. Well, do you want a nuclear power plant next door to you? Do you realize that your microwave oven is your own little box of radiation? I know, your argument is that it's not nuclear radiation—it's "low energy, non-ionizing radiation.'' Right? So what? Why do you need a constant source of low-level radiation in your home? For convenience? I'm sorry, but that's just one more example of how the ''fast food, no time for cooking'' mentality has really got us by the throats. These ovens exist because of laziness and ignorance of the facts. The manufacturers have marketed microwaves to us as ''an indispensable modern convenience,'' and *no one* has bothered to caution us of their dangers. So what if you can cook a frozen chicken in four minutes? Is it worth having a potential source of radiation poisoning in your home? *Are they dangerous? Yes!* Leading natural hygienists, particularly Dr. Virginia Vetrano of Austin, Texas, have been warning against the hazards of microwave radiation for decades.

A microwave oven is like a fallout shelter in reverse. It's a tight little box designed to keep radiation in! If it's a perfect, tight little box, then the radiation won't get out—but it's *not*. Radiation *does* leak out, especially around the door and seals. These leaks are so prevalent that government standards have actually been set to determine ''acceptable leakage'' rates. Now, who do you suppose that is designed to protect? You or the manufacturer? And who is checking to see how much *your* microwave is leaking? Any government inspectors show up lately to do that for you?

Listen! **THERE IS NO SUCH THING AS A SAFE DOSAGE OF RADIATION.** Dr. Karl Morgan, a researcher on the effects of radiation on human health, has stated, ''From 1960 to the present, an overwhelming amount of data have been accumulated that show that there is *no safe* level of exposure and there is no dose of radiation so low that the risk of malignancy is 0.''* The concern about microwave ovens is *not* that the food becomes radioactive. *Any* cooking destroys at least some of the vital nutrients in food. It is just that microwaving destroys them faster. The main reasons for concern have to do with *you!* Your body has no way to warn you to protect itself when it is being affected by radiation. We have sense organs that warn us of the dangers of other poisons, but we get no warning when we receive doses of radiation. We cannot feel them, taste them, or smell them. *They are deadly silent!* Nor do we have some kind of warning device to inform us of their cumulative damages. The health effects may

*Mike Benton, ''Radiation in Your Kitchen,'' *Lesson 51, The Life Science Health System*, Austin, Texas: Life Science.

not be evident for years, by which time it is too late to remove the cause. Some of the suspected effects from microwaves are interference with heart pacemakers; damage to sensitive body cell tissue, especially in the developing fetus; eye damage, including cataracts; and nervous exhaustion.

The real problem is that *nobody knows* how dangerous microwave ovens may be. The so-called "safe" standards for microwaves that have been set by our government are industry-biased. Dr. A. H. Frey has discovered that the human nervous system reacts to microwave exposure that is *300 times below* the levels the government has declared safe. If you are voluntarily going to invite that kind of abuse into your home—your comfortable surroundings—at least know this: Older microwaves leak more than new ones, due to general wear and improper servicing. Damage through shipping or use is possible, so be alert. Objects should never be inserted between door seals. Use of scouring pads, steel wool, or other abrasives can cause more leakage—clean only with mild detergent. Stay at least an arm's length away when the oven is in use, and keep your eyes away from the door. Still want one?

Maybe none of these arguments overrides that of convenience, so if you are going to use one, check it regularly with a microwave leakage detector (available at Radio Shack) to determine the extent of leakage. And remember that, in addition to all the above-mentioned health hazards, there is a far greater issue: Do you want nuclear power plants all over this country? Do you believe any increase in convenience is worth the threat of power plant disasters or the burden of nuclear waste disposal? I don't. Non life-threatening forms of energy are what we need to support and get behind. The more we buy the "convenience" of nuclear appliances, the more deeply entrenched the nuclear industry will become. Presented with the question "Since microwave is so groovy, do you want a nuclear power plant in your backyard?" I know what *my* answer would be!

It will probably come as no shock to you to learn that the levels of radiation coming off your television are *definitely* harmful when added to all of the other X rays we have in our lives today. Just before he died in 1960 from cancer *caused* by X rays, Dr. Emil Grubbe, the world's foremost expert on radiation, gave an interview in which he answered the question of what television radiation could do. With one arm gone, several fingers missing from his other hand, and his nose and chin eaten away, he said, "Look at me. Or imagine some small child helplessly dying of leukemia. Even if television radiation itself is below harmful levels, I say it has to be harmful when added to all the other X rays we have today. The television manufacturers don't think of this. Subject a man to atomic tests, medical X rays, plus the normal cosmic rays in the air from space, then throw in four hours a night of exposure to radiation six feet from a TV and you have a pretty grim picture. *But I don't think television is safe even by itself!*''

The government has set a ''safe'' level of TV radiation. Now, I know what you are thinking. Safe for whom? Us or the industry? It's the same old story. ''Safe'' is supposed to be sixteen kilovolts. Most televisions operate *way above* that level—the amount of radiation increases with size and color. There are enough X rays produced by the television tube to cause the manufacturer to place warning tags on all new tubes for repairmen. Why is the consumer not also warned? No information is allowed to reach the public on subjects like these. It's too costly to the industry. According to the International Commission on Radiation Protection, no one should receive more than five rem by the age of thirty. We get one rem for each year that we watch TV! By age thirty that's *thirty* rem! Mothers are unknowingly allowing their children to watch TV for *hours* every day and are not even told what I am now going to tell you: **THE GREATER THE DISTANCE FROM THE SCREEN THE LESS HARM WILL BE DONE. MOVE THOSE KIDS BACK FROM THE TV!** At least six feet is where you should *start*. With twelve out of a hundred children being born with birth defects, pregnant women should be warned that the potential danger to the fetus is very great, since the human cell is most vulnerable to X-ray damage during cell division. So there you have it. Television carries with its benefits some very substantial risks, doesn't it?

There's one more thing you should know. Since our government first enacted safety levels for exposure to X rays in 1968, *they have been lowered eight times*—and they are still 1000 times higher than accepted levels in the Soviet Union. No one knows anything about the cumulative effects of this silent killer. All we can do is have as little of it around us as possible in our homes. At least have the wisdom not to just leave the television on all day, whether it is being watched or not. I'm not kidding! Some people do that! The best way to counteract home radiation or what you receive from computers and copiers in the office is to get outside in natural light as much as possible. To all you parents who repeatedly find yourselves saying to your kids, "Turn off that TV and go outside and play!"—you're right on the money!*

Your home is your retreat. Whatever is there must be purposefully there to support your well-being. It is easy to eliminate caustic chemicals that you have been using excessively. It is easy to rearrange your room so that your distance from the television is safer. And there are other easy measures you can take to insure that your home is a healthful place to be.

You know, we are by nature an outdoor species. Long ago we spent much more time outdoors than we do today. Our sense organs still respond to the beauty of the outdoors. Our legendary or actual paradises are full of plants and flowers. These lift the spirits and calm the mind. Bring them into your home. Fill it with plants and flowers whenever you can. We live in symbiosis with plants. They take in the poisonous carbon dioxide we give off and break it down to provide the oxygen we need to breathe. Living plants will actually help keep the air in our home pure. A weekly flower budget, even a very modest one, will provide impressions of natural beauty your body craves *biologically*.

In your garden you can do more. Plant trees! They cleanse the air. The rain forests that keep our planet oxygenated are being destroyed at a frightening pace. By the year 2000 only *10 percent* of those forests will remain! Help to counteract this insanity by planting trees wherever and whenever you can. Plant flowers, which you can cut for your house. Plant a vegetable garden. All this is an investment of your time and energy directly in *you*.

Color has far more of an effect on us than we realize. Different colors impact the different energy centers in our bodies. For example, *red* stimulates sexual energy. *Orange and yellow* aid in digestion. They are cheerful and radiant and affect us like the sun. *Green* touches our hearts and is full of love, harmony, and peace. It soothes emotions. *Blue* affects the lungs and breathing. *Purple* is inspiring, spiritual, and etheric. It supports quiet and meditation. *White* is the color of higher levels of consciousness. Intense colors excite intense reactions. Soft (muted but not weak) colors are calming backdrops for a soothing existence. Use colors consciously

---

*For an eye-opening discussion on the effects of radiation, see Dr. Virginia Vetrano's work described in "The Greatest Health Discovery," Natural Hygiene Press, Chicago, Illinois, pp. 177–186.

in your home. They have a greater impact on your health than you realize.

Music affects us much the way color does. Tranquil soft music can be very soothing. Loud and abrasive music can act as a form of pollution. Plants subjected to hard rock 'n roll wither, while those treated to soft classical music thrive. Use music appropriately and not unconsciously. It can really help you feel good. Music was one of the healing elements employed in the temples of Asklepias. Use it to *improve*, not undermine, your health.

A QUIET MOMENT NOW AND THEN

For some the pace of modern life is too hectic. It sets the mind reeling and rippling. Clear thinking becomes difficult. Emotional reactions are sudden and uncontrolled. Sleep is restless. Digestion is disturbed. Relationships are draining. And all because the mind is on overload.

Our mind is the screen on which we view life. It is like a lake. If the lake is calm we can see clear through to the bottom; we can see the shiny quarter someone has tossed into it. When the lake is full of waves and ripples, that same quarter looks like a giant fish lurking on the bottom. It is the same with our mind. If it is calm, we can see what our life is about. We can understand our relationships better and we can see what we must do with our work. If our mind is in chaos, we lose control of our direction. Little quarters become giant fishes. Small incidents become major problems. Life seems full of hassles and disturbances.

Quieting the mind is a wonderful practice. It's like turning off the computer for a while, disconnecting from all the sources of input we are normally connected to. All day long we are bombarded with a never-ending stream of input. Input and demands are coming from our mates, our children, our employers or employees. We're under siege as we go in traffic from one place to another. During our waking hours our minds and thoughts are racing at a nonstop, breakneck speed. We live in a world of distressing background noise. Everyone has experienced something like the grind and squeal an electric saw makes while a tree is being cut down. Although we actually become accustomed to the sound, once the sawing stops we experience the relief of sudden quiet. The same relief can be experienced when you treat yourself to a quiet moment each day, an interval that refreshes, strengthens, clarifies, and renews.

People think such moments are only for the spiritually inclined. In truth, these moments are a gift to humanity that we *all* have the ability to enjoy. *Anyone* can reap the benefit of a few quiet, meditative moments. Simply sit comfortably in a chair, your feet on the floor, or sit directly on the floor, with your legs comfortably crossed. Fold your hands palm to palm in your lap and close your eyes. You will first notice that your mind is squealing and jumping like a puppy at the end of a leash. No way can you get it to quiet down. The more you force it, the more it resists, because you are using the mind to try to quiet the mind. It's like telling the nuclear industry to regulate itself. Sure!

The nature of the mind is to race. It doesn't want to be harnessed or trained. It likes to be in control. So you must be patient. Rather than forcing it, surrender to it—let it do its thing. You simply go somewhere else. When it blasts a thought at you, like a child crying for attention, tell it, "Not now," and instead focus your energy on your breath. Listen to your breath going in and out of your body. *Feel it*. Watch it with your eyes closed. You can even give it a sound if you like—it actually does have a sound: *HOM* as the breath goes in, *SA* as it goes out. Repeating these sounds inside yourself with each inhalation and exhalation will help you to ignore the shenanigans of your mind, and eventually it will learn to calm down. You can also use the breath to cleanse your inner being. On each inhalation, breathe in **LOVE**. On each exhalation, breathe out whatever negative emotions you may sense: **ANGER, JEALOUSY, HATRED** or the feelings of **TENSION** they create. Since "the Kingdom of God lies within," use this exercise to sweep that kingdom clean and fill it with God's love. The longer you do this regularly the more calm your mind will become. Eventually it will flow effortlessly with your breath. Your breath will slow and become very gentle; your mind will become more and more still. This is when the brain rests and heals. It is said that twelve minutes of this deep, restful state is equal in body and mind rejuvenation to a whole night's sleep.

Few people realize how surprisingly difficult it is to sit in a thought-free state for even *one* minute. It may sound easy, but simply try it right now, and see if you can sit for one minute with a completely still mind *totally* free of any thought whatsoever . . . How did it go? See what we mean? As you do this, you may find that in the beginning you only get a few seconds that are completely thought-free, but you will *feel* them. When the mind is still, even for a few seconds, it's like the cool peace at the bottom of a well. You get a glimpse of a totally restful state of being. Build from these few seconds to a minute or two to as long as eight or ten or twelve minutes. For many people it can take a long time, even years, to accomplish this, but the *daily practice* to bring about each little increment will bring indescribable benefits. What benefits exactly? You will find yourself much more capable of coping with the demands of daily living. You will find yourself less irritable, less tense, less critical, and more loving and accepting of others in your relationships. You will be less inclined to over-react to situations and more capable of judiciously observing them before taking appropriate action, plus you will be less demanding on others and feel more complete and self-sufficient.

To begin to include daily quiet moments into your life-style, start with five or ten minutes a day and work up to twenty-five or thirty minutes. Discipline yourself to sit for a predetermined length of time, whether you get a glimpse of the thought-free state or not.* Sometimes you will, sometimes you may not. Do this when-ever it's convenient, in the early morning is a good time because your quiet moment will compose you for the rest of the day. If morning isn't possible, take some time during a break at work, before dinner, or before retiring. If you do it at the same time every day, your mind will come under control even faster, since it will learn to expect the discipline of your regular, quiet moment.

Quiet moments help you to become more loving, creative, and productive in your daily life. They will counteract the stress of daily living and help you to put yourself and the world around you into perspective. Once you have developed the habit of sitting quietly *every* day, a day without quiet time will not seem complete.

---

*Set a little timer, first for two minutes, then increase to five, then seven, then twelve. The peaceful composure you will experience as a result may encourage you to increase to twenty, twenty-five, then thirty minutes. If the timer goes off and you want more, reset it.

PART

III

Special
Concerns

CHAPTER 14
Animal Products

HARVEY:

Flim-flammed, short-changed, underhanded, fleeced, bamboozled, hoodwinked, duped, boondoggled, swindled, hornswoggled, conned, Tommy-rot, hocus-pocus, mumbo jumbo, bill of goods, malarkey, gibberish, poppycock, hooey, balderdash, deception, snow job, misleading, hogwash, chicanery. Guess what they all have in common? They are all words that can be used to describe what has been done to or fed to the public in the selling of animal products. Animal products are all meats (including fish and chicken), dairy products, and eggs. They are the high-protein foods that cost the most and are the hardest to digest, and yet we are continually admonished to eat more and more of them. We are being pushed to eat several times more protein than our bodies can possibly use. *Animal products are killing us.*

In **Fit for Life** we presented two chapters on animal products that created quite an uproar. Some dietitians and nutritionists practically had coronaries when they realized someone had finally decided to tell the truth about some of the most destructive and worthless of all foods eaten in our diets. Quite frankly, in those chapters we only gave *part* of the story. We didn't actually let on how harmful these foods really are. We weren't sure people were ready for it all, so accepted is the propaganda that animal products actually have some benefit. The idea was to start slowly, first to warn the *public*, which is far more willing to hear the truth than are the "experts."

Notwithstanding dietitians and nutritionists who will say anything to protect their funding from the meat and dairy industries, great numbers of people have already begun seeing through the propaganda smoke screen and eating fewer animal products—and feeling enormously healthier. People's allergies are clearing up. Children are having fewer colds and ear infections. Arthritis and gout sufferers are reporting less pain. Blood pressure is lowering. Those suffering from respiratory ailments are getting relief. Folks are generally feeling better without so much animal product in their diet.

ANIMAL PRODUCTS WILL MAKE YOU SICK!

Ladies and gentlemen, animal products are very much worse than you could ever imagine. The pain and suffering caused by these "foods" is incalculable. They can be linked to practically every major disease we suffer from today. There is so much evidence to back up what I am saying, that it's truly amazing more people have not managed to see the obvious. Both commonsense arguments and corroborating literature in journals and textbooks abound, yet those with vested interests have the unmitigated gall to actually express outrage at our pointing out their products' cost in human destruction. Before this chapter is over, I'm going to express a little outrage of my own. But where the industries are outraged about decreasing profits, I'm outraged about the suffering their billion-dollar money makers have visited on the innocent public. How dare they pretend that they're not aware of the mountain of evidence incriminating their products.

Before going any further, I want to make perfectly clear that I do not think that *everyone* in the business of producing and selling animal products is aware of the negative aspects of these products. Unlike, for example, the tobacco industry, where there can simply be no doubt that their product kills people, there are members of the meat and dairy industries who *truly* believe that their products are valuable. Unfortunately, they are gravely mistaken.

Don't think for a moment that I'm not aware of the controversy of what I'm writing about here, but be certain of one thing: After the storm that was raised by self-interested, misinformed dietitians and nutritionists over what was written in **Fit for Life** on dairy and flesh foods, there is no way on earth we would allow one word of this to appear that could not be backed up. I will prove to you that what I am saying about the harmfulness of animal products is accurate by two measures.

First, by the greatest enemy of the animal products industries and dietitians, common sense. *They can't stand common sense.* It drives them nuts. You see, they can confuse the issues and confuse the lay person by throwing around a lot of talk weighted down with multisyllabled words and half truths. They haven't yet devised a way to trick people into forsaking their common sense.

The other proof comes from the scientific journals. Ironically, *all* of our contentions are backed up by their own journals, *and the dietitians and nutritionists are not even aware of it!* Can you imagine? It's like a burglar's denying having stolen a gold watch to a judge and jury while wearing the watch on his wrist. Personally, I would just as soon not cite the scientific studies because, quite frankly, *anyone* can prove *anything* they want. Throw enough funding money at dietitians and they'll prove in a week that eating old carpets is better than food. Ever hear of a book entitled *How to Lie With Statistics*? Researchers can manipulate statistics to make any point they wish. Benjamin Disraeli, a prime minister of England in the nineteenth century, once said, "There are three kinds of lies: lies, damned lies, and statistics." However, the dietitians and nutritionists are so adamant in claiming there's "no proof in the literature" that it will be kind of fun to prove my contentions using their own precious journals. Besides, the publisher insisted on scientific backup. Throughout this chapter you will see number references in parentheses next to statements made about animal products. These are references to bibliography entries, books and articles detailing the facts we present here. (The bibliography entries are all numbered for your convenience.)

One more point before proceeding. Although I'm building a case against animal products, I am not trying to convince you to discontinue all animal products from your diet overnight. That may be too unrealistic. Remember, ideal versus the real. I haven't *totally* removed animal products from my diet, and I have been eating this way for seventeen years. The purpose is to make you aware of the situation—sort of like "know your enemy." There is a way of including animal products in your diet so as to suffer the least amount of harm possible, and it is simply foolish not to take advantage of that information.

What if you had to swim across a channel for some reason?

Would it make much sense to you to plunge into the water not knowing how far you had to go, in what direction, or what the currents were like—plus you're not even a very good swimmer? Now, under those conditions you might still make it through sheer luck and a reliance upon your instincts for survival, but wouldn't it make more sense to take certain precautions to minimize the danger? That's how it is with eating animal products. I am not suggesting you avoid them altogether, but rather that you realize they present a clear and definite danger and take steps to decrease your risk of harm.

Ever hear of high blood cholesterol, arthritis, or osteoporosis? Of course. Who hasn't? Consider this. If it were not for animal products, you would never even have *heard* of these three problems, let alone know what they are. The *only* reason they exist is because of the consumption of animal products. Shocking? You bet! Preventable? Absolutely! An exaggeration? No way! And these are just a few of the problems, a fraction of the health problems I am going to cover, all associated with the consumption of animal products.

Every area of the academic community, from the American Cancer Society to the World Health Organization to the American Heart Association to the National Institutes of Health, is imploring us to cut down on fat and cholesterol and increase our fiber intake, right? This is no surprise to anyone. Animal products are *very* high in fat, *very* high in cholesterol, and very *low* in fiber. This is not speculation. *This is fact.* Animal products are exactly the opposite of what we are being told to consume.

Cholesterol is a substance unique to animals and humans. It is secreted by the liver and is necessary for many functions of the body. Actually, many people think of cholesterol only in a negative way. However, the human body secretes about 2000 milligrams of it daily, and the body uses it in *all* of its tissues.

The body will secrete its needs daily whether or not you take any in with food, because *only its own* can be utilized. Cholesterol taken in via the diet, as you may already know, is a severe health hazard. Remember, *you can find cholesterol nowhere else but in the tissues of animals. It is not to be found in plant life!* (98) Get it? If people did not eat animals or animal products, there would never be a cholesterol problem. Studies show that while animal protein raises blood cholesterol, vegetable protein actually lowers it! (350) Want to cut down on your cholesterol? Cut down on your animal products, and increase your consumption of vegetables. It's plain common sense.

By the way, ever hear of gallstones? They are caused mainly by that same fatty waste product, cholesterol. (52, 165, 294, 339) And in societies where cholesterol levels are kept low, heart disease is also very rare. (98) Saturated fats from animal products raise cholesterol levels and increase your chance of dying of a heart disease. (28, 232) Cholesterol and the highly saturated fat in animal products contribute to atherosclerosis as well. (147, 273) One ten-year study showed conclusively that heated milk is a primary contributor to all forms of heart disease. (30, 237) The high fat content of animal products also contributes to high blood pressure, or what is called hypertension. (75, 232, 299) As saturated fat is lowered in the diet, blood pressure goes down. (316)

Uric acid is one of the most potent poisons known and high-protein foods, especially flesh foods, are a major source of uric acid. When autopsied, all victims of leukemia show a high uric acid level in their blood, *which decreases on a low-protein diet.* (205, 292) Uric acid is responsible for both gout, an extremely painful and deforming type of arthritis, and uric acid kidney stones. Both are prevented *and* healed with a low-protein diet. (59, 94, 423) Calcium kidney stones, very painful and the most common type of kidney stone, are also the result of a high-protein diet. They, too, can be prevented by lowering animal product consumption. (113, 328, 389) Protein is the most difficult food for the human body to deal with, and because of the strain imposed by processing excessive protein, the liver and the kidneys are overworked and they enlarge. (187) It has been shown that people experiencing kidney or liver failure improve dramatically when a low-protein diet is taken. (161, 207, 213, 265, 406)

When uric acid crystals settle in the joints, you get the excruciating misery of arthritis. (135, 170, 223) There is no question but that animal products are also a major contributing factor to the development of arthritis. A thirty-year study in Scandinavia showed an indisputable link between milk and arthritis. (6) One carefully conducted study described a patient with serious rheumatoid arthritis who improved dramatically when dairy products were removed from his diet and relapsed immediately when they were reintroduced.* This evidence makes it very clear indeed that dairy

General Practitioner, September 17, 1982, page 55.

products are a major culprit in this excruciating, agonizing malady. Both heart and arthritis sufferers show dramatic improvement when they decrease the amount of dairy products in their diet. (146, 281) Arthritis is rare in societies where low-protein diets are eaten. (46, 47, 356) So, it is never too late to do the right thing.

If dairy products are a contributing factor to arthritic conditions, then when you eliminate or cut down on them, you eliminate or cut down on the arthritis. The high fat content of animal products is also implicated in the development of diabetes. And it has been amply demonstrated that a low-fat, high-fiber diet can actually lessen the need for insulin. (27, 39, 185, 274, 349, 368) Marilyn and I have seen this over and over in our practice over the last decade. Diabetes sufferers have shown marked improvement, needing less and less insulin as they lower the amount of animal products in their diets. Tinnitis, or ringing in the ears, is another malady caused by the high fat content of animal products. (361)

Cancer. There's something about that word. It's ugly. It's scary. It's unnerving and frightening. Something happens when you hear the term—visions of something gruesome, involving pain, helplessness, and anguish. Even though twice as many people a year die from heart disease, people fear cancer more. *Animal products cause cancer.* Absolutely no doubt about it. It's not an issue of whether they do or not. They do! The issue is just how much. In my opinion, if by some stroke of cosmic good fortune animal products were entirely removed from our diets, cancer (other than smoking-related cancer) would cease to be a problem. I can't quite prove that yet, but I'm working on it. However, what *is* proven is that, because of their high fat, high cholesterol, low fiber content, animal products cause their share of cancer, among which are cancer of the colon, breast, liver, kidneys, prostate, testicles, uterus, and ovaries. (31, 86, 106, 183, 184, 235, 250, 270, 326, 407, 420)

Colon cancer affords us a perfect example of what I'm talking about here. Ten years ago when we tried to tell people of the link between colon cancer and diet, no one was particularly interested (mind you, Natural Hygienists spoke of the link over half a century ago). (9, 10, 81, 85, 118, 201, 337, 373, 374, 375, 379) But, after President Reagan's difficulties with cancer of the colon, all of a sudden *everyone* became interested, and now organizations such as the National Cancer Institute and the American Cancer Society are finally pointing out that this link does indeed exist—

that colon cancer can indeed be *prevented* by good diet. As a matter of fact, studies prove that diets highest in animal fats and cholesterol coincide with the highest rate of colon cancer (24, 71, 97, 104, 248, 249, 387, 388) while other studies prove that a high-fiber diet prevents it. (74, 182, 235, 248, 302, 395)

THE CASE AGAINST MEAT

Ever eat a dead dog? How about a dead puppy? (They're a lot more tender.) Some of you, I'm sure, are wrinkling your face in revulsion and saying, "What do you mean, eat a dead dog?" But how does one determine which animals killed and eaten are or are not okay? People eat dead chickens, and dead pigs. People eat dead baby cows. Why not dead baby dogs? Actually, in some places in the world, dogs and puppies are considered a great delicacy. Some people look upon us as barbarians for eating baby cows. Of course, when you order this "food" in a restaurant, you don't ask for baby cow parmesan. It's called *veal* parmesan. It's given another name so that you don't have to feel disgusted or ashamed when you order it. Clever? Actually, if more people knew what veal really was, they would probably stop eating it on the spot, because *barbarism* is a mild word to describe the torture and inhumane abuse necessary to produce this "delicacy."

If you like animals—I don't mean to eat, I mean as friends— you may want to skip over the next few pages, because they are a bit harsh. Calves chosen for the "veal factory" live for four months at most. During that time they are put through a living hell in order to supply people that "fashionably white," tender veal. Veal producers take calves immediately after birth (one day) and place them in individual stalls in the veal factory building. Calves will never see their mothers again. The stalls are barely larger than the calf, which is often tied at the neck to restrict movement. This is so that there is no muscle development and the meat stays nice and tender. Like other young animals, calves like to prance and frolic in the open. This a "vealer" never does.

Throughout its confinement the calf is fed "milk replacer," a mixture of dried skim milk, dried whey, starch, fats, sugars, mold inhibitors, vitamins, and antibiotics. It *never* tastes its mother's milk. These replacers are extremely high in fat to cause the immobile calves to gain weight rapidly. That extra fat just can't wait to get to your arteries. The calf is kept on a totally iron-free diet —iron would normally be in its natural food—so its flesh is totally anemic. That keeps it white. The stall contains no straw or other bedding, for the calf would eat it, giving it some iron, which would darken its flesh. Heavens, we couldn't have that! The unfortunate animal can often be seen trying to eat its stall or licking nails or any other metal around it in an attempt to get some iron. Oh yes, the barns where calves like this are kept are *pitch dark*. The darkness helps keep them quiet.

This abuse goes on for about fifteen weeks, at which time the calves weigh about 330 pounds and are ready for slaughter. Actually, producers would like to keep them longer to fatten them up a little more, but by this time they are so severely anemic and unhealthy that with any more of this treatment they would sicken and die. So, right before they die of disease, they're whisked off to be butchered and brought to your table ever so tastefully prepared: sautéed with just the right amount of parmesan cheese and bread crumbs. Bon appétit!

Dead calves are not the only things we rename to keep from feeling queasy when we eat them. Ever have strips of a dead pig's belly? Bacon. How about chopped up dead cow? Hamburger. And let's not forget various and sundry dead cow and pig parts, wastes scraped from bones and loose scraps chopped up and stuffed into a casing. Hot dogs. There's no reason to rename an apple or a piece of watermelon, is there? Some people will take umbrage with the language I'm using, but I'm being literal with a purpose in mind. It is to help reinforce the point that we are not, by design, flesh eaters—not physiologically and not psychologically.

I've already half *proven* that we're not psychologically equipped. Break out your common sense for a moment. Did you not find the language and description of the last few paragraphs at least a little offensive? *That is because it is not in your nature to eat a dead animal.* If just reading about it offended you, how would you come by dead animals if they were not slaughtered for you? Would you even *consider* killing a calf with your own hands then slashing it open with a knife and wading through the blood and guts to carve out your favorite portion? Then, of course, you would have to deal with the carcass before it started to rot and stink. What would you do with it, especially if you had no refrigeration? Bury it in your back yard? If we really were predisposed to the eating of flesh, you would salivate with anticipatory delight over the prospect of getting to tear into an animal. Moreover, like *every naturally designed* flesh eating animal on earth, you would eat it *raw*. How does that appeal to you? Could you tackle a pig, somehow kill it, and bite right into it and eat it? Your natural aversion to capturing, killing, slaughtering and eating another living creature whole and raw should make you realize that psychologically we are not flesh eaters. And it is even easier to prove we're not physically designed to eat flesh.

The history of our species is very clear. We developed as eaters of plant foods, not as flesh eaters. (14, 29, 223, 250, 266, 279, 297, 306, 330, 394) Our teeth are not designed for the rending and tearing of flesh. Do you have fangs? Look into the mouth of a shark or a wolf and you'll see what kind of teeth you would need in your mouth if you were a flesh eater. Our saliva is totally different from that of a flesh eater. Ours contains an enzyme designed solely for the purpose of digesting the complex carbo-hydrates found in plant food. Flesh eating animals have no such enzyme. Their saliva is highly acid for breaking down concentrated protein. Ours is alkaline. A flesh eater's stomach will secrete ten times more hydrochloric acid than ours. This concentration readily breaks down flesh. Flesh eaters also have the capacity to eliminate huge amounts of cholesterol, and they have the enzyme uricase for breaking down uric acid. Our liver can process but a small amount of cholesterol, and we do not possess the enzyme uricase. The digestive tracts of flesh eating animals are short, about three times the length of their torso. This allows for the rapid expulsion of decomposing, putrefying flesh. All plant eating animals have long intestines, about eight to twelve times the length of their torso, in order to allow sufficient transit time to digest and extract nutrients found in plant foods. Nope. Any way you look at it we're not flesh eaters.

I realize that a sufficient number of people have successfully been terrorized into believing that, without eating high protein foods *every day*, they will suffer from a protein deficiency. Of course, the fact that you don't get much protein from eating protein foods is not something the meat and dairy industry play up too much. They would much rather people remained under the delusion that human protein is built from animal products. If you take a bite of a chicken, that is chicken protein, *not* human protein. If you take a bite of a pig or a steer, it is pig or steer protein, not human protein.

Protein is built from amino acids. This is too short and too meaningful a sentence to say only once. **PROTEIN IS BUILT FROM AMINO ACIDS!** There is not a physiologist on earth who would tell you differently. That is no more at issue than whether or not the sun is hot or water is wet or interest rates are too high.

The fact that amino acids are the building blocks for protein is the reason why elephants, water buffaloes, oxen, horses, rhinoceroses, gorillas, and other animals of strength and endurance have not become extinct because of protein deficiencies. Even cattle, which we are presumably supposed to eat until the meat oozes out of our ears, don't eat animal products, and they suffer from no protein deficiencies. Ever wonder about that?

"What about lions?" you ask. "They eat zebras and turn it into protein. Why can't we do that, too?" First of all, lions' digestive tracts are *designed* to transform flesh into protein and glucose, and the number-one prerequisite for being able to do so is that they eat their zebra meat *raw*. (Ever see a pride of lions barbecuing their dinner?) When eaten raw, the amino acid chains comprising zebra protein are easily broken down and reassembled into lion protein. When cooked, amino acids fuse together, making the protein unusable. That is why carnivorous animals fed only cooked meat become sickly, diseased, sterile, and unable to reproduce. Even the task of converting raw zebra protein into lion protein is so energy consuming that lions sleep twenty hours a day. Orangutans eat only fruit and sleep only six hours.

I suppose if you're willing to eat your steer, pig, and chicken meat raw and sleep twenty hours a day, your system *might* be able to transform it into the human protein you need. But why not get your amino acids (protein) from the source that your digestive tract is biologically adapted to utilize? *Fruits and vegetables.* **EVERY AMINO ACID NEEDED TO BUILD HUMAN PROTEIN IS TO BE FOUND IN FRUITS AND VEGETABLES.** I see a couple of the more backward-thinking dietitians over in the corner "pshawing" this. Fine, don't believe me. Just go arm wrestle a silver-back gorilla, who is three times our size but *thirty* times our strength. They eat nothing but fruit and bamboo leaves and can turn your car over if they want to. Where are they getting their protein?*

*The entire subject of protein and amino acids is discussed in much more detail in chapter 9, "Protein," in **Fit for Life**.

THE CASE AGAINST DAIRY PRODUCTS

It is outright misrepresentation and commercialism to perpetuate the ridiculous belief that we can't meet our protein needs without eating animal products.

I'd sure love to watch those of you who disagree chase down a rabbit, tear it apart with your teeth and hands (if you could catch it), and devour it raw: blood, guts, bones, skin, flesh, and all, just as any genuine, self-respecting flesh eater would. And after finishing off the rabbit, I'd like to watch you go out into a pasture, get down on all fours, and suck the milk out of a cow's udder to wash the dead rabbit down. That's a little repulsive, too, isn't it? Why? *Because it is not our natural inclination.* If you didn't get the milk from your own mother's breast, *it's too late*! The fact is that the majority of people on earth react to cow's milk by getting sick. (121) It's an insult to nature's grand scheme to go to another species for milk.

It slays me how some people are always trying to figure out a way to do things in opposition to nature's design. And they always use some half truth in an attempt to justify it. For example, have you seen the big billboards and full-page magazine ads showing several different dairy products with a caption that reads, "Calcium, The Way Nature Intended It"? They left off two very important words: *"For Calves"*! Calcium, the way nature intended it for calves! Cow's milk is for calves! What's so hard to grasp about that? Once weaned, even a calf won't drink milk—of its own kind or of any other animal, either. They're too innately smart to try circumventing nature's grand plan. Too bad we're not!

The exquisite magnificence of nature is simply too exceptionally splendid, too marvelously perfect for us to have the arrogance and effrontery to dare trying to second guess its grand purpose. There is a reason why *all* mammals have milk available at the birth of their young. It is because each species' milk is uniquely beneficial for *that* species. That's nature! That is why two things are true for *every* mammal on earth except us:

1. They do not consume the milk of another species. That would mean crossing over their biological adaptation, and they don't do that. (Remember, we're not talking about pets or animals in zoos, whom we have managed to pervert as much as ourselves.)

2. Once weaned, *no* animal ever again consumes milk. Milk is the food designed by nature to feed *the young* of the species. It is specifically designed for the rapid growth of an infant. That is what it is for! It is idiocy to insist we continue drinking it after infancy, to drink it into our eighties, if we can get that far. The ridiculousness of it is lamentable. Are we actually to believe that when our mothers finish cows should take over?

How is it that the species with the most sophisticated brain, the greatest intelligence, and the unique ability to reason is too dense to see this simple truth? And then there's the ironic fact that **DAIRY PRODUCTS ARE DISEASE-PRODUCING.** They're harmful. They *cause* suffering. They're the perfect thing to eat if you want to be sick and have a diseased body. The dietitians and nutritionists who are mouthpieces and cheerleaders for the dairy industry, telling you that dairy products are a good food, should hide their heads in shame—not only for leading the innocent public to believe that dairy products are actually valuable, but also for failing to keep abreast of the field about which they are *supposed* to know something.

To say that dairy products are a good food for humans is evidence of unpardonable ignorance of the facts. There is simply too much evidence proving dairy products to be a clear and present danger. I can understand this faulty thinking from someone not in the health field, but for someone in the health profession, which is looked to for reputable advice, to mislead people because of laziness or ignorance or pride or financial gain or *all four* is beneath contempt. It is criminal outrage to sell off the health of our population for the almighty dollar. And, as you will see, the evidence is not just now coming to light; it's been known for *decades* just how harmful dairy products are. I've already presented evidence describing the diseases that high-fat, high-cholesterol animal products (including dairy) can cause. And there is much more proof, confirmed by common sense and scientific literature.

Cow's milk is designed to quickly create a huge, big-boned animal with four stomachs, and there's no way humans meet those criteria (although, unfortunately, I have seen some people who are starting to look dangerously close). Consider this: Cow's milk is designed to take an infant calf, weighing 90 pounds at birth, to a weight of 2000 pounds in only two years. Human infants weigh 6 to 8 pounds at birth and will attain a weight of only 100 to 200 pounds in *eighteen* years! Eating dairy products is eating a food designed by nature to make you very big, like a cow, very fast. If you're presently eating dairy products, I hope you're not trying to lose weight. You'd have a better chance of putting out a fire by throwing kerosene on it. But there is so much more that is harmful about dairy products that I hardly know where to start.

Cow's milk causes more mucus than any food you can eat—thick, dense mucus that clogs and irritates the body's entire respiratory system; mucus that coats the inside of the body and prevents the fluid operation of the system; dense, gluey mucus that places a tremendous burden on the eliminative faculties of the body, clogs the delicate mucous membranes and invites disease. Hay fever, asthma, bronchitis, sinusitis, colds, runny noses, and ear infections are all primarily caused by dairy products. Dairy products are *the* leading cause of allergies. (36, 37, 73, 153, 264, 377) Practically every book, every paper, every study that discusses allergies implicates dairy products. There simply is no question of its role in this area.

In addition to many other sources, this is borne out by two of the most eminently qualified researchers into the effects of dairy products. Both are medical doctors and have most impressive credentials. Dr. William A. Ellis, nearly eighty years old, has researched the effects of dairy products for over forty years; Dr. N. W. Walker, the author of eight books, researched nutrition and healthy living for eighty years and passed away in 1985 peacefully of natural causes at age 109. Both of these learned gentlemen have made only the most derogatory statements about dairy products. They have also reported the heart disease it causes—as well as severe chest pains. As Dr. Ellis points out, it has been known for 200 years that cheese is a major contributing cause of headaches. A study published in *Nature* magazine in July 6, 1974, shows that a protein found in many cheeses is responsible for migraine headaches. I have seen hundreds of people who stopped having headaches after discontinuing dairy products or simply by cutting back on them.

Do you have children? Has your child ever had an ear infection? Considering that they are thought to be a *normal* part of childhood by the medical profession and dietitians, I would be surprised if you said no. If your child did or does suffer from ear infections, I would be willing to give *any* odds that he or she eats dairy products or formula or both. In seventeen years I have yet to come across even *one* child who suffered from ear infections who did not eat dairy products. Here's how you can verify what I'm saying and at the same time save your precious child from further suffering: Remove all dairy products from the child's diet or dramatically cut down on them and watch what happens. After an initial period, during which the child may still have a runny nose and perhaps another ear infection as the body cleanses out the residue mucus, the runny nose will go away and stay away, and no further ear infections will occur. We have seen it happen literally *hundreds* of times. A child's body is very fast to react to positive changes. Stuffed-up runny noses, and ears that hurt to the point of tears are *not normal!*

Of course, you may be saying, "But, what about calcium?" You have been carefully manipulated and hundreds of millions of dollars have been spent to get you to have just that reaction. Worry not. I will address that issue shortly and allay your fears. And fear is exactly what is wielded against you to get you to consume dairy products in the first place. Think of it. What better advertising ploy is there than to get you to think that without a certain product you will suffer deficiencies, pain, and misery? Fear is an effective ploy that has been used for decades to get people to act a certain way to achieve a desired outcome. Most frequently the outcome is bad for your health but good for business.

A case in point: During the mid-twenties, when there was a lot of smallpox vaccinating going on, quite a few people opted not to vaccinate themselves or their children because of the number of deaths that the vaccinations were causing (similar to our present-day swine flu fiasco). So the best strategy known was used. Fear. The following declaration by Dr. John P. Keller, Commissioner of Health of Milwaukee, Wisconsin, appeared in an article in the *Wisconsin Medical Journal* of November 1925:

> Since people cannot be vaccinated against their will, the biggest job of a health department has always been and always will be to persuade the unprotected people to get vaccinated. This we attempted to do in three ways: First, by education; Second, by fright; and, Third, by pressure. We dislike very much to mention fright and pressure. Yet, they accomplish more than education because they work faster than education, which is normally a slow process. During the months of March and April, we tried

education and vaccinated only 62,000. During May, we made use of fright and pressure and vaccinated 223,000 people.

Remember, dairy products are high in cholesterol and fat, and contain *no* fiber—a bad combination according to everyone and anyone who knows anything at all about nutrition. Strange, isn't it, that dietitians and nutritionists so adamantly praise dairy products, *knowing* that high-fat, low-fiber foods are counter productive. What further proof do they require? Whose needs are they looking out for, anyway?

Despite overwhelming scientific fact, basic common sense, and clear logic, successful advertising by the dairy industry and the promptings of dietitians and nutritionists hired by them have somehow convinced us that calves' food is essential for human survival.

There are two elements in dairy products that have to be broken down by enzymes in the body: lactose and casein. Lactose is broken down by the enzyme lactase, and casein is broken down by the enzyme rennin. By age three or four rennin is nonexistent in the human digestive tract and, in all but a small number of people, so is lactase. The term *lactose intolerance* is thrown around as if it were some rare occurrence that manifests only on occasion. In fact, *over 98 percent of the population is lactose intolerant*, for they have no lactase. But instead of recognizing this as part of nature's grand scheme and discontinuing foods that demand lactase (all dairy products), the pharmaceutical companies get right in there and start advertising chemical preparations that you can ingest to help break down the lactose. As if the public were not already ingesting enough drugs, (OVER 25 MILLION PILLS AN *HOUR*) more have to be produced to help us move something through our bodies that doesn't even belong there in the first place. Mother Nature does everything in her power to help us recognize that.

Casein is the protein component in milk. It is a very thick, coarse substance and used to make one of the strongest wood glues known. Glue sandwich, anyone? There is *300 percent* more casein in cow's milk than in human milk. The by-products of the bacterial decomposition of casein end up in thick, ropelike mucus that sticks to mucous membranes and clogs our bodies. The human body plainly has *no* digestive mechanisms to break it down. We referred earlier to Dr. N. W. Walker, recognized throughout the world as an authority on this subject and an expert on the glandular system.

His studies convinced him that the growth of goiter in the throat and other dysfunctions of the thyroid gland were the direct result of casein from cow's milk. He specifically pointed out that the problem is considerably *compounded* when dairy products are pasteurized! (We'll discuss the hoax of pasteurization shortly.)

For years ulcer sufferers were advised to consume milk to ease the pain. Natural Hygienists voiced their disbelief of such absurd advice from the beginning, knowing that acid-forming foods are the *worst* thing for an ulcer sufferer, and all dairy products except butter are acid forming. The Natural Hygienists were at first scoffed at by the elite credentialed health "experts," but check with medical professionals or dietitians today and they will now agree with the very hygienists they used to attack. Dairy products aggravate ulcers. (171, 199, 272)

Ulcerative colitis is another extremely painful and uncomfortable ailment. Frequently it is a precursor of colon cancer. Dairy products not only contribute to colitis, but removal of dairy products from the diet results in a dramatic improvement of colitis. (317, 382, 419) And, as stated earlier, dairy products, in common with all other high-protein foods, are a major contributing factor to colon cancer.

A recent study in Italy indicates that death from prostate cancer is about 60 percent higher in the north than in the south. Frequent consumption of milk and cheese was found to be a risk factor. (370)

Sudden infant death syndrome (SIDS) is a particularly heartbreaking tragedy. A small, innocent newborn baby goo-gooing and gaa-gaaing one moment is dead the next. While SIDS can't be blamed on any one cause, dairy products are unquestionably partially to blame. (100, 242, 280, 390) I realize that bit of information will not make mothers very happy, especially those who have unfortunately lost their child to SIDS, but the evidence is there and it must be looked at.

Actually, the list of ailments that can be linked to dairy products is so extensive there is hardly a problem it doesn't at least contribute to. One book that presents a most convincing and thorough indictment of dairy products is *Don't Drink Your Milk*, by Oski and Bell. Included in the host of diseases and maladies the authors attribute at least in part to dairy products, many of which have been discussed here, are Lou Gehrig's disease and multiple sclerosis. Multiple sclerosis is most frequently found in areas of the world where children are raised on dairy products rather than breast milk. (7, 21) A low-animal fat diet used for thirty years by a medical doctor at the University of Oregon has dramatically helped multiple sclerosis patients. (367)

Were it not for modern technology, all mammals would simply feed their young, and, once weaned, *all* would then go on to exist on the foods they are biologically adapted to. In the wild, milk drinking is not an issue; it is only an issue for that one mammal too ''smart'' to trust nature's plan. Of course, a big business is looking out for its profits and doing what it can to perpetuate the myth that cow's milk is an appropriate food for humans.

Before he became a highly paid consultant on nutrition to the National Dairy Products Company, Professor E. V. McCollum stressed the fact that milk is *not* an essential in the diet of man. (See the earlier editions of his book *The Newer Knowledge of Nutrition*.) He pointed out that the inhabitants of southern Asia never drink milk. Their diet is made up of rice, soybeans, sweet potatoes, bamboo sprouts, and other vegetables. According to Professor McCollum, these people are exceptional for the development of their physique and endurance, and their capacity to work is exceptional. They escape skeletal defects in childhood and have the finest teeth of any people in the world. This is a sharp and favorable contrast with milk drinking peoples. Unfortunately, the professor found it expedient to delete these facts from all editions of his work published subsequent to his becoming a consultant to the National Dairy Products Company. Truth must be suppressed when and if it threatens profits and salaries. (336) This is the sad truth of life in the U.S. Again, the health of the people is sacrificed for the almighty dollar.

THE PASTEURIZATION FRAUD

What if I were to tell you that there exists a special bomb that, if dropped during wartime on a city where fighting was going on, would kill only the enemy and leave our allies unscathed. Would you believe me or think I was lying? What if I were to tell you that I could take a food with some good ingredients and some bad ingredients and heat it to a temperature so hot that it would kill the bad (our enemies) and leave the good (our allies) unscathed? Would you believe that? Lies are odd things. If you tell one big enough, loud enough, long enough, and often enough, people will come to believe it as truth. Indeed they will. *Indeed they have!* Because a great big, whopping lie has been told very loudly, very often, and for a very long time and the public has come to accept it as truth. What's the lie? It's the second example given above —pasteurization.

Anyone who tells you pasteurized milk is safer than raw milk is either out and out lying or exhibiting the most classic example of how far in the sand someone is willing to bury his or her head for the sake of some funding or a paycheck. Pasteurization is plainly and simply one of the biggest hoaxes ever to have been foisted on an unsuspecting people. There is enough evidence proving this to be true to easily fill this book many times over. Pasteurization has been so convincingly sold that the very people it hurts jump to its defense. What is most galling is that the people responsible for pasteurization actually accuse others of what they themselves are guilty of. Remember those old westerns in which the villain would commit a dastardly deed then cause the hero to be blamed, actually leading the indignant townsfolk against the hero to have him brought to justice? The villain was the most outspoken accuser. When I was a kid watching those things on television, I'd become so frustrated that I'd yell to whoever would listen, "Hey, no fair, the bad guy did it and he's blaming the good guy!" The poeple behind pasteurization must have *written* those scripts.

The truth is that the problems associated with drinking milk are much more pronounced with pasteurized milk than with raw milk, and still the pasteurizers are pointing an accusing finger at others. Hey, no fair!

Let me be clear on one thing: I don't think milk, raw or pasteurized, should be consumed by *anyone* interested in a healthy life, but the idea that pasteurized is somehow superior in some way to raw is too absurd for words. Take any food or plant abounding with life and heat it to intense temperatures and what is the result? *It dies!* Enzymes, the life principle of every living cell, are killed at 130 degrees. Milk is pasteurized at over 170 degrees. Subject a slice of watermelon to 170 degrees and there will not be anything of value left in it. It will be killed. Subject a plant from your yard—a rose or a violet—to 170 degrees, and it will meet the same fate, death. Subject a handful of fresh sprouts teeming with life to 170 degrees and you will get the same results.

It's the journey's end, curtains, the portals of no return, the Grim Reaper, DEATH!

When milk flows from a cow's udder, it is alive with the raw materials of life for the calf. Pasteurize the milk at 170 degrees and the same thing happens to it that happens to the watermelon or the plant or the sprout. *It is made dead!* As we demonstrated in chapter 8, **DEAD FOOD CANNOT SUPPORT LIFE.** Pasteurization kills.

The entire purpose of pasteurizing milk was ostensibly to supply a *clean* product. In the late 1800s, as the demand grew for more and more milk, it was becoming dirtier and dirtier. People were becoming sick, even dying, so there was a big push to *clean up* milk. But the opposite of dirty is *not* pasteurized; the opposite of dirty is *clean*. Pasteurized milk is not automatically clean. It can be as dirty as any other kind of milk. The problem, at least with raw milk, is that if it goes bad, it immediately sours and you throw it away. When it is pasteurized, it can also go bad—but it doesn't sour. *It rots!* It turns putrid, and there isn't a dairy farmer on earth that doesn't know that. Unfortunately, when it's pasteurized, you can't *tell* when it's beginning to spoil! So the chances of drinking contaminated pasteurized milk are much greater than when drinking raw milk. Pasteurized milk is rancid *long before* it develops an obvious odor.

The need for pure milk was no small issue. People were clamoring to clean up the dairies. Understand? They wanted *the dairies* cleaned up so they could supply fresh, clean, *raw* milk. People had been drinking raw milk for hundreds of years, and they liked it. They opposed this newfangled idea of pasteurization. They didn't want anybody messing with their milk. They just wanted it cleaned up. But, if it were pasteurized, supposedly the issue of cleanliness would be resolved. People did not like the heated milk because it did not have the same flavor. It tasted awful.

The death knell for raw milk came when those with business and marketing talents realized the advantages of having milk that would not sour. Hey, hey! They could produce more milk, store it, even *ship* it, and it wouldn't go sour. This was major good news—for business. Not for people's health. Of course, it wouldn't make sense to ask people to go along with pasteurization because it was good for business. So the push for pasteurization came under the guise of killing off all the malevolent beasties in the milk, making it healthier. Never mind that when the bad was killed so was the good. The people *still* didn't want pasteurization. They didn't like the taste and didn't trust the idea of it. So it was big business versus the people. Guess who won? Take your time. Don't rush. I know what a tough question that is.

Pasteurization began in 1895. The worry of cleanliness was no longer an issue because, with the heating of milk, cleanliness was no longer considered necessary. Not that you couldn't get raw milk—you could. The Medical Milk Commission, a group of physicians that inspected and "certified" raw milk to make sure it met very rigid standards of safety, was established. By 1930, clean *un*pasteurized milk was readily available throughout the country.

Interestingly enough, the dairy industry itself also fought compulsory pasteurization. They fought it in court—and lost! (41) But they've gotten over it now and they're pretty happy about pasteurization after all. Why not? In less than a hundred years the milk industry has come from almost total obscurity to become the Goliath of the food industry. And they owe it all to pasteurization. Guess who else was against pasteurization. *The dietitians!* Honest! Realizing that commercial interests were only concerned about shelf life and not about unadulterated milk, they *strongly* opposed pasteurization. Where are they today? Well, they haven't left the side of the dairy industry. They were there fighting pasteurization with the industry when they *knew* it was wrong, but now that things have worked out—financially, that is—they're ferociously supporting the very process they used to assail. So you see, they once actually knew what they were talking about.

Before continuing, let me share a few statements made by the people who were trying the best they could to protect themselves against pasteurization during the 1930s.

These notes are taken from the *Vaccination Enquirer*, a periodical that was published in England from the early 1900s through the mid-1900s. The first is from April 1, 1932. "Pasteurizing made milk dangerous and not safe. Pasteurizing might be necessary, it might even be good, but it could never make bad milk into good milk." In an editorial in that same issue: "Is it not appalling to reflect that bureaucracy and medical despotism have marched hand in hand to the point where a citizen, for the first time in the history of the world, may be unable to procure natural milk drawn directly from a healthy cow under all clean precautions and will have to consume only milk which has been treated and doctored in accordance with the changing medical dogmas and prescriptions of the hour. We can only hope our friends in Parliament, though reduced in number, may find the means to offer a determined, and may we hope, successful opposition to this monstrous and insufferable innovation.'' Wasn't exactly welcomed with open arms there, now was it?

The following quote was taken from the same periodical, the *Vaccination Enquirer*, from June 1, 1938. A correspondent wrote, ''It is amazing to me that so much professional propaganda should be devoted to discrediting raw milk which, provided it is clean, must be the state in which nature has given man its maximum virtues. Proof of this comes within my own knowledge. Salt Coates Town Council some years ago, in a fit of enthusiasm, started a milk factory from which they sold only pasteurized milk. In due course, there was an epidemic of trouble amongst infants in the town who were being fed on this milk. Mothers and doctors were at their wits end as to the cause until a general return to raw milk, straight from the farms and retailed in the town, coincided with thriving children. Needless to say, the pasteurizing plant soon disappeared but such evidence is perhaps too simple to impress scholastic minds worshipping theories.''

Another article in the June 1, 1938, edition cited a letter to *The Daily Telegraph*: ''The Honorable Mrs. Lionel Guest, who had kept cows for ten years in Canada and ten years in England, says cats and dogs, unless almost starving, refuse pasteurized milk. Even rats will not drink it willingly and they are not famous epicures. Practically all pasteurized milk is stale milk disguised. It never sours properly but gets rancid. Nowadays too, cows are inoculated with so much anti-this and anti-that that the milk is made nasty.''

From the issue of March 1, 1937: ''[The Cattle Diseases Committee] reported that the reduction of the Vitamin C content of milk due to pasteurization may have serious effects on young children if uncorrected by the addition of fruit juice and that pasteurization is supported by the whole weight of great commercial interests who cannot dispense with it.'' As you can see, they knew why it was being done.

One last quote, from the issue of September 1, 1939: ''Dr. Marie Stopes had a very fine article on milk in *The Daily Mirror* dated 9 June, 1939. It read partially, 'A chain of circumstances has resulted in a recent push for pasteurization which is an acute menace to everyone in the country. Big commercial interests are behind the pasteurization. Only individual efforts stand up against it, so naturally the public is being made ready to accept what I quite seriously describe as a pernicious poison. It may not injure you rapidly, but it will do so in due course. That pasteurized milk does not even go honestly bad is one of its dangers. When fresh milk goes bad, you know at once that it is bad by its taste and smell. Commercial interests are of course pushing for pasteurization, for to them it means the legalized right to sell stale milk. After pasteurization, it is supposed to be safe. It is not. I quite sincerely describe it as a pernicious poison.' '' They knew what was going on, as did a lot of people in the United States, yet you know who won out.

Dr. N. W. Walker, the 109-year-old gentleman referred to earlier, was adamantly opposed to pasteurization, calling it commercialism and calling the claims that it prevents disease "unmitigated falsehoods." In his book *Diet and Salad Suggestions*, he reported 12 *deaths* attributed directly to pasteurized milk in San Francisco in 1928. In 1927, in Montreal, Canada, 533 deaths occurred from pasteurized milk.

Dr. William Ellis, who has researched the subject for forty-two years, says that pasteurization destroys valuable enzymes, making pasteurized milk much worse than raw. One ten-year study proved conclusively that pasteurized milk was a primary contributor to all forms of heart disease. In 1945 there were 450 cases of infectious disease caused by raw milk. There were *1492* caused by pasteurized milk. (257) In June 1982, more than 170 people in three states in the southeast United States developed an intestinal infection causing severe diarrhea, fever, nausea, abdominal pain, and headache. Over 100 were hospitalized. The cause? Pasteurized milk. (34)

Pasteurized milk is frequently touted as essential for good teeth. A study with rats whose tooth decay process is biologically identical to human teeth indicates otherwise. The rats were separated into three groups. The first group received a standard rat chow made by Purina. They averaged less than one cavity for their entire lifetime. The second group was fed a very heavy refined sugar diet. They averaged five and a half cavities per rat. The third group was fed pasteurized milk, and they had nine and a half cavities each, *almost twice that of the sugar-fed group*! (359) In the *Lancet* during the 1930s, it was reported that children's teeth are less likely to decay on a diet incorporating raw milk rather than pasteurized. (168) In the same journal, it was reported that chilblain, a very prevalent malady that causes terrible itching and rashes in children, was practically eliminated when their milk was not pasteurized.

And again in that same journal, it was reported that *resistance* to tuberculosis increased in children fed raw milk instead of pasteurized to the point that in five years only one case of tuberculosis had developed among them, whereas in the previous five years, when the children had been given pasteurized milk, fourteen cases of tuberculosis had developed. Another study in 1933 demonstrated statistically that children's growth was significantly greater when they drank raw milk than when they drank pasteurized milk. (211)

Dogs fed pasteurized milk developed mange and other disorders. Litters fed on raw milk thrived. When an English physician fed puppies and kittens just pasteurized milk, they died. Puppies and kittens fed on raw milk thrived. (336) But here is the one that tops them all: *Calves fed on pasteurized milk died before maturity in nine out of ten cases*. (245, 344) Calves! The very animal the milk is designed for—the *only* animal it is designed for—can't live on it if it's pasteurized. Now, you think *that* over for a while. Pasteurized milk kills.

There is one long-term study that so clearly proves the disease-producing nature of pasteurized milk that I've saved it for last. Not only was it conducted by someone enormously well respected and well known for his clinical studies, but also the nature of the study leaves no doubt as to the destructiveness of milk that has been heated. The study is the same one we referred to in chapter 8—the study conducted by Dr. Francis M. Pottenger on 900 cats. Please reread the results of this study (on page 111), which conclude with a devastating indictment of cooked food. If you recall, the animals were fed only two foods, either cooked or raw. I intentionally did not mention what the two foods were so the impact here would not be lost. The two foods were *meat* and *milk*. When these were given raw, the animals thrived. When the same foods were cooked, cats became diseased and died.

Here comes the knockout blow. *Even when the meat was left raw and only the milk was heated, the same symptoms of degeneration occurred!* Dr. Pottenger conducted another test with three infants. One was breast-fed. One was fed raw milk. The third was fed pasteurized milk. The first two infants were healthy and developed normally. The third was sickly, small, and developed asthma at the age of eight months. (336) These findings cannot possibly leave any doubt in the minds of anyone willing to look at the evidence *honestly* and objectively. Pasteurized milk is dangerous and destructive. It causes disease. It has not one redeeming quality. All it does is mask spoiled milk so that big business can make some *big* money.

Of course, the public is not told that pasteurization is necessary in order to satisfy commercial interests. No! They have to be convinced that it's healthier—or, better yet, scared to the point that they actually demand it be pasteurized. How's that for irony? People have been duped into demanding something that destroys their own health. A carefully orchestrated smoke screen has been used to scare people into thinking that pasteurization actually affords them protection from something as common as salmonella. People have been led to believe that this is some sort of horrific entity residing only in raw milk and will "do you in" if you get any in your body. Well, that's a big fat load of bull. First of all, salmonella is just about everywhere. It's in your carpeting. It's in your hair. It's in your nose. And it is in your digestive tract. It is also in a great deal of your food. In fact, call up the Center for Disease Control in Atlanta, Georgia, and ask them where it is most common. They will tell you in meat and in chicken. So you are probably eating some salmonella every day if you're not a vegetarian.

Secondly, pasteurization is no guarantee that salmonella won't be in your milk anyway. In October 1978 there was an epidemic of salmonella food poisoning in Arizona. It affected sixty-six people and was caused by *pasteurized* milk. The bacteria level was twenty-three times the legal limit. And the Center for Disease Control reported that the milk had been properly pasteurized. (262)

Nature intended all milk to be consumed raw. Every animal in nature consumes it that way—except us, of course. The way it flows from each specific animal's breasts (or udder) is the way the Grand Creator designed it to be consumed. To pasteurize it is to adulterate it and strip it of its value. **DAIRY PRODUCTS, IF EATEN AT ALL, SHOULD BE CONSUMED RAW—BUT CLEAN!** If raw milk is "certified" as clean, it can be *safer* than pasteurized, because pasteurization does not mean clean, it means *heated. A pasteurized product can still be dirty.* Dirty milk means just that. It could have hair, soot, dust, dirt, dung, perspiration, or small insects in it. Pasteurization will not remove any of these. Dirty milk, raw *or* pasteurized, is a clear danger. The real issue should be cleanliness, but the real issue has been buried under an avalanche of self-serving propaganda. It is an insult and an affront to the public's intelligence to suggest that nature's purpose and intent is wrong and that the dairy industry and the "health" professionals it employs are right—that nature's purpose is somehow inferior to that of the dairy industry. All the talk and confusion and statistics and scare tactics and blustering of the "experts" will never alter the fact that nature *cannot* be improved upon, and to perpetuate the myth that it can is arrogance and ignorance of the highest order.

WHAT ABOUT CALCIUM?

Now let's address the burning question that is on the tip of everyone's tongue: "Where do I get my calcium? Do you expect me to let my bones shatter like dry twigs from osteoporosis?"

You'll be interested to know that a multibillion-dollar industry has been built around the issue of calcium. Fear and misinformation are being spread like a bad rumor. Be aware that everything you're hearing about calcium is *not* accurate, nor is it altogether honest. In just the last two or three years, as a result of major media coverage, the issue of osteoporosis has grown from an occasionally discussed subject to a raging monster. Women, in particular, have been made to feel that without taking extra calcium into their bodies every day, they can *count* on suffering from osteoporosis sooner or later. The dairy industry has spent many millions of dollars telling people that the best, most surefire way to prevent osteoporosis is to drink at least three eight-ounce glasses of milk a day, plus load up on as many other dairy products as can be crammed into the stomach. They tell you that for the sole purpose of assisting you in achieving a high level of health. And, if you believe *that*, perhaps you'd like to invest in a land development project being planned in the southern Everglades.

There are many ironies in life. There are many in the field of health. There are many in this book. But here is the irony to end all ironies. We are ceaselessly being beseeched to consume dairy products to combat osteoporosis, while **DAIRY PRODUCTS ARE A MAJOR CAUSE OF OSTEOPOROSIS!**

I know, it's too bizarre to believe, yet there is indisputable evidence to corroborate this most disturbing revelation. I am not just making it up. There is a *huge* body of scientific data that directly conflicts with the one-sided, self-serving propaganda being circulated by the dairy industry. Of course, I can totally understand the industry doing and saying anything it possibly can to perpetuate this flagrant distortion of the truth. After all, business is business. What I find absolutely inconceivable is that dietitians and nutritionists, who *should* know better, also insist that dairy products help overcome osteoporosis. This is an outrage. Could so many of them truly not be aware of the *many* studies reported *in their own journals and textbooks* proving otherwise? That is too preposterous to believe.

There are three issues of importance concerning osteoporosis: (1) What is it? (2) What causes it? (3) What can be done to prevent it?

First, what is osteoporosis?

Your bones are made up of a number of elements. The two most prevalent minerals in bones and teeth are calcium and phosphorus, which are deposited into a protein-rich material to form the structure of bone. Calcium is lost from the structure of the bones for various reasons. It literally leaves the bones. Over time, if a sufficient amount is lost, the bones become porous and brittle and can break with the least provocation. A sneeze can break a rib. Going over a bumpy road can cause a hip fracture. Even a friendly hug can cause a bone to break, so fragile do they become if sufficient calcium is lost. Think of a plank of wood—strong when solid but if worm-eaten, you can break it by barely tapping it. So it is with bones deficient in calcium. It is as if they were worm-eaten.

Osteoporosis is an extremely serious problem for a great number of people. Between 15 and 20 million people are affected by it in the United States. (99) Some 15,000 people *die* from hip fractures alone each year.

Osteoporosis has become a $4 billion industry in the United States. The calcium supplement pushers are in heaven. Practically out of the clear blue sky comes this windfall of millions of women who have been whipped into a frenzy of fear, clamoring for calcium. All of a sudden calcium supplementation is the latest selling tool for products. It used to be "new and improved"; now it's "with calcium added"—magic words to make the cash registers ring. You can get antacids with calcium, laxatives with calcium, soft drinks with calcium, bread with calcium, cereal with calcium, flour with calcium, vitamin pills with calcium. I'm waiting for one of those car salesmen who come on television screaming, "Hurry on down and take advantage of these prices!" to conclude with " . . . and, the first five hundred people to buy a car this weekend will get a sack of powdered calcium thrown in." As you will see shortly, these calcium supplements do more harm than good.

What causes osteoporosis? As is true with many other afflictions, there is no one cause. There are many variables that together contribute to the end results of impairment. And so it is with osteoporosis. It would be just grand if osteoporosis could be avoided by one simple measure such as adding calcium to the diet. Although on the surface that would seem to be just the solution, it's not. In fact, studies have shown quite clearly that so long as the factors that cause calcium loss from the bones are continued, even very high doses of calcium supplements have no benefit. (17, 25, 90, 143, 234, 260, 269, 329, 362, 405, 416) Think about it. A multimillion-dollar industry is out pushing calcium supplements when the evidence is already in: *They don't help*! In fact, they hurt! Most of these supplements are cooked bone meal or dolomite, and many contain harmful amounts of lead, arsenic, mercury, and other toxic metals. (309)

The body's need for calcium is filled quite easily, believe it or not—a lot more easily than most people realize. Once that need is met, that's it! Adding more doesn't help. If you have an eight-ounce glass and a full pitcher of juice, once you've filled the glass to the brim it won't take any more. That's it. No exceptions. If you continue to pour the juice into the full glass, it will only spill onto the floor and be wasted. That old saw "If a little is good, a lot is better" is a bunch of flotsam. Yes, it would *seem* to be so, and that seemingly apparent formula is precisely what the supplement pushers use to get you to load up your body with more calcium than it can possibly use. But, unlike the spilled juice, which is just lost or cleaned up, the excess calcium in the body has some *very* serious consequences. It's been shown clearly that when calcium is lost from the bones, it is not just eliminated from the body. This calcium in the body is picked up by the blood and deposited in the soft tissues—the blood vessels, skin, eyes, joints, and internal organs. Calcium combines with fats and cholesterol in the blood vessels to cause hardening of the arteries. The calcium that ends up in the skin causes wrinkling. In the joints it crystallizes and forms very painful arthritic deposits. In the eyes it takes the form of cataracts. And in the kidneys it forms hard deposits known as kidney stones. (108, 117, 204, 249, 310) So don't think that taking extra calcium is an innocent precaution. It's not! It's disease producing!

So what does create the problem of osteoporosis? Several influences are to blame.

TOBACCO. This does not surprise me in the least, considering that tobacco so negatively affects so many other aspects of health. Why should it be different in this case? You see, one of the crucial roles calcium fulfills is to maintain a proper acid–alkali balance in the body. Minerals, including calcium, are needed to neutralize excess acid. Smoking is an exceedingly acid-producing habit. It is so important for the integrity of the body that this acid be neutralized that calcium is actually drained from the bones and teeth to meet this need. (110, 354)

ALCOHOL. Alcohol impairs calcium absorption by affecting the liver's ability to activate vitamin D. Vitamin D is important in the metabolism of calcium. The more alcohol you drink, the more you hinder your body's ability to build up and maintain healthy bones. (60, 354)

CAFFEINE. This drug, found in coffee, tea, soft drinks, chocolate, and many over-the-counter drugs, causes twice as much calcium to be excreted (eliminated from the body) as normal. This has been demonstrated in several studies. (146, 172, 243)

SOFT DRINKS. The culprit here is phosphoric acid, added to many soft drinks to keep bubbles from going flat. It is made by treating phosphorus with sulfuric acid. Does that sound like something you'd like to have come in contact with the sensitive lining of your stomach? Sulfuric acid, yum! Just another little caustic something brought to you by your friendly, concerned, and caring soft drink manufacturer.

It is important to understand that calcium does not act on its own in the body. The body uses calcium in concert with other minerals. Phosphorus plays a vital role. There should be a two-to-one ratio of calcium over phosphorus taken into the body. High-phosphorus diets cause a substantial rise in the level of phosphorus in the blood. In an effort to maintain the proper ratio of calcium to phosphorus in the blood, the body responds by removing calcium from the bones and releasing it into the bloodstream. If calcium did not buffer the excess phosphorus, the subsequent acid level in the blood would place one's life in danger. (In addition to soft drinks, guess what two other food groups have the most phosphorus? Right! Meat and dairy products! In fact, meat has twenty times more phosphorus than calcium. (146) Good old animal products. Cheeseburger, anyone?)

SALT. This acid substance is often a principal constituent of animal products, to say nothing of the tons of it we add to our own food and/or have added for us by the food processors. In one journal I found the perfect statement: "The equation is a simple one. The more sodium [salt] you take in, the more calcium you excrete." (298)

ANTACIDS. Some antacids contain aluminum, which causes an increase in calcium excretion. Those who are popping these "relief agents" throughout the day should be aware that they are causing a further calcium deficit.* (125) Also, hydrochloric acid helps absorb calcium in the stomach and antacids neutralize hydrochloric acid. (144) There's another good reason to start combining your foods properly.

INSUFFICIENT EXERCISE. It has clearly been shown that exercise increases bone mass, while lack of exercise causes bone loss. Of this there is no question and many studies prove this to be the case. (12, 18, 19, 120, 142, 173, 277, 352, 415) Exercise will even rebuild bones already affected by a loss of calcium. Bones are *alive* and react to exercise just as muscles do—they become stronger. Exercise and activity exert pressure upon the skeleton, and that in turn stimulates the formation of new bone. For more on exercise, refer to chapter 10.

---

*Antacids that contain aluminum include Rolaids, Amfogel, Digel, Gelusil, Maalox, Mylanta, Riopan, and Someco. There may be more, so check the labels. Of course, you can start to combine the foods you eat properly and thereby eliminate a need for any of them in the first place.

LACK OF SUNSHINE. Vitamin D plays an exremely important role in bone metabolism. Since the best source of vitamin D is sunshine, it doesn't take a lot to figure out that getting a little sun each day or so sure couldn't hurt your chances of preventing osteoporosis. (134, 146, 198, 210, 249)

THE NUMBER ONE CAUSE OF OSTEOPOROSIS. Now we come to the last cause of osteoporosis, the *major* cause, far and away more hurtful than any of those mentioned so far. This is truly the knockout punch, the crowning insult, the coup de grace, the death blow. Have you figured it out yet? Yes, it's that harbinger of disease: **animal products.** Had the people of this country not been so harassed, scared, bullied, threatened, bulldozed, coerced, intimidated, strong-armed, browbeaten, terrorized, and bludgeoned into gorging their bodies with hugely excessive amounts of protein from animal sources over the last half century, the last part of this chapter would not be necessary, because you would never even have heard of osteoporosis. Flesh foods and dairy products are the main reasons you *do* know what it is.

Because of propaganda fueled by commercial interests, we Americans are simply consuming far more protein than our bodies require, and *anyone* who has taken the time to look at research on the subject knows this to be true. Right now the World Health Organization's suggested minimum daily protein requirement is about 40 grams a day. The RDA is about 55 grams a day. On an average, Americans are now taking in over 100 grams a day! (53, 223, 250) The shocker is that it's been shown that we can fare very, very well indeed on *less than 30 grams per day*! (119, 166, 175, 186, 223, 225, 250, 251, 313) The World Health Organization and the RDA recognize this, too, but they nearly double that figure to add a "margin of safety." The margin of safety adds about 30 to 50 percent to our real needs to compensate for any *possible* needs that *some* may have for more protein. This is then doubled, and the result is that *everyone* is told to consume more than *twice* the protein actually needed by the body. It has been proven that far less protein is necessary to sustain life, and it is quite simple to verify.

Unfortunately, the idea that we need so much more protein is based on tests conducted three-quarters of a century ago on rats. (276) These same tests, long since disproved, are still the basis for today's ridiculously high recommendations. When weight is taken into consideration, an adult rat requires three and a half times more protein than an adult human. (68) The protein concentration in the breast milk of rats is ten times greater than that of human breast milk, which is only 2 percent protein. (49) *We are not rats!* That notwithstanding, we are admonished to stuff ourselves with much more protein than we need every day and, of course, we are led to believe that animal products are the best source of protein, when it has been demonstrated over and over again that a diet totally devoid of animal products can supply us with all we need. (1, 2, 15, 32, 65, 85, 92, 112, 122, 126, 167, 176, 178, 191, 209, 211, 212, 228, 250, 282, 303, 322, 383, 418)

Here's the killer, and I do mean *killer*. What do you think happens to all the excess protein? First, it is broken down into amino acids, some of which are metabolized in the liver and excreted through the kidneys as urea. With the urea and amino acids excreted into urine go large amounts of minerals. (324) One of the minerals lost is calcium! **STUDIES SHOW THAT THE MORE PROTEIN YOU CONSUME, THE MORE CALCIUM YOU LOSE!** (17, 25, 64, 88, 105, 146, 177, 179, 203, 233, 234, 241, 249, 250, 393, 405, 409)

One of today's greatest researchers into the effects of animal products on every aspect of our health, including osteoporosis, is John A. McDougall, M.D., Assistant Clinical Professor at the University of Hawaii School of Medicine. Dr. McDougall has not received nearly the recognition he deserves. His two books, *The McDougall Plan*, and *McDougall's Medicine*, should be required reading for anyone entering the health professions, to say nothing of the lay person. Between these two books he has over 1600 references to back up his work, which is some of the most eye-opening material you'll ever read on this subject. Why isn't his name more widely recognized? For one thing, he's not on the payroll of the National Livestock and Meat Board or the National Dairy Council.

In Dr. McDougall's words,

> The calcium losing effect of protein on the human body is not an area of controversy in scientific circles. The many studies performed during the past fifty-five years consistently show that the most important dietary change

that we can make if we want to create a positive calcium balance that will keep our bones solid is to decrease the amount of protein we eat each day. (20)

In 1930, the first study was published that showed that in humans, a diet with a high meat content caused the loss of large amounts of calcium and a negative calcium balance. (247) And yet, fifty-five years later, our learned medical authorities are still pondering the cause of osteoporosis.

I know thousands of people must be asking, "Why aren't the authorities reading these studies if they are, in fact, in their own journals?" We are constantly wondering the same thing.

To me the simple, commonsense arguments are far more important and of far more impact than all the scientific studies combined. As I said before, you can manipulate statistics until they say whatever you want them to, but common sense hits you in a place that *can't* be manipulated. Eskimos consume one of the highest protein diets in the world. They sometimes consume over 400 grams a day. Eskimos also have one of the highest incidences of osteoporosis in the world! (244) They are already stooped over in their mid-twenties.

When one considers that this fact is reported in the *American Journal of Clinical Nutrition*, the nutritionists' *own* journal, it kind of makes you wonder what the dietitians and nutritionists who insist we have to eat lots of protein to avoid osteoporosis have been doing with their time and who's paying for that time. Those "experts" who insist that dairy products *must* be eaten for calcium or our bones will crumble like dry leaves might want to skip over the next couple of paragraphs—unless, of course, they can keep from going into convulsions at the prospect of having to tell the truth about dairy products.

The people of the United States consume more dairy products than any other country in the world, a whopping 75 *billion* pounds a year. That is more than 300 pounds for every man, woman, and child in this country. That's a lot of mucus. Here's where we might lose a few of our "experts," because you'll need some common sense to appreciate this. If dairy products really did help avoid osteoporosis, we should have *none*—or precious little—considering the astonishing amount of dairy products we consume. But despite the public's consuming astronomical amounts of dairy products, osteoporosis is getting *worse*. Why? It's right before our eyes. Year after year we consume billions of pounds of dairy products yet we have more osteoporosis than ever before. It doesn't take a Ph.D. to draw some fairly incriminating conclusions about the so-called benefits of the dairy products we've had stuffed down our throats over the years. How much more obvious could it possibly be? If you smashed your thumb with a hammer and it became all purple and sore, what would you think of someone who told you to smash it again to make it feel better?

Now, this will have to shake some of these dietitians out of their world of self-deception and into the world of reality. When the problem of osteoporosis is studied worldwide, one is struck by the fact that the highest incidence of osteoporosis is in countries where dairy products and calcium supplements are consumed in the greatest quantities (the United States, Sweden, Finland, and the United Kingdom). The incidence of osteoporosis is lowest in the countries where the least amount of dairy products is consumed (the Asian and African countries). (231, 385, 386, 396) Where protein consumption is highest, osteoporosis is most common. (231, 357, 385, 386, 397) A number of studies have been done among the Bantu women of Africa. They consume less than half the protein of Americans and have a life-style demanding large amounts of calcium (nursing up to ten children in a lifetime), yet osteoporosis is almost unknown among them. (357, 397, 398)

In researching this chapter, I could not help but be shocked at the enormity of the evidence indicting flesh foods and dairy products as the number one cause of osteoporosis. It astounds me that whoever is responsible for keeping the truth of the matter hidden from the general population has managed to do so for so long. And calcium supplements simply make the situation *worse*! (90, 260, 269, 329, 362) It's clear as clear can be that the calcium depleting effects of protein are not lessened even when *large* doses of calcium are ingested. **OSTEOPOROSIS IS NOT DUE TO A DEFICIENCY OF CALCIUM IN THE DIET!** (17, 25, 177, 179, 203, 233, 308, 405) I repeat: **OSTEOPOROSIS IS NOT DUE TO A DEFICIENCY OF CALCIUM IN THE DIET.** There can be no doubt about it. The "literature" is very definite in revealing that calcium deficiencies due to insufficient calcium from a *natural* diet simply do not occur. (157, 285, 369, 396) Spreading the fear that one can't get sufficient calcium without the consumption of dairy products is an unpardonable fraud, a lie perpetuated in the quest for profits rather than out of a genuine concern for people's health.

Where do you get calcium?

Calcium is found in all foods that grow from the ground. They easily supply a sufficient amount of calcium to meet the requirements of both growing children and adults. **CALCIUM COMES FROM SOIL THAT PLANTS ABSORB AND INCORPORATE INTO THEIR STRUCTURE.** Animals consume the plants and absorb the calcium. *That's where the cow gets calcium!* Cows don't consume dairy products and yet they have all the calcium they need. How is this? How is it that cows have no difficulty whatsoever in meeting all of the calcium requirements for themselves *and* their young without ever having to consume even one glass of milk? When confronted with commonsense questions like this, the dietitians who steadfastly insist that we can't also get calcium from the plant kingdom break the land speed record shifting to another subject! It's been established clearly that green leafy vegetables are a prime source of utilizable calcium in human nutrition. (16, 26, 146, 249, 336, 416) In addition, all raw nuts and seeds, grains, beans, fresh fruit, dried fruit, and vegetables have calcium. Statements that we can't meet calcium needs by a diet devoid of dairy products are outright fibbery, unqualified falsehoods, out and out lies! Remember, researchers have determined that calcium deficiencies don't occur among individuals on a natural diet.

Don't be misled by shameless commercial interests. No animal anywhere in nature consumes dairy products after weaning . . . and osteoporosis is not an issue in the wild. Osteoporosis is unique to the human species. The only exceptions are animals *under the care of humans.* (286)

As a point of interest, besides phosphorus, which we discussed on page 258, another mineral much involved with calcium utilization is magnesium. Magnesium is needed for the absorption of calcium. It is used by the body to transport calcium to the bones. If you had to cross a river and had no boat, you couldn't get to the other side. Even if you brought ten more people to the shore with you, you still would be in need of a boat. The extra people would do you no good. There would just be eleven people stranded instead of one. So it is with magnesium and calcium. Without the magnesium to transport the calcium to the bones, you can swallow a bucketful of calcium to no avail. It will circulate in the body, with no "boat" to take it to its destination, and settle in the soft tissues, causing the many problems described earlier.

The body needs twice as much calcium as magnesium, but most people consume far more calcium than that. Because there is so much more calcium in our diets than magnesium, it's been shown that, when the average person's total calcium intake is *lessened*, more calcium is actually utilizable because of the closer balance with magnesium. How does that grab you? A *low*-calcium diet may actually help guard you against osteoporosis. Too much calcium, on the other hand, blocks the absorption of magnesium. (204) And dairy products, which are high in calcium and phosphorus, are a very poor source of magnesium. (Too many people, no boat!) *Studies also show that an increase in dietary magnesium raises both calcium and magnesium levels.* (70) This is because the increase of magnesium puts its relationship with calcium into a better balance. Then, *without* increasing calcium intake, the calcium in the body is more efficiently utilized. (146, 179, 195, 249, 250, 259, 416)

Another extremely important factor in calcium utilization is a substance called calcitriol.* This substance circulates in the body and controls and protects calcium. Low-calcium intakes raise circulating levels of calcitriol and improve the efficiency of calcium absorption. High intakes of calcium *depress* calcitriol formation so the calcium is inefficiently used. (177) That is why calcium deficiencies are so rare throughout the world wherever calcium intake is low. So this big push to get you to consume so much calcium is actually aggravating the problem, and contributing to osteoporosis. With all of the variables discussed in this chapter which play a role in the calcium/osteoporosis connection, to suggest consuming dairy products for more calcium as a preventative measure represents a lack of understanding of the situation that borders on idiocy.

One other mineral employed to scare you into consuming more dairy products than you can use is iron. Iron is in many fruits, all green leafy vegetables, corn, beans, wheat and many other vegetables. One recent U.S. study points out that, while there is iron in milk, only 5 to 10 percent of it is available to the body, and infants fed on cow's milk can actually suffer iron deficiency anemia.**

*This hormone is produced in the body as a result of Vitamin D absorption.
***Pediatrics*, Volume 75, 1985, page 182.

I know a lot of people are wondering why health professionals and industry have chosen to ignore the direct link between animal products and calcium loss and osteoporosis, instead condoning and recommending calcium supplements that have been shown to be useless. Look at the expense of meat, dairy products, and calcium supplements. If huge numbers of people were to find out the truth and start to rely less and less on these products and more and more on natural sources of calcium—fruit, vegetables, nuts, and seeds—it would present great economic hardship to these industries. I know it's sad that it has to come down to profits versus health, but we are talking here about a monumentally vast amount of money. Let us not be naïve. People will compromise themselves for the old green stuff, and there is no better example of that than the attempt by the dairy industry and it's hired mouthpieces to convince you to continue using its products despite a mountain of evidence proving they contribute to osteoporosis!

CUT DOWN ON DISEASE!

As I stated earlier in this chapter, representatives from the dairy industry have expressed outrage at our contention in **Fit for Life** that dairy products may not be as good a food as we've been led to believe. Now that I have shown that dairy products are worse than not good, *they are downright harmful, dangerous, and disease producing*, I'd like to see if this outrage is anything more than an act, a smoke screen calculated to mask their commercial motives in pushing a harmful product on people while feigning indignation when confronted with their chicanery.

Dairy products are implicated in all respiratory problems. Every *unbiased* researcher and authority on the effects of dairy products agrees on this point.

Over 30,000 children under the age of five die of respiratory disease each year. Fifteen thousand of these unfortunates die in the first month of life. Over 5000 die in the *first week* from respiratory disease syndrome (RDS), or what is called hyaline membrane disease. For children under three years of age, it is the number one cause of death by disease in the United States.

From my seventeen years of work in the health field, I am unequivocally certain that the massive amount of dairy products that pregnant women are routinely terrorized into consuming is the cause of this national tragedy. Huge amounts of excess mucus coat infants' little lungs and prevent them from developing properly. Ever wonder why it's necessary to have a suction tube at every birth to suck the thick mucus from the infant's throat and nose immediately upon delivery so it can breathe? Babies born of women who do not consume dairy products during pregnancy *do not* need this suction, because their breathing passages are clear. The January 1960 issue of *Lancet* (page 230) identifies the substance "muco-protein" in the lungs of infants who die of RDS. (93) This thick mucousy protein is precisely what develops in the body when dairy products are consumed, and studies show that the delicate little lungs of these infants are coated with it. In my opinion, this substance would not be there if the mother-to-be drastically cut down on her dairy consumption during her pregnancy.

I challenge the dairy industry—*I dare* the dairy industry—to prove me wrong. With a minuscule, infinitesimal percentage of the hundreds of millions of dollars they spend on advertising to convince people to consume their product, they could easily prove it one way or the other. They could set up a simple test, monitoring one group of women consuming as much dairy products as the nutritionists who represent the industry suggest, another consuming half as much, and a third group consuming none. It is my contention (and that of other experts in the field) that the first group will have the most difficulty giving birth and the highest percentage of RDS. The second group will have less, and the third group will have the least.

I'd like to see the people who run this industry stop hiding behind the clever verbiage of their paid nutritional experts and stop pretending to be offended by legitimate concerns over their products. If they want to be outraged about something, let them be outraged about *their own role* in this tragic matter.

Mark my words. The dairy industry will either ignore this, make light of it, or accuse *me* of something instead; they'll *never* take me up on my dare as long as there is even a remote chance of jeopardizing their cash flow, dead babies or not.

Remember, I am not suggesting that you discontinue all animal products. If you ultimately do that, great! But for now just consider cutting down and think of yourself as in transition. The reason you will find animal products included in the menus in this book and in **Fit for Life** is to learn how to eat them so they present the least amount of harm possible. What is most important is your direction, *not* the speed at which you achieve your goal. As long as you are making some progress, you are improving your health—no need for guilt, recrimination, or frustration. Considering the evidence in this chapter, *please do something* about decreasing the amount of animal products you eat. The only reason you may not want to do so is that you are totally unconcerned about the possibility of developing cancer, leukemia, heart disease, heart attack, high blood pressure, high cholesterol levels, diabetes, arthritis, multiple sclerosis, thyroid impairment, goiter, ulcers, gout, kidney damage, liver damage, migraine headaches, gallstones, kidney stones, SIDS, tinnitis, asthma, allergies, ear infections, bronchitis, sinusitis, or osteoporosis.

SPECIAL NOTE: When I first started to research this chapter, my idea was to cite *every* study I could find showing the harmfulness of animal products. To my amazement, there was so much more material than I expected that I quickly realized it would be impossible to do so. If I wanted to cover everything, I would need a book *several* times larger than this one. Please do not think I am exaggerating merely for effect. There are enough studies to easily fill *three* books the size of the one in your hands. Quite frankly, I was stunned. I knew animal products posed a danger, I just didn't realize how *much* evidence there was supporting that contention or for how long it's been known even to traditional science (Natural Hygienists, of course, have known of the dangers for ages).

Is there a doctor or dietitian or nutritionist or member of the meat industry or member of the dairy industry who would like to continue insisting that animal products are not dangerous, acting as if all this information did not exist? If you are *genuinely unaware* of the mammoth amount of evidence proving otherwise, I invite you to go to your nearest university medical library and look in the *Cumulated Index Medicus*. This directory, a publication put out by the Department of Health and Human Resources, is so massive and so comprehensive that it is truly staggering. Twenty to twenty-five volumes are published *every year*, containing all studies worldwide pertaining to health issues. You can look back over several decades under the subject headings "Meat" and "Milk"; look under the subheading "Adverse Effects." There you will find listed the many hundreds of research studies on the subject and the journals in which they appear.

Those of you who are still unconvinced, don't attack *me*. Take your complaints to the myriad researchers whose work I refer to. I'm sure they'll find your position most interesting. Better yet, do the people of this country a huge service and bring yourself up to date on this subject.

One day in the future *everyone* will be as aware of the harmfulness of eating animal products as we today are aware of the necessity of physicians' washing their hands before delivering a baby. Why not get a head start and catch up with those who have been warning people against the consumption of animal products for over a century? Take a position that will begin to decrease the amount of suffering NOW!

The first twenty-five years of my life were spent eating animal products a minimum of three times a day. I was fat, sickly, tired, unmotivated, in pain, and constantly contending with one health problem or another. The last seventeen years have included a minimal amount of animal products (raw butter and sour cream), and my life has been totally free of all those past ailments. Thousands of others have turned their lives around in similar fashion either by cutting out animal products altogether or by dramatically decreasing them, and **SO CAN YOU!**

CHAPTER 15
For Our Children

HARVEY:

Our most precious resource, our treasure—our future—is our children. The enormous concern Marilyn and I feel for them is truly our most driving force. Our children deserve to be loved, nurtured, and protected against what seems at times to be an all-out assault on their well-being. The pure, sweet innocence of children is a gift from God that nourishes us, a delight that warms our hearts as nothing else can. We, as the guardians of their health until they are old enough to fend for themselves, have an awesome responsibility *and* obligation to supply them whatever will best ensure their health and vitality.

If an adult looks over different approaches to living and, after weighing all the possibilities, decides to lead a life in which most of the elements of health are ignored, that is that person's inalienable right. But there is no right to impose those values on children, who are totally dependent upon the judgment and guidance of their guardians.

These are duties of ultimate importance. Whether our children are going to be healthy and happy or constantly afflicted with one malady after another rests almost entirely on our shoulders. This can be a heavy burden to bear at times. Working conscientiously at doing the best for a child can be extremely difficult. With our children constantly confronted with every conceivable unhealthful product under the sun, at times even the most dedicated parent becomes so frustrated as to take the easy way out, giving in to the ceaseless onslaught of inferior possibilities. This "Oh, hell, I give up!'' attitude is precisely what many advertisers prey on. That's right. There are people who spend endless hours concocting things to entice our children into wanting, even craving. That they may do harm is not even an issue to them. It's what will sell and at what price.

You've already learned how important food is in our lives, as the building material of our bodies. In no circumstance is food selection more important than during the formative, growing years of a child. We can tell how well our children are being nourished by how well they are feeling, how well they are performing.

Our children should be glowing examples of the glory of vigorous health. The fact is that *twice as many children are limited today in their activities by chronic illness than twenty-five years ago!* Children are now subject to strokes. Ninety-eight percent of youngsters have at least one factor that predisposes them to heart disease. Seventy-five percent are much too fat. Forty-two percent have cholesterol levels above the "acceptable" level. In 1954, 58 percent of our children could not pass a physical fitness test. When the same test was given in 1978, 86 percent failed. In 1983, 99 percent of our children could not pass, could not qualify for the Presidential Physical Fitness Award. Things are getting progressively worse.

George Allen, former coach of pro football's Washington Redskins and now chairman of the President's Fitness Council, said he is "appalled by the situation. A lot of boys and girls today can't even run a mile in thirteen minutes. Think about it! Most adults can walk a mile in eleven minutes without straining." At the heart of the problem, according to Allen and other authorities on fitness, is that school children are not receiving the proper instruction on exercise and nutrition. No kidding!

Talk to practically any pediatrician and he or she will tell you that the constant fevers, colds, diarrhea, ear infections, runny noses, and coughs suffered by our youth are "common childhood maladies." Weak, frail, sickly children have become so prevalent that our health advisers, our "experts," wave off these problems as *common!* They should *not be* common. That they are is a tragedy of colossal proportions. These "common" problems of childhood are warnings from the body that things are not right. Rather than having the sense to recognize this message from the body and taking proper measures to correct the problem, they are made light of and the children are given some drug to suppress the symptoms.

The problem with suppressing symptoms and failing to address causes is that the cause becomes progressively worse and worse. Our cherished children, our most adored and beloved young ones, should be bursting with life. They should be the absolute embodiment of life. They should be gloriously alive. Not only are they *not* the picture of health and vitality that they should be, but they suffer from every malady possible: heart disease, obesity, diabetes, colds, pneumonia, fevers, digestive diseases, poor eyesight, bad teeth, lethargy, and the list goes on and on. The crowning insult is that the number one cause of death by disease of our children is cancer. *Cancer!*

What dastardly crimes have our innocent young committed to deserve such a horrific experience during their most tender years? It is being done to them. Let me give you three quick examples to help you understand that the food processors in this country will stop at nothing to continue poisoning your child for profit. They're after children as infants, as preschoolers, and once they're in school. Even in the face of overwhelming evidence of health damage, they lobby against changes, exerting every effort to continue. Only when forced by law to stop will they actually stop—I hope.

The first example is a tragic series of at least 130 cases in which babies failed to grow and fell ill after being fed infant formulas that were deficient in some nutrients. In 1980 Congress enacted a law establishing minimum nutrient levels, quality control, and other standards for infant formulas. Although the FDA issued proposed rules to carry out the law, newly appointed FDA officials delayed implementing those rules and complied with requests of infant formula manufacturers to *drastically weaken the regulations*. Why on earth would they do that? These are the people you depend on to supply you with the *only* food your child may be eating. *They fought to keep it inferior!* And my friends, they won—if you want to call it winning. The altered rules were finally issued in April 1982 and took effect in July 1982. According to an FDA memorandum, the way the rules were rewritten "basically reflects the modifications proposed by the industry." Nice.

The second example has to do with Gerber and Beechnut, two of the nation's biggest baby food manufacturers. There are three types of food they make for kids: strained baby foods, slightly more solid junior foods, and toddler foods. In the 1970s Gerber and Beechnut were forced by public pressure to stop adding dangerously high amounts of salt to their baby and junior foods because of the effect it would have on high blood pressure later in life. But since they weren't specifically told to lower it in toddler foods as well, they didn't. And in 1984, the Center for Science in the Public Interest had to take them to task again for that. You must be very clear with these people—''I don't want *any* of my kid's foods treated with dangerously high levels of salt, even my toddler's.'' By the way, in 1984 Beechnut was the recipient of the New York State Department of Agriculture's largest fine ever, $250,000. Beechnut was selling apple juice for the kiddies labeled ''100 percent pure'' apple juice. Turns out the liquid contained synthetic additives and little or no apple juice. These aren't cars they're lying about, not televisions or toasters. *This is your child's food!*

The third example is a case of trying to sneak some inferior flesh food into your child's stomach. In January 1985 the United States Department of Agriculture suspended two poultry companies from providing food to the Federal School Lunch Program on the grounds that the firms falsely represented that their products met government specifications. Evidently Cal-Pacific Poultry and Beaumont Poultry, both in California and under the same management, were using unauthorized stamps to falsify production dates, thus concealing the true age of the meat. Yuck! Send your kid off to school for some rotten chicken meat. There are so many cases like these of big business looking out for their profits rather than your children's health that it's downright nauseating. *It's going on all the time*.

I don't want to make it sound as if there's no hope. On the contrary, there is no question that the situation can be turned around. Indeed, in many instances it *is* being turned around by those concerned enough to take the appropriate steps necessary to protect their loved ones. No one but no one can love your children as much as you, and no one can be more counted on to protect them than you. The only way they will be spared misery and blessed with the gaiety and liveliness they deserve is if *you* protect them, and one of the best measures you can take right now is to start protecting them from what is probably the most violent assault against their well-being today, the junk food industry.

Before going on we must rename junk food, at least for the purposes of this book. The term *junk food* is so frequently used that it has practically become passé. It no longer has any real meaning. It is even joked about. It certainly is no joking matter. In this book we will call it "dead" food, since that is what it is. Let's not beat around the bush.

Let's define a dead food: typically, a very highly processed food that has been stripped of all nutritional value, is high in salt, sugar, and fat, and meets *none* of the needs of the body. Sound like something you would like to raise your kid on? No? Well, the dead food industry would like nothing better. They spend millions of dollars to hook you and your children, and they hire "experts" whose prized credentials are for sale to the highest bidder to convince you that their offal is not so bad.

Dead foods are more than just something to eat. They represent money, profits, and high-powered advertising. More than half the foods eaten by a typical American are dead foods. That's over 700 pounds of dead foods a year. This does not count substandard foods such as meat, alcohol, or white bread. Since dead foods have no food value, why do people eat them? Because they are highly visible, heavily advertised, and the foundation of the nation's food business. Dead foods exist for the simple reason that they are so enormously profitable.

It's a well-established fact that the lowest profit item in most grocery stores is the produce—you know, the *real* stuff that keeps us alive. Packaged, processed dead foods have the highest markup. How perverse. What will help you the most and is actually better for you costs the least, but people eat far more of the products that do the most harm and cost the most money.

Look at the potato, an easily grown, highly nutritious food containing vitamins, minerals, and *all eight* essential amino acids. What does it cost? Twenty-five cents a pound? Take the same potato, boil it in oil, kill off anything of value, add salt and preservatives, package it in a colorful bag, give it a catchy name, and you have potato chips that sell for ten or twenty times the cost of the original potato. Talk about sticking it to the public with potatoes. Ever hear of Betty Crocker's Twice Baked? It is an insult to the intelligence, to say nothing of the noble potato. Aside from a small amount of tortured potatoes (dried, of course, meaning processed, meaning worthless) there are about *thirty* other ingredients: chemicals, chemicals, chemicals, BHA, BHT, monosodium glutamate, corn syrup, chicken fat, lard or beef suet, and on and on. Then you add the milk, eggs, and butter. A *real* potato has practically no fat. Twice Baked has loads of fat. Here's the rub. Instead of buying an honest to goodness potato, baking it, and getting some value from it for about twenty-five to thirty cents a pound, you can buy a five-ounce box of Twice Baked for a $1.19, or $3.81 a pound. Tricky.

The reason dead foods are so expensive is that someone has to pay for all that packaging and advertising. That someone is you. Without advertising there would be no dead food industry. If we never saw it splashed before our faces, we sure as the Dickens wouldn't know anything about it. And since dead foods meet no nutritional needs and our bodies have no innate need for them, we would simply reach for something our bodies could use when we were hungry.

Who do you think the dead food industry goes after most aggressively? Why, your little darlings, of course! Why not? They are the most helpless members of society, having no understanding whatsoever of the word *nutrition* or the importance of eating wholesome foods. What they know about food they get from television programs and advertising, and they are pounced upon with a vengeance. Some of the slickest advertising and marketing people are hired to *get your kids*! Snag 'em and don't let go. Attract them, tantalize them, and *hook* them! A few months back my son asked me if I'd like to watch a "Charlie Brown" special with him— "It's a *whole* hour, Dad." It ran from eight to nine in the evening. I sat down with him with a pen and paper and I wrote down the commercials that were aired during that time. There were eleven. Nine were for highly sugared, highly processed dead foods like candy, breakfast cereals, sodas, and the like. *Nine in one hour!* Even my son realized that he was being manipulated. He said, "There they are, trying to hook me on sugar again. Right, Dad?"

BREAKFAST CEREALS— AN ASSAULT ON YOUR CHILD'S HEALTH

Breakfast cereals are a textbook example of successful cashectomy. In the late 1800s Dr. John H. Kellogg ran a sanitarium for vegetarians in Battle Creek, Michigan. In 1895, at a time in history when people ate tremendous amounts of meat, convinced that fruits and vegetables were "dirty," Dr. Kellogg, searching for a healthy substitute for meat, invented "corn flakes." This was a relatively pure product—merely untreated, unprocessed corn, ground, liquefied, heated, and dried. Dr. Kellogg, who had a genuine concern for people's health, would cringe in shame and embarrassment (to say nothing of rage) at the present-day perversion of the cereal he developed.

You know how corn flakes are made today? First, corn kernels are soaked in lye. *Lye!* The same caustic, corrosive substance that will burn the skin right off your body. It's used in making rayon, soap, *and* breakfast cereals. Then, the kernels are hit with a blast of steam, after which they are ready to be soaked in a flavoring syrup, which is mostly refined white sugar. Then they are dried until hard and run through huge rollers that flatten them with seventy-five tons of pressure. After that they are toasted, heated, and flaked and are ready to be doused in a chemical bath of preservatives and additives. What started out as a real live grain of corn has turned into an agent of death.

Go into your local grocery store and see what takes up more shelf space than any other food item. It's breakfast cereals. When you realize that they're nearly all made from the same basic ingredients—corn, wheat, rice, and oats—you can see that the manufacturers have to use some pretty imaginative marketing ploys to convince you to buy their particular product over the dozens and dozens of others. All are vying for your dollar.

Before showing you some of their sales strategies, let's first take a look at the ingredients in this "highly nutritious" product. I can't talk about all of them because there are too darn many. So I will choose one from the Kellogg's line, Fruit Loops. I hope this doesn't cause Dr. Kellogg to squirm in his grave too much. (Follow along with *your* favorite.)

By law, one side of the cereal box has to list "nutrition information." You can bet your empty calories that it wouldn't be there if it weren't required by law, but even so the manufacturers have done a superb job of making the list barely understandable. It's a mish-mash of grams (g), milligrams (mg), one-ounce servings, equivalents, and many multisyllable words. Down at the bottom of this list you will see "carbohydrate information" listed in grams (g). Everything is in terms of a one-ounce serving, which is 28.35 grams. There are two listings: (1) complex carbohydrates and (2) sucrose and other sugars. In Fruit Loops there are 13 grams of sugar, meaning over 45 percent of the cereal is sugar, making it the number one ingredient. That's right. More than whatever corn, wheat, and oats the cereal has. If by now there is anyone left who is not aware of the dangers of processed, refined white sugar in the human diet, I would indeed be shocked. Its use has been associated with so many different diseases and metabolic disturbances that it would be difficult to discuss them all in this chapter.

During the refining process, sixty-four food elements are destroyed in sugar. All the vitamins, minerals, enzymes, amino acids, and fiber are gone, leaving only empty, non-nutritious, harmful sucrose. It has virtually *nothing* of value. When you eat it, your body must take vital nutrients from healthy cells in order to deal with it. For a real good education on how sugar ushers you to an early grave, there are two books you should read: *Sugar Blues* by William Dufty and *Sweet and Dangerous* by John Yudkin.

So far, we have 45.85 percent sugar. Next is 12 grams of corn, wheat, and oat flour. Not corn, wheat, and oats, but the highly processed *flour* of each. That's 42.3 percent refined flour. Guess what? *Over 88 percent of the cereal is refined sugar and starch!* Let me repeat that. *Over 88 percent is refined sugar and refined starch!* For your kid? Every day? Lord have mercy. What's the other little under 12 percent? Well, there's some hydrogenated vegetable oil, a somewhat polite way of saying saturated fat; salt; artificial colorings; some butylated hydroxytoluene (BHT), brought to you by our friendly chemical company for the purpose of preventing hydrogenated vegetable oil from going rancid; and some synthesized, inorganic, artificial vitamins and some inorganic minerals. This is not food. This is a very bad, sick joke. Please don't be fooled by the manufacturer's flashy ploy of saying "NOW FORTIFIED OR ENRICHED WITH ESSENTIAL VITAMINS."

The dead food pushers are constantly trying to figure out new routes to the entrance to your wallet. This is just one more cheap trick. They *know* that their products have no nutritional value, since all of the original nutrients have been heated, rolled, puffed, squeezed, and sugared out of existence. So, to ward off attacks by detractors, they try adding something back in. They add inorganic fillers, which are chemicals just like the other additives and preservatives already laced through the destructive foods. These cannot be utilized by the body the way any naturally occurring element can. They in no way replace or serve the same function as do the vitamins, minerals, and coexisting nutrients in living whole food. The scheme is to get you to believe that the addition of some synthetic nutrients miraculously transforms an adulterated, overly processed conglomeration of dead food and chemicals into a nutritious healthy food. Will new seats and a new coat of paint transform a broken-down jalopy into a well-functioning car?

In the process of milling and refining, over twenty-six essential elements are damaged or removed from the flour. The "enrichment" process puts back a tiny, *unusable* percentage of these. If someone took $26 out of your pocket, kept $22, and gave you $4 in counterfeit money, would you consider yourself "enriched"? So there you have it: a mixture of refined sugar, refined starch, saturated fat, salt, and a bunch of chemicals to keep it all together. Talking about chemicals, want a shock you'll never forget? Open a box of Fruit Loops and immediately stick your nose in the box and take a good smell. You will not believe that some people actually let their kids eat that stuff. It smells like a chemical spill, absolutely *sickening*, which is precisely what it is in the body.

Dr. Edward A. Taub told me about an unpublished experiment using Fruit Loops several years ago at a West Coast university. A box of Fruit Loops was put into a cage with some rats; the rats ate the box and left the Fruit Loops. Just take a sniff and you'll see why.

Advertising is what gets people to eat foods that even rats avoid. We're talking serious money here, about 4.5 billion dollars in sales. The industry uses the most underhanded, despicable ploys possible, whatever methods they can to get the kids to want these dead products. It's beyond cheap giveaways and talking animals and happy clowns. They've taken to naming these abominations after the cartoon characters the kids watch. So there are multi-colored, sugar-soaked, chemical-laced cereals called Strawberry Shortcake, Smurffberry Crunch, Donkey Kong, Mr. T, CP3O's, G.I. Joe, Cabbage Patch Dolls, PacMan, ET, Rainbow Bright, and Ghost Busters. I find this particular ploy to be the most contemptible. Our children's little impressionable minds look at these characters on their favorite morning television show as heroes. The ever alert food processors pay a fortune for the right to put these heroes on boxes of swill disguised as food. There oughta be a law.

Parents all over the country have taken a stand against drug pushers. They've joined together to get these entrepreneurs of death out of their neighborhoods and away from their schools. The only way the pushers of dead food are going to leave your child be is if you stop paying them to make more of their junk. The number one reason parents buy these things is because they're convenient—they save time. But your children deserve all the time necessary to see to it that they receive live food that hasn't been tampered with so they can lead happy pain-free childhoods. If you stop buying these high-profile, low-value dead "foods," they will go away. They will only be around as long as there is a demand. *Demand excellence*, not second-rate processed and refined products incapable of meeting the needs of a growing child's body.

There is another consideration to be taken into account with regard to eating these cereals. What is usually poured over them? Milk! Milk does not remain a liquid in the stomach. During digestion, whenever a liquid is consumed, what leaves the stomach first is the water. What is left in the case of milk is a coagulation of thick, dense curds that demand intense digestive activity to break down. The curd is a very concentrated protein. The cereals are starches, so you have a totally incompatible food combination that spoils and rots in the stomach. Adding fruit to the cereal and milk makes for an even more abysmal combination that can only build disease while robbing your child of his or her energy. When children eat these cereals and milk, all of their energy must go toward dealing with this incompatible mixture in the stomach; they are left with no energy to cope with other demands being made on them. It's no wonder that so many children are whiney and difficult to handle.

In the *Los Angeles Times* I found an easily missed little article entitled "Study of T.V. Ads Shows Stress on Sugary Foods" buried in the paper. It reported that in the first nine months of the year it was possible for a child watching television on weekend daytime programs to have seen more than 5500 commercials for cereals, candy, and other sugared items, and just *one* for vegetables! As astronomical a number as that is, consider that it is only for the first nine months and only the weekend programs. No telling what the number would be if they tallied up *all* those ads for the full year.

Of course, the sugar industry will do absolutely *anything* to bring a bit more respectability to its product. Since consumption is actually down 25 percent since the early 1970s (thank God), the sugar industry went on a $2 million radio and print campaign using the slogan "Use Real Sugar If You Know What's Good For You." They will *say* anything, they will *do* anything, and they will hire whoever will serve as a mouthpiece for them. Their favorite scheme is getting nutritionists, of all people, to go on the road and praise sugar. It is such a blatant incongruity that someone with nutritional "credentials" would speak well of a poison such as refined processed sugar that it stuns the intellect. Imagine the beer industry paying the head of MADD (Mothers Against Drunk Drivers) so much money that she would actually defend a moderate amount of drunk driving. Imagine the NRA (National Rifle Association) hiring someone whose kid was killed in a robbery with a legally purchased gun to speak in defense of the "right" to buy a gun out of a magazine ad. Now imagine the sugar industry paying nutritionists to *defend* sugar consumption. In truth, you don't have to imagine that one, because it is happening all the time.

Without knowing the speaker, who would you guess made these statements: "I would recommend that most people could healthily double their sugar intake daily. People say that all you get out of sugar is calories, no nutrients. There is no perfect food, not even mother's milk." "Sugar should be called fun food not junk food."

Yes, someone actually said those very words. Was it the head of the sugar industry? Was it the president of the breakfast cereal industry? Perhaps it was the head of the confectioners industry?

You might as well give up. You'll never guess. It was Dr. Frederick J. Stare, *the founder of the Department of Nutrition at the Harvard University School of Public Health*. I know. I couldn't believe it either. Dr. Stare has received retainers from the Cereal Institute and the Kellogg and Nabisco companies and has testified before Congress on behalf of the breakfast cereal and sugar industries. Starting to get the picture?

In an address on food faddism published by the Sugar Research Foundation on May 16, 1951, Dr. Stare is quoted as saying, "I should certainly say before closing that the food industries, the Sugar Foundation, the Nutrition Foundation, and a number of other food companies as individual companies have certainly done a lot in helping to support basic nutrition and a lot in helping to support our department [of Nutrition at Harvard], for which we are certainly appreciative." Between 1950 and 1956, according to *Open Letter II* of the Boston Nutritional Society (January 22, 1957) these same groups contributed almost a quarter of a million dollars to Dr. Stare's Harvard Department of Nutrition. *Fresh air. I need some fresh air!*

It is encouraging to know that not everyone is as stupid and gullible as some of our nutritional "experts" would like to think. In September 1983, on the nationally televised "Donahue Show," another of these so-called "authorities" in the field of nutrition got a rude awakening after trying to lay some of his flapdoodle about sugar on the audience. Dr. Victor Herbert must have thought he was talking to a bunch of nitwits. Either that, or he was so used to being taken seriously because he had "acceptable" credentials and "M.D." after his name that he forgot to think. He was defending sugar for some reason and practically got hooted off the stage when he tried to tell the audience—with a straight face, mind you—that some tests had been done that showed sugar actually *calms* kids down. After the gaffawing died down, an irate member of the audience stood up and said, "I'm a school teacher and the worst week of school to teach is the week after Halloween. With all that sugar in their systems, they go nuts." Then Dr. Herbert attempted to defend his asinine position, explaining himself in terms that no one in the audience could understand. Fortunately, Donahue saved him and went on to another subject. I must admit that watching him squirm while trying to defend himself against this more enlightened audience was enormously encouraging. Thank goodness, people are no longer willing to believe just anything merely because it comes from the mouth of an "expert."

THE TRAGEDY OF CHILD CANCER

The earlier reference to cancer being the number one killer of our children is a sobering one. This is not something to be taken lightly. It's happening and each of us *must* do whatever we can do to protect our children from this tragedy. We cannot depend on science or medicine to help us in the area of cancer. As much as they would like us to believe they are "winning the battle" against this most horrible affliction, they are not. In fact, medical science is slowly losing its grip on cancer altogether. Regularly, big, confusing headlines like "Drugs Used Alone As Cancer Cure Told" are splashed across the paper. They are designed to lull us into thinking progress is being made. But later in the article, in much smaller print, we find, "The *cured* patient died of pneumonia."* Ever see the cartoon where two pallbearers are standing

*This is not made up. The article actually appeared in the *Los Angeles Times* on February 2, 1979.

over a grave site and one says to the other, "Well, at least he didn't die of anything serious"?

After billions of dollars, years of research, misleading proclamations of progress, and *millions* of deaths, the "proven" methods of treatment have proven only to be unsuccessful. Talk of progress is just that, talk! *The New England Journal of Medicine* is one of medical science's most prestigious journals. What do researchers who have studied the problem have to say about their findings in this journal? It is not encouraging. The authors of one particular paper set out to assess the overall progress against cancer during the years 1950–1985. Their conclusion: "These data taken alone provide no evidence that some thirty-five years of intense and growing efforts to improve the treatment of cancer have had much overall effect on the most fundamental measure of clinical outcome—death. Indeed, with respect to cancer as a whole, we have slowly lost ground. Incidence of cancer is also increasing, suggesting a failure to prevent or control new or current causes of cancer." In another paragraph they state, "The main conclusion we draw is that some thirty-five years of intense effort focused largely on improving treatment must be judged a qualified failure."* Can anything be more clear? In closing, they state, "The reason for this failure needs to be carefully assessed, but in the meanwhile it may be that our approach to cancer needs to be changed." The authors suggest that for future application "The most promising areas are in cancer prevention rather than treatment."

That is what Natural Hygienists have been saying for *three quarters of a century*. There's a lot of talk about prevention, but not enough is being done.

I don't know about you but I've seen the treatment firsthand. It's ugly, it's painful, and it's *not* working.** I must give you one example of cancer treatment that is used both on adults and on our precious children. It serves as a representation of the futility

---

*One of the coauthors of the report cited here was John C. Bailar, who was editor of the *Journal of the National Cancer Institute* and worked for the NCI for twenty-five years!

**Dr. John Cairns of Harvard also states that the battle against cancer is being lost. In his words, "My criticism is that cancer treatment and research is giving the public an endless succession of breakthroughs and solutions that aren't really that at all."

and desperation of much cancer treatment. In many instances treatment is in direct opposition to the dynamics of the human body. More often than not, I think, treatments are attempted simply because medical technicians have to do something or people will start to ask questions about where exactly the billions of dollars are going. All too frequently treatments are so outrageous and such an affront to our common sense that it is a wonder that they are continued.

All wars have their monstrous modes of destruction and suffering. During World War I, the Germans introduced and used nitrogen mustard gas against United States and allied troops in Belgium. This abominable weapon caused heavy casualties. Those who did not succumb to the gas suffered violent blistering of the lungs, skin, eyes, and intestines. Many who did not die were left permanently disabled. All types of medical treatment failed, and autopsies later showed that the gas had even destroyed lymph tissue. The use of this ghastly poison was banned by the Geneva Convention of 1925. Since that time certain countries have been using it anyway. In 1984 it was revealed that Iraq was using mustard gas against Iran. The Reagan Administration strongly condemned the practice. The Soviet Union has been accused of using mustard gas in Afghanistan. ''ABC News Closeup'' did a story on Afghanistan called ''Rain of Terror.'' It reported extensive evidence that people were indeed dying of mustard gas poisoning. People's lungs were so badly burned and blistered that they were coughing up gobs of blood. In a statement about the use of nitrogen mustard gas, a United States State Department spokesman said, ''There can be no justification for its use by any country.''

Let me set a scene for you. A woman is in a doctor's office with her dearly beloved teenage son. A nurse comes in, wraps a rubber strap around the boy's scalp line and says, ''This will help minimize hair loss.'' The mother is breathing erratically in nervous anticipation. The boy rolls up his sleeve and the nurse ties a tourniquet tight about his elbow. As he makes a fist, she pokes his forearm, feeling for an adequate vein, one that has not been hardened by the trauma that is part of chemotherapy. As the boy squints with the insertion of the needle, his mother tries to stifle a gasp. The first drug to flow into his arm is Oncovin. Its acrid odor quickly triggers nausea in the boy. The nurse instructs him to take some deep breaths. The second syringe contains only about three tablespoons of liquid, but it looks like a quart and just the thought of it being pumped into his veins adds to the boy's nausea. As the nurse removes the last needle and leaves the room, the boy's eyes meet his mother's. He tries to smile; she sheds a tear and says, "You okay, baby?" He nods yes, but his face contorts. His mother calls his name as he runs to the sink, his stomach exploding in deep retching. The *eight-hour aftermath* of this treatment has begun. The nurse returns with a cup of cold water; the boy vomits again. As he and his mother walk hand in hand to set the date for the next treatment that he will get—every ten days—the boy's face shows no relief. He knows that the physical side-effects of the therapy will mar his entire day, and the emotional scars will remain with him for a lifetime.

Have you made the connection yet? The second drug that threw the boy's body into such violent turmoil was *nitrogen mustard gas*. Yes, the very same nitrogen mustard gas that caused people to cough up parts of their bloody lungs during wartime, the same nitrogen mustard gas outlawed for use during war, the same nitrogen mustard gas that everyone from the President on down has expressed outrage over.

How do you feel after reading this? Is your common sense screaming out in indignation? If it's not, it's on vacation somewhere. The scenario you read was not made up out of my head for impact. It was written by the boy who went through it.

On September 21, 1946, the *Journal of the American Medical Association* published the first scientific paper on the use of chemotherapy in cancer. It had the simple title "Nitrogen Mustard Therapy." I don't care what kind of mumbo jumbo some "credentialed" doctor in white smock and stethoscope utters. My instincts and my common sense scream out in shock and outrage at the suggestion that the same abominable substance used to kill can be used to heal. The mere fact that the body will be locked in excruciating pain and agony for *eight hours* should be sufficient evidence that the body is struggling to protect itself from such a hideous concoction. If the patient dies, the cancer is blamed. If the patient manages to survive, the treatment is given the credit.

The idea of condoning a substance so inherently vile and deadly for use in a person's body because the person is *sick* is too impossibly ignorant to be believed. Yet the idea is actually defended by our medical "experts," who have somehow managed to rationalize in their minds that it could be helpful. What would you think if you were to read an advertisement for this book that invited you to learn about the elements of health—food, air, water, exercise, rest, nitrogen mustard gas, etc. You'd have to wonder if you weren't reading *Mad* magazine. **THE ELEMENTS OF HEALTH ARE WHAT ARE NECESSARY TO SUSTAIN LIFE, WHETHER YOU ARE IN A STATE OF HEALTH OR ILL HEALTH.** If you wouldn't poison a healthy person with nitrogen mustard gas, then you surely must not poison a sick person with it either. I can assure you of one thing without any possible doubt: If nitrogen mustard gas had not been created for use during wartime, it *never* would have been thought of for use in the treatment of cancer. It is being *tried* on patients simply because it is there. It's the same reason the Department of Energy is trying to treat our food with radioactive waste: It's just lying around, so we might as well use it for something. Right!

What is my point with all this talk about cancer and its treatment? Since we know more of our children will die of cancer than any other disease, we must truly take preventive steps *now* so our precious children will never have to be treated with nitrogen mustard gas—or anything else. I know there are many factors that play a role in this dread disease. Certainly diet is among the most important. There is no reason a child's diet cannot be improved, and there is no better time to do it than right now. It has become painfully obvious that we cannot depend on medical science to lessen the incidence of cancer or deal with it successfully once it has been detected.

The greatest protection your child will ever get will come from *your* efforts. Protection against the sugar-laced, chemical laden dead food pushed by food processors is protection against cancer. Your child needs it. You can do it, and there is no better expenditure of your time.

CHAPTER 16

Our Children Have the Right to Be Fit for Life Too

MARILYN:

One of the questions that has come up most frequently since we wrote **Fit for Life** has come from mothers everywhere: ''How do I know if this program is a good idea for my children?''

My heart goes out to these women. Concerned mothers have been incredibly victimized and confused by masses of contradictory nutritional information coming at them from all sides. That we as mothers have lost the instinctive knowledge we once had and that all females of the other species on earth possess—the instinctive knowledge of how to feed our offspring—is frightening evidence of how far we have been pulled from our true biological heritage. You can be sure that for millions of years our ancestral mothers had no questions whatsoever about the care and feeding of their children. There is no way that we could have survived as a species if they had not *instinctively* known how to raise one healthy generation after another. Our young ancestors had to be fleet of foot and strong enough to climb and walk long distances. They lived outside most of the time and spent long hours in the sun, wind, and rain.

Today there is clearly cause for concern, particularly in light of the present proliferation of processed and dead foods into every corner of our children's lives. I know that I don't have to describe it for you. As caring parents, you are, I am certain, deeply and painfully aware of the direct link between these dead foods, which are known poisons for our children, and the sorry state of health that so many of them are experiencing. We know what the situation is: The processed food industry concentrates on addicting them to dead, chemicalized foods so they will eat them from morning until night. In spite of the efforts of many aware parents to eliminate dead foods from their children's diets, advertising continuously pushes these poisons on the kids.

Even school lunches are now served to our children by the dead food industry, who, with the help of the dietitians and nutritionists they hire, have sold the United States Department of Health and Human Services a bill of goods claiming to bring in a more nutritious meal at lower cost. Ha! This more nutritious meal consists of hamburgers, french fries, pizza, and hot dogs. You can walk down any street in America and get that same meal from your choice of any number of fast food stands. It is predominantly made up of denatured fillers and saturated fat! When the United States Department of Agriculture made the unexpected and encouraging proposal that peanut butter, nuts, and seeds be substituted for meat in the school lunch program in order to lower our children's intake of carcinogenic fats, we learned about an interesting rule. Evidently, this rule requires that meat *must* be served to children. I wonder who was responsible for that. As a parent I ask—and I know some of you ask with me—how we as a nation can afford to subsidize foreign wars if we cannot afford to provide nourishing, high quality foods for our children's school lunches? What good are our present expenditures in arms development? Should we not be more concerned about developing strong future generations of Americans? Can they be strong if we cut corners on the quality of their food? **INFERIOR FOOD YIELDS INFERIOR HUMAN DEVELOPMENT.**

Some have questioned whether the **Fit for Life** program is a sound, nutritional approach for children. One answer to that comes from ten-year-old Gina Barlotta of Columbus, Ohio, who wrote to us on July 28, 1986.

Dear Mr. and Mrs. Diamond,

My mom and dad bought your book about seven months ago. They usually don't buy books for dieting or weight loss but they bought your book because it makes sense. They read through it and decided that we should start eating this way.

Mom and Dad also told us what salts, sugars, and

meats do to our arteries. My baby sister, who's five years old, knows what it does by memory. We'll be riding in the car and she'll start telling us what it does.

Every now and then we'll go to Dunkin Donuts or Baskin Robbins, but "at least we don't do it every day." That's what Patrice (my five-year-old sister) says.

Natalie (my nine-year-old sister) usually didn't eat a lot of vegetables. Now that we are eating this way she likes almost every vegetable (except lima beans)! As a matter of fact nobody in our family likes lima beans except Dad.

In Columbus there's a health food store. We go there maybe once a week. I don't know if they're based on your book but they're against meats and dairy products. You can buy fake milk or carob covered peanuts there. Mom buys the fake milk for pancakes. We use wheat flour for the pancakes also.

Even though people don't think your way of eating is right, lots of people out there do think it's right, including us.

Yours sincerely,

Gina Barlotta
Aged 10

Accepting the fact that **Fit for Life** is appropriate for children —which it is, having been endorsed by many doctors, including two of this country's most forward-thinking pediatricians, Dr. Edward A. Taub and Dr. Robert S. Mendelsohn—how do we then tailor it to our children's life-styles? First of all, since cancer is the greatest killer of children and so much cancer has been directly linked to diet, let's look at the dietary recommendations for cancer prevention from the American Cancer Society:

1. Eat more high-fiber foods such as fruits, vegetables, and whole-grain cereals.

2. Include dark green and deep yellow fruits and vegetables rich in vitamins A and C.

3. Include broccoli, cabbage, brussels sprouts, kohlrabi, and cauliflower.

4. Be moderate in consumption of salt-cured, smoked, and nitrite-cured foods.

5. Cut down on total fat intake from animal sources and fats and oils.

6. Avoid obesity.

7. Be moderate in consumption of alcoholic beverages. (Applicable in that many children's cough medications contain outrageously high proportions of alcohol.)

Every one of these seven recommendations is included in **Fit for Life**.

These dietary recommendations from the American Cancer Society are prefaced by this comment: "There is evidence that diet and cancer are related. Follow these modifications in your daily diet to reduce the chances of getting cancer." This is encouraging and tragic at the same time. It's encouraging in that they clearly show us that **CANCER IS IN OUR CONTROL**. It's tragic in that for *eighty* years, while Natural Hygienists were pleading for people to understand the relationship between diet and cancer (and all other diseases for that matter), those in charge of treating and preventing disease vehemently denied the relationship and actually had the audacity to threaten and intimidate the advocates of Natural Hygiene. Now that the correlation can no longer be denied, given overwhelming supporting evidence, we are finally given a cancer prevention diet. How many lives could have been saved if these recommendations had been published sooner?

But look! Look at what is out there in the public sector for kids to eat! Why is there not more pressure against the fiberless, unfresh, fatty, salted, and sugared foods being pushed on our children? Are school lunches in accordance with these anticancer, diet recommendations? They most certainly are not! Why does the American Dietetic Association, which is solely responsible for the school lunch program and the food served to our sick children in hospitals, totally ignore the recommendations in the cancer prevention diet?

Who are they worried about protecting—the industrial profiteers or our children? Does the FDA oblige the food industry to adhere to the anticancer diet recommendations when it comes to food produced for children? They don't in any way! Do the medical doctors and nutritionists who are supposedly in charge of our well-being, cry out in outrage at the way our kids are being fed? Isn't it perfectly obvious that it is completely up to us as parents to protect our children from the social and economic forces that do not cherish them as our most valued and important resource? We as parents must take control and stand up for the right of our little ones to be healthy.

Obviously, it is up to us to take control of our children's nutritional welfare. It has *always* been up to us, but many have not known what to do and so have left it up to the children, who have become the innocent little consumer victims of the dead food industry. The time has come to regain control and protect the innocent, who are so desperately in need of our protection. Let's start to do so for *their* sakes, and as quickly as we possibly can. So if you are wondering if **Fit for Life** is appropriate for children or are confused because some special interest doctor or nutritionist has said it isn't, check it against the anticancer diet. It satisfies (and then some!) every recommendation, with the bonus that it takes body physiology into account so that stomachaches and pains now experienced by your child as a result of wrong food combinations will be things of the past. It will provide you with a formula for integrating more fruits, vegetables, and whole grains into your child's diet as you decrease fatty animal products.

Several years ago we were contacted by Dale and Martha Kirstine, a lovely couple from San Juan Capistrano, California, who had gone on our program, then called the Diamond Method, after reading about it in the *Star* newspaper. Dale lost thirty pounds and found he no longer suffered from acute hypoglycemia and allergies. Martha went from a size 14 to a size 6. Their two beautiful young daughters also went on the program with them, and that, Dale told us, was the *real payoff*. Therese and Lorie were at that time in a grade school for children with learning disabilities. After they had been on the program for six weeks, their teacher contacted their parents to ask if there had been any changes in their home life. Dale and Martha explained that the girls were following a new way of eating. The teacher replied that their work at school was showing marked improvement, and she invited Dale and Martha to come and give a talk to other parents about the Diamond Method. Both girls were subsequently able to leave the special school and enter regular school. When I chatted with Dale and Martha recently, they told me that, three years later, both Therese and Lorie are still doing good work in regular school and have a complete understanding of the effects of eating wrong on how they felt and on their performance.

If you are a parent, there are certain important guidelines for applying **Fit for Life** principles to your child's life-style that I feel will make your life easier. To begin with, **DO IT FIRST FOR YOURSELF.** Start *your* day with fresh fruit until noon. Properly combine *your* lunch and evening meals. Cut down on dairy products and beef. Have starches like potatoes, pasta, and whole grains as your main course in the evening from time to time instead of any flesh food. Always eat fruit on an empty stomach and never as a dessert. Substitute fresh fruits and vegetables or raw nuts for sugary snacks, although once in a great while, if you must, a "sweet" at tea time (4:00 P.M.) is okay. Try to cut out sodas and substitute fresh fruit and vegetable juices. Those are simple changes, and once you have implemented them (and you don't have to do it all overnight) you will start to look and feel fantastic! That feeling will fill you with confidence; you will exude enthusiasm and *that* is when it is appropriate to begin to implement some of these same changes in the lives of your children. It is harder to change them before you have changed yourself.

Changes in children's diets must be made without pressure or regimentation. I know how you feel. You want to take everything that is poisoning them out of their lives at once! You want to start fresh, turn over a new leaf. You are filled with frustration and fury against dead food processors who make poison for profit and sell it to your kids! I know all those feelings! But you have to accept the facts. If your children are typical American kids more than a few years old, drinking sodas, eating candy, and loving their visits to the dead food restaurants, you have to accept that they have reached a certain level of addiction to most of what you might wish to eliminate. *Nothing can happen overnight.* It took a while to get them where they are, and it is going to take a while to get them to where you want them. **BUT THE BEAUTIFUL THING ABOUT KIDS IS THAT THEY REALLY WANT TO FEEL GOOD.** They really notice the difference very fast in their energy. When stomach pains from bad food combinations and the headachy feelings from sugar that they have learned to live with all their lives go away, they like that! So please, the most important aspect of making your child fit for life is *patience*. If you turn it into a battle of wills or a nagging situation, they will come to associate food with tension rather than with love and pleasure, and you will be doing them and yourself a great disservice.

If your children are little, younger than three, it is easiest. Cut down on dairy for them and watch all kinds of respiratory problems, colds, and ear infections, clear up. Substitute fresh fruit juices and fruits (but expect one initial mucousy discharge from the nose—a cold or some coughing—when you first make the change). I can guarantee you that some nutritionist or television doctor will quote me out of context on this and tell you that I am saying that when kids go on the **Fit for Life** program they get sick, *but I am not saying that!* When you cut down on cow's milk and cheeses and yogurt and ice cream, their little bodies, which have been clogged up from foods that they cannot efficiently metabolize, will sing for joy and spew out all that is clogging them. That stage will pass quickly, and your children will be practically "cold-free" from that point on, *if* you keep them away from dairy. This last line, I would wager, will *not* be quoted! Children of all ages, especially young ones, need fresh, whole, living foods to grow fast, to develop whole, living bodies.

There should be a study done on the relationship between cow's milk and toilet training. In my experience children who don't have cow's milk train easier and earlier. Nerve impulses simply do not transmit well in a clogged up little body and the learning process can be retarded for this reason. Common sense! This is not a food that will improve intelligence! It is a food designed for a sweet but small-brained, *unintelligent* animal! During one of our recent book tours, a young mother in Denver told us that her four year old suffered from regular bed-wetting. After reading **Fit for Life**, she took her off milk and the bed-wetting stopped. Once in a while after that when she would have milk, the bed-wetting would reoccur. This was not due to the liquid intake alone, because the child was having juices instead of milk. Maybe that's not "scientific" enough for some people, but it's certainly worth considering if you are a mother who is sick and tired of wet diapers and sheets. Our son, who *never* had cow's milk was totally toilet trained at the age of one year.

Give them mother's milk as long as you can. They know when

they have had enough and will usually stop on their own between the ages of one and three years. Remember, mother's milk is the food designed by nature for the human young. It is perfectly balanced for them, containing only 2 percent protein. Supplement mother's milk with *fresh* fruit juices, nut and seed milks, and *fresh* fruit for as long as you can before you introduce cooked vegetables.

Mothers, once you have finished breastfeeding or even as a supplement to breast milk, you can give your children delicious, easy-to-make, high quality nut and seed milks. Make them from raw almonds, filberts, sesame or sunflower seeds or from a blend of the four. Nut and seed milks are an age-old source of fine nutrition used by the American Indians, Europeans, Asians and Africans long before dairying became a profitable industry. It is a practice we ought to resurrect for the sake of our children. Nut and seed milks have been used for decades by Natural Hygienists in this country and are highly recommended for children and adults by countless hygienic practitioners. Excellent sources of usable calcium, protein, vitamins and minerals, they have none of the scientifically proven harmful side effects of cow's milk. From nut and seed milks you can make delicious ice cream substitutes— creamy nut milk shakes—by adding fresh fruit and frozen bananas, all done in a simple blender or a Vitamix. Our children have been drinking almond milk for years, and they adore it sweetened with a little maple syrup and blended with a handful of strawberries. If you have a Champion juicer, you can make wonderful frozen fruit ices for your children as ice cream substitutes. The recipes are included in **Fit for Life**, and some are repeated in the recipe section of this book for your convenience. (I personally drink sesame milk regularly.) Try it! It's great!

As for the practice of giving little ones cereal at an early age, which most pediatricians and nutritionists still recommend, know this: Your children have no ptyalin, the enzyme necessary to break down starches, until around the age of eighteen months. They cannot metabolize starches before then. That's another reason why we see so many little Americans with clogged or runny noses. Bread, cereal, potatoes, and all cookies and chips will clog them up. Keep them on fruits and vegetables as long as you can. They do not need nearly the variety we feel they must have. Don't introduce a whole bunch of new foods at once. One at a time with several days spacing is fine. Children are little people; *they need real people food.*

Stay away from starchy, salty, dead "baby" foods. Take their fruit and blend it for them fresh until they have enough teeth to chew. Make blended salads. Blend avocado with a little water. They will love the fresh, real flavors and they will thrive. When you feel the need to add cooked food, blend fresh steamed vegetables—for example, carrots, string beans, zucchini. You can add a little butter, if you like, but you don't have to. That just teaches children that they "need" butter. The longer you delay introducing cooked foods, the better. Introducing cooked foods too early leads to allergies and childhood obesity.*

Remember that mother's milk is only 2 percent protein, and avoid giving children animal protein for as long as you can. *Never is best*. They are getting probably much more than 2 percent protein in the fruits and vegetables and all of the whole grains that you will give them later on. *Leukemia and intake of animal protein are related, without a doubt*. Children get the amino acids for building protein they need in the right proportion from fruits and vegetables. Again, nutritionists will take issue with this, but that is because they have no sense of the true nature of human physiology. We don't *eat* protein for protein. We *build* protein from amino acids, which are plentiful in the plant kingdom. They have bought profit-oriented propaganda coming from studies funded by the industries they represent. They are pushing that vested interest propaganda on you, and that hurts you and it hurts your kids.

Fruits and vegetables are the most ideal foods in a young child's diet. Wait as long as you can to introduce starches, and start with cooked potatoes and yams. Creamy blended soups are also wonderful baby foods. Add crackers and breads and grains after age eighteen months, if you can wait that long.

If you don't teach children to eat sugar, they won't crave it. If you teach them that a treat is cherries or blueberries or watermelon rather than a cupcake or cookie, then they will not become sugar addicts, and as they grow sugar intake will be more controllable, a once-in-a-while, take-it-or-leave-it situation.

I know how hard it is in this society to keep children away from sugar. It is all around them. It was not always easy for us but Beau *never* had any sugar until he was five years old. Now aged eight, perhaps he will have some once a month at a party. He'll

*See "Baby Shouldn't Be Rushed to Eat Solids," *Los Angeles Times*, September 13, 1984.

have a little and that will be all he'll want. Sometimes the next day he feels "yucky" and he knows why.

Once your child is past the age of three, making changes can be more complicated. You then come up against addictions, which can become more serious as the child becomes older. Most parents expressing concern about their children's diets are usually preoccupied with sugar abuse. I have found that, with many children between four and twelve, a good heart-to-heart talk about the consumption of sugar, sugar addiction, and soda addiction can be very helpful. Children like to participate in decisions being made about their lives. They have a lot more common sense than we realize. It is also important for them to understand that Mom and Dad are concerned and are trying to find ways to help them be healthier. If you decide to talk to your child about all of this, make sure first of all that the scene is conducive to real communication. Don't try to have a heart-to-heart talk while you are driving and your attention is fragmented, with Johnny in the back seat peering at the back of your head. Make sure that you are relaxed and have a block of uninterrupted time during which you can really share your thoughts and feelings and hear what your child's reactions are to them. If you have more than one child, it might be best to do this with each one individually. Eating habits are a very personal issue.

I am suggesting this strategy to you because I had to use it myself with Beau after he had been in school awhile and he was around six and one-half years old. He was watching brightly packaged candy, cookies, and sodas pass him by right and left. Kids were relishing them. The wrappers were pretty. The candies were neat shapes and sizes and colors. He felt left out. He wanted to know firsthand for himself what these things tasted like. Early on, Harvey and I had made a pact that we would never deny him anything he really wanted to try, so home could be his safe zone, a place where *everything* was okay. Thus, he would never feel he had to hide himself from us to experience something he felt he needed to experience.

It started out this way. He just wanted to know what some of these unfamiliar things tasted like. He wanted to experience them. Our words were no longer enough. Of course, we wished it could be otherwise but we acquiesced. So Beau had a taste of this one day, a taste of that another day. A few days later, there would be something else he wanted to try. This went on for a few weeks, and I noticed that what had started out as a taste was fast becoming a "may as well polish it off" situation. I was witnessing my child's growing addiction to sugar. I realized that, for the first time in his life, his strong little body was under attack from a poisonous chemical that would suck the minerals right out of his bones. His smooth little disposition and even temper from birth was fast dissolving into a fretful edginess that I had witnessed in other children but never in him. It made me sick. So we had our little talk. While we talked, I got down to his level, so that we could see eye to eye, and I stroked his head and his arms to support my verbal communication with physical contact.

This is how our conversation went:

"Beau, I know that you are very curious about candy and cookies and I know that the kids make it look so good at school and on TV that you want to try it."

"Yeah, because they like it so much, I want to know what it tastes like."

"And I've let you taste a lot of it, haven't I?"

"Yeah . . ."

"But the thing is, I've been having a hard time lately, thinking about letting you have this stuff. It's bad for you; it is poison! It has processed sugar in it. It makes your bones so weak you can't grow up strong, and there are lots of other poisonous chemicals in it. And I don't even *know* what harm they will do to you. But there are a lot of chemicals that damage your brain or your eyes or give you cancer and these could do that. And chocolate is so bad it keeps some people from having babies when they grow up. And you know you haven't been feeling as well as usual lately. Also candy has dye in it, and a lot of those dyes are poisonous."

"Well, why do they make them?"

"Beau, the people who make these things make them so they can earn a lot of money. They don't make them because they are good for children. They are bad for children, and they know they are bad. But they care more about money."

"Well, I think they are doing a bad thing, but my friends don't know that and they eat them."

"Here's the thing, Beau. Your friends don't know how bad they are and their mommies don't know how bad they are, but *I do*, and when I say you can have them, I feel so sad because I am letting someone hurt you. I am letting you be hurt by someone who doesn't care about you. I love you too much to let you be

poisoned. I can't let anyone poison you, even if the poison is in a pretty package. I have to keep it away from you because I love you so much.''

''Well, maybe I won't have so much anymore.''

''Well, darling, if you do ask me for it all the time, I will have to say *no*. Do you know what I mean when I say no about candy and stuff like that?''

''You mean you love me.''

A conversation like that with your child can be a lot more effective than ''laying down the law.'' It may not put the situation completely to rest—sugar addictions are strong—but you can always bring it back to your love for the child. **YOU ARE NOT DENYING YOUR CHILD ANYTHING BY SAYING NO TO SUGAR FOODS; YOU ARE GIVING YOUR CHILD LOVE.** Children sense that. They are smart. Subliminally they know all those sugary foods are bad for them, and when you say no your love for them is subliminally reaffirmed.

At the natural food stores—and soon, we hope, in the supermarkets—you will find healthful, sugar-free alternatives: sweets, cookies, better sodas, and cereals. Now obviously, these foods still need to take a back seat in your child's diet to more whole, living foods like fruits, vegetables, whole grains, and mother-made foods replacing all the packaged stuff. But these more healthful alternatives make good substitutions for poisons. You will be able to recognize the ingredients: butter,* whole-wheat flour, honey, peanut butter, almonds, maple syrup, graham flour, carob, peanuts, dates, cornmeal, oats, granola, cream, etc. Read a popular candy bar label or the label on packaging for soda, cookies, or a sugar cereal. Read it *if you can*, I should say. You will not recognize much of what you read as food ingredients. There will be processed sugar and chemicals and dyes and additives and preservatives and, dear parents, *these things are not food*. They are killing our children—slowly, in most cases, but surely, in all cases. If you stop buying them and demand *real* food, the food manufacturers will have to meet your demands or go out of business.

One more little illustration about substituting real for synthetic. In the spring of 1986, we did a segment with Beau on the ''Merv

---

*Butter, unlike other dairy products, is not acid-forming because it contains little or no milk solids. It is neutral, being a fat rather than a protein.

Griffin Show.'' Now, Merv is an incredible person who cares very much about people. He loves children and he took to Beau right away. Beau brought his lunchbox to show Merv what he eats at school. In it was a Gypsy Boots Bar, made from dates, peanut butter, coconut, peanuts, carob, butter, etc. It is good and it is *real*. Merv took a bite and smiled one of those magic smiles he is so famous for. He loved it! Beau loves it! We all do! For several weeks after that show, Beau had to share his Gypsy Boots Bar with four or five friends every day at school. They had seen him on television, and when they heard about a candy bar that was good for them, they wanted it. After that show, we received quite a few letters from mothers wanting to know where they could find Boots Bars. We are presently working to market a totally nutritious, sweet bar that will have candy enthusiasts of all ages swooning.

Sugar addiction is the hardest problem to deal with if your child is really hooked. Everything else is easier. In working the **Fit for Life** program into the lives of grade school children it is important to be flexible, understanding, forgiving, and patient. If your kids have been used to the typical American diet—hamburgers on buns, chicken and noodles, cheese and bread, pizza, ice cream for dessert, fruit as a snack after meals, drinks with meals, heavy breakfasts, lots of processed and dead foods—there is going to be a lot to change. Remember your goals when the effort at implementing change seems to get overwhelming. You just want to get more whole, real, living food into your child's life. Set the example yourself, and don't expect any miracles to happen overnight.

The best place to start is with breakfast. I know what many parents feel. After years of thinking that big breakfasts are important, it is hard enough to make the change for yourself, let alone for your child. But with over 75 percent of our children overweight, we've got to let their elimination cycles work for them; we've got to allow their bodies to *naturally* cleanse themselves of toxic buildup or they will be fat and they will be sick. Some kids don't like breakfast. Good! Stop forcing it on them. But have them make the fruit concession—''Okay, no breakfast, but I do want you to eat some fruit.'' Tell them why: ''Fruit is fuel for your brain. It will give you energy during the morning at school.'' If your child is a breakfast eater, you may have to start with fruit, but if that is not enough, you may have to offer other foods until he or she gets used to the lighter, high energy feeling of just fruit

in the morning. Just *make those foods real*. The ideal breakfast includes fresh juice or a smoothie, two kinds of fruit, some celery or lettuce, and ½ ounce of raw nuts. Or offer some hot steamed vegetables—better real corn than corn flakes. Keep frozen vegetables like peas and corn and lima beans on hand, but you should know that freezing destroys about 30 percent of the nutrients in food. For this reason, it is not good to rely on frozen vegetables *exclusively*. If your child is a cereal freak and won't go for the vegetables, try granola (honey- or date-sweetened) with almond milk or apple juice. These are delicious, albeit still too heavy for the morning. But you will see, you can phase them out slowly. A piece of whole-grain toast, a toasted bran muffin, or some other fresh baked muffin is also good, especially on the weekend. But always *after* a fruit plate or salad.

Speaking of the weekend, when breakfast might be more of a ceremony, you can try fresh homemade Coconut-Apple Granola, made from apples, coconut, almonds, etc. Or try French Toast with Maple Syrup—the bread is soaked in almond milk instead of egg. (Both dishes are deliciously innovative, and I have included recipes for them in the back of this book.—see pages 375 and 430.) But please, start with a beautiful bowl of fresh fruit, and don't have the other stuff sitting around under the kids' noses first thing in the morning. If all they see is the fresh fruit and you sit down to enjoy it with them enthusiastically, they may fill up on it and not want anything else. Then you can happily chalk up one more day for an elimination cycle that runs unhampered, cleaning built-up toxic waste from their bodies. If you pack them off to school after a fruit breakfast, pack more fruit for their morning snack, maybe even some sun-dried fruit. Remember, **FRUIT IS THE ONLY FOOD THAT WILL GIVE THEM ENERGY WITHOUT TAKING ENERGY.** Once they make the transition from heavier foods to fruit in the morning—a process that can take from a few days to a few weeks to months—they will have much more energy to work in the morning, since a heavy meal is not draining their energy reserves. If you are worried in the beginning that "they will be hungry" add some raw nuts to their lunchboxes, just in case.

Here are possible items for a typical lunchbox for Beau, and I know many other mothers who use this basic format:

1. Some fruit peeled and sliced in a thermos cup or bagged whole.

2. A wide-mouthed food Thermos filled with hot potatoes sautéed in butter and mixed with corn, peas, or string beans or all of the above. I usually keep lots of vegetables that have already been steamed in the refrigerator, so it's really very easy to reheat this main course for lunch. (Steamed vegetables should not be kept for more than two days, however.) Beau is a potato man, so a hot potato dish at lunch is perfect for him, and he never asks for anything else. (Kids will eat the same thing over and over if they like it.) You could easily substitute vegetable pasta or rice for the potatoes— with vegetables. On days when it seems Beau might be getting a little stuffed up, the wide-mouthed Thermos serves well as a cold receptacle for a lettuce salad with cherry tomatoes, sprouts, and his favorite dressing, or a simple vegetable soup.

3. Along with either the hot potato lunch, the salad or soup I add celery sticks or a carrot or sliced cucumber. On salad days, Beau gets all three.

4. On hungry days, a toasted bread and butter sandwich.

5. A dried fruit and nut bar or raw almonds for an afternoon snack—or a good cookie.

6. I also provide a Thermos of distilled water, so if Beau's thirsty he won't be attracted to drinking the inferior juices made from concentrates, which are usually served at school.

I know what you're thinking. You are wondering how you can possibly get all of that into a child's lunchbox. You can't! You will have to go out and buy a *workman's* lunchbox in order to get it all in. Don't laugh! Just do it! There are also insulated nylon lunch containers that work very well. You'll see how easy it is once you get into it, and it sure feels good to pack your kids off with real food instead of a lot of dead stuff.

When we first sent Beau off to school, he felt "different" and was treated as "different" at lunchtime. We kept telling him that it was a "good different" and that eating healthy food was a gift not to be taken lightly. It didn't take long for the other kids to come around to the view that that nice crisp watermelon, those mouthwatering cherries, and that big Thermos full of buttery potatoes and corn were not such a bad idea. I found myself packing extra celery, carrots, or little tomatoes for him to share—and you've already heard about the Gypsy Boots Bar episode. At camp this summer we followed the same regimen with Beau. After a few days watching Beau eat his yummy potatoes, another kid in his group told him he was lucky. And I recall a friend of his who always ate your basic hamburger/hot dog fare coming over and, after having a meal with Beau, saying, "You're lucky, Beau. I wish my mom had the same 'cook brains' like your mom."

Getting back to school lunches, Mom, most kids really don't care all that much for bologna. Most of them kind of accept it as a fact of life, like bedtime. Complex carbohydrates at lunch are the way to go—potatoes, pasta, rice, or whole-grain breads. Children only get energy from fruits and these carbohydrates, or starches. Protein at lunch will slow them to a dead halt, especially if you mix it with bread. If you do have to pack a sandwich, pack one that is properly combined or make a Goodwich (see pages 410 and 411). Improperly combined lunches will sap children's energy and have them reaching for sugar to pep themselves up artificially the way you may reach for a cup of coffee.

At dinnertime *properly combine* your child's meal. If chicken is the main course, serve it with vegetables and a salad. Don't make potatoes, rice, or noodles that night, and don't offer any bread. If you are having pasta or rice, serve those as a main course with vegetable sauces and a salad. Potatoes can be a favorite main course with most kids. Make them baked, broiled, roasted, mashed with gravy, as hash browns, or even french fried *on occasion*.

The Goodwich is a great replacement for the dead food children are so typically addicted to. I know kids who eat them every day. Learn how to make Goodwiches. Your whole family will love them. Substitute Tomburgers (page 408) for hamburgers. The recipes are included in the back of this book together with many easy economical meal ideas that your children will love.

I have alluded to this point before but I think it bears reinforcing: *Feeding children does not have to be made into a complicated, difficult undertaking.* I know that many, many mothers have become dependent on the "convenience" foods that are available, like frozen dinners and canned and packaged foods, to say nothing of how many rely almost totally on fast food restaurants to feed their children. That is a *major* mistake! Each time you opt for that kind of convenience you are making a dead food choice for your child. You know, in the last generation these foods barely existed.

Our mothers were raised on food prepared by our grandmothers. When packaged, canned, and frozen foods became available, they were a once-in-a-while "occurrence" when Mom wanted to give herself a break. Now they are the norm, not the exception. We and our parents had the opportunity to eat far more real, unadulterated, homemade food than do the children of this generation. And that is the reason cancer and heart disease are now so prevalent among the young, who should not even be diseased in any way but are chemically poisoned daily by all the chemicals in all the processed, dead foods.

Please understand that nutritious home cooking is so much easier than you realize. Just use fresh ingredients, real butter, and as little chemically adulterated food as possible. Kids love bowls of strawberries, quartered oranges, or plates of sliced melon, peaches, plums, or cherries. I hear them in the supermarket begging Mom for strawberries. She says they are too expensive then reaches for an equally priced package of processed food. We need a new way of thinking on this issue. With processed foods we pay for processing, packaging, and shelf life, which all equal dead food and doctor bills, not nutrition. **REAL FOODS ARE DOLLAR FOR POUND MORE ECONOMICAL AND FULL OF NUTRITION.** When you start to emphasize the fresh fruits and vegetables of the season in your meal planning rather than packaged foods and meats, you will see your food bills go down. It is more economical to eat real food!

Kids love simple foods. There is a six-year-old child who visits us regularly. I make him pasta—usually vegetable or whole grain—and he "wolfs it down." His parents are amazed. At home he won't touch pasta, but they always have meat or tomato sauce and cheese on it. Frequently we impose our adult need for more "flavorful" foods on kids who couldn't care less. They love buttered baked potatoes and corn on the cob. They love string beans that they can eat with their fingers. Lots of kids love hot, still crunchy steamed broccoli that they can dip into melted butter, and many love artichokes. Whole-wheat garlic bread is a winner. Hot corn tortillas with butter or avocado and sprouts make good, nutritious snacks. So do raw nuts. Mashed avocado as a dip for corn chips with carrot and celery sticks makes a great lunch. Kids love mashed potatoes and gravy for dinner. They love tomato or avocado sandwiches for lunch. Make your meals simple with pasta, rice, or potatoes as a main course and see how your kids take to them. *They will*. They will also love soup as a main course with hot cornbread or biscuits and salad. If you have kids who won't eat salads, try putting little fried potato croutons or macaroni in them. Have salad ready with a dressing they like—Thousand Island is usually a favorite—and when they say they are "starving" for dinner, sit them down to the salad first while you finish preparing the rest. It will soon be gone, you'll see! If they like cheese but you are trying to cut down on it, put small cubes of it in their salad.

I have tried to include many kid-tested recipes in the recipe section. Try some of them with your kids. Don't make a big deal over doing so or put out any great announcements like "From now on we are going to eat healthy food!" That can sound too threatening and may prompt resistance. What matters to them is that this food is *good* as well as being healthy. Add a few new recipes a week to your repertoire without pressuring yourself or them. You'll be appreciated because the food will be good, and your caring will speak through it.

If you have teenagers, of course you can't force them to make changes in their diet. But you should know that we have had many letters and comments from teenagers who are extremely excited and enthusiastic about the results they have had with **Fit for Life**. The most you can do with teenagers is present the information to them in a nonthreatening way and allow them to make the changes at their own pace—and support them in doing so.

The best piece of news is the statement made by Henry C. Ross, director of dining services at Bucknell University in Pennsylvania. He told an interviewer that "about 500 of the 2000 students he serves daily prefer a vegetable-oriented lunch or dinner." As a result, the college has installed a special dining room that serves soup and salad for lunch. Ross said that cooks on his staff have found it hard to believe that students prefer vegetables to meat. "The students still like desserts," Ross said, "but the accent is on health. Fresh fruit tops the sweets list."

What an encouraging trend! For the future health of people in this country, this report, in *real* terms, is more meaningful than any of the "medical breakthrough" headlines we are constantly exposed to in the press. With an increase in the number of editors and reporters who are aware of the incredible impact of the ageless, simple truths of Natural Hygiene, reports like this, instead of being buried in the back of the paper, will begin to make front-page headlines. Our young people are demanding *for themselves* the foods that will keep them strong and disease-free! We should all take a break and dance a jig!

Although the women's movement has been positive in ways many of us cannot yet fully assess, one tragic result has been that mothering, which encompasses providing safe nourishment, has fallen from the position of high respect that it deserves. Far too many young mothers, feeling that they are inadequate in comparison to their "professional sisters," are searching for a way to feel validated even though that validating activity is right under their noses, looking to them helplessly for the attention it deserves. What could be more validating than assisting in the continuation of a healthy species through the gentle, constant, and tender care that the female of our species is so well equipped biologically to supply. It is far more important for our survival than promotions and bonuses. A society that values those over mothering and thereby forces its women into the workplace at the expense of their children is a society that cares little for its young. In my opinion, **A SOCIETY THAT DOESN'T CARE FOR ITS YOUNG HAS NO FUTURE.**

It is sad for young mothers to be under pressure to leave their families and enter the work force when their children still need them. Until children are in school and have reached the age of independence, mothering is a full time and enormously *worthy* profession. Once a woman has fulfilled that responsibility, she is far more capable of providing whatever further contribution she has to make to society than one who is trying to do everything at once and winds up exhausted and full of guilt for doing neither job well.

You may have friends who simply don't grasp the importance of making the effort to feed their children properly. They say they just don't have time to do it. To them it is more important that their nails remain perfectly manicured than that they prepare wholesome food for their children. Or they may feel that tennis or art lessons are more important. The time that mothers refuse to spend feeding their children properly is time they will ultimately spend worrying about how they will get better when they have lost their health. In a society where 75 percent of the children are overweight, where cancer is the major cause of death of children, and where almost all children have at least one symptom of heart disease, no activity could possibly be more important than the proper care and feeding of those children. The time that mothers refuse to spend doing this may even end up being hospital time. There is no way to get around it. You either do it right the first time when you have the chance or *you and your child* pay the heavy price later on down the line.

Why should kids be sick? They are young and should be clean and strong. *Those who don't wish to take the time to keep them well are actually making them sick.* Mothers of America, come on! It is our job to take care of the children of America. We have the natural, inborn, magnificent ability to do so. The mothers of no other country in the world are raising their children on junk food! We have become lazy and complacent and *we've got to wake up*! Don't listen to anyone who tells you that anything else is more important! Do it and be proud that you do! *It is an act of great love.*

CHAPTER 17

Detoxification— What to Do During a Crisis

MARILYN:

In chapter 5 I talked about enervation and its effect on the body. I explained that when we have depleted our nerve energy supply, all body processes begin to suffer. The elimination of the toxic debris of cell metabolism, which is normally a routine and ongoing process, drastically slows, and the body begins to retain within its pristine boundaries the poisonous waste that should be eliminated. In addition, digestion, absorption, and assimilation are less efficient. Without adequate nerve energy to carry on these functions at their full potential, the body carries them on at a below normal rate. Some of the toxic waste generated from food that is not adequately digested or that has spoiled in a sluggish digestive tract is absorbed into the body, and this further adds to an already toxic condition.

The human body, however, is able and equipped to defend itself against the "auto-intoxification," or self-poisoning, brought on by enervation. It does this in the form of chronic crises. We will have a cold or we will run a fever. We may get a sore throat or diarrhea. We may be headachy or irritable. This is the way the body takes control. It knocks us off our feet by making us so uncomfortable that we will cease all activity, lie down and rest, and turn over to its greater intelligence whatever energy remains for an expulsion of this life-threatening, poisonous waste. Remember, **ENERGY IS THE ESSENCE OF LIFE**, and it is spent on every body process and activity of our daily lives. Remember, too, that **THE ONLY WAY ENERGY CAN BE BUILT BACK UP OR RECOUPED IS THROUGH REST AND SLEEP.**

So when you feel unwell, when you are "broke" in terms of energy, if you are not wise enough to rest, sleep, and allow your body to make new deposits in its depleted energy bank, your body takes over and forces you into bed with a cleansing or detoxification crisis.

Once a detoxification crisis sets in and your body forces you to allow it to eliminate poisons that cannot be held in any longer, there is an important understanding that you must have. You must understand first that you are not "sick." You have not "caught" anything. You are actually witnessing a most miraculous aspect of human existence: the ability of your body to maintain its health and integrity by ridding itself of that which is harmful. Of course, it is able to do so! It is able to develop from a tiny ovum to a full-grown adult. It is able to reproduce. It is able to maintain a myriad of bodily functions simultaneously. How can it be possible, given these abilities, that it would not be able to care for and defend itself? When we overdo—when we eat too much, work too hard, take into our bodies too many harmful substances from the air, food and water, when we are excessively emotional or overactive sexually, and when we sleep too little—our bodies are forced to take control and counteract the state of enervation that we have brought on ourselves and the toxic condition that accompanies it. *What you do* at this time will greatly affect your overall health and determine whether you will be increasingly stronger or increasingly weaker as time passes in your life.

If you support the detoxification crisis by allowing it to pass naturally, you will be stronger and less prone to other crises in the future. If you thwart it, the crises will come regularly as the body endeavors to complete the unfinished cleansing process. Let's look at this last statement in a bit more detail.

How can you support a detoxification crisis? The answer to that is what this book is about. **IN BOTH HEALTH AND ILL HEALTH, YOU MUST PROVIDE FOR YOUR BODY THAT WHICH IT REQUIRES BIOLOGICALLY.** These are the simple elements of health we have been discussing—air, water, food, rest and sleep, sunshine, exercise, and positive emotional influences. These are the age-old health-restoring elements that have never been "discovered" by medical science because there was no money to be made from them. They are the simple hygienic measures that will improve your health without *any* harmful side effects. Certain of these elements are more important when we are in a crisis than when we are not. These are rest and sleep, fresh air, pure water, the food we eat, and our relationships.

First and foremost in importance are rest and sleep. Detoxification has been brought about by enervation, and the symptoms we are experiencing, whether they be simple fatigue or sneezing, coughing, aches and pains, and so on, are the body's ways of telling us that our batteries are low, our bank accounts are overdrawn, or, in real terms, that we are *out of energy*. When these symptoms tell you that you are out of energy, for health's sake listen! **YOU CAN ONLY BUILD ENERGY THROUGH REST AND SLEEP**, and when you have built enough, the crisis will have passed. Therefore, when you are detoxifying, please give your body a chance to rest! If you do, it will recoup its energy, and before you know it, it will once again be carrying on all the bodily functions at a normal rate and you will be feeling fine. If you deny your body rest at a point when it most needs rest, the crisis will drag on and your vitality will be low for a much greater length of time. The body will not be able to rid itself of all the poisons that have accumulated as a result of enervation, so the process will be incomplete, and during this crisis you will be laying the foundation for another one. Remember that *all* activity drains energy. When you are detoxifying, cut back on every activity possible and rest in a quiet, comfortable room. Modern living doesn't allow for us to do so easily, I know, but that is what is wrong with modern living and that is why we are not in possession of the high level of health and energy that we should be experiencing.

It is obvious that most people totally ignore the importance of rest as a factor in health, and this must be changed. We used to receive calls all the time from friends in the entertainment business who were following the **Fit for Life** program and couldn't understand how they had "come down with" a cold or the flu even though they were "eating so well." We always asked, "How much rest are you getting?"

"Rest? What's that? You know how busy I am. I barely have time to sleep!" (what with this film or that record deadline or all the meetings, dinners, and social obligations that are part of that industry).

Getting one of these people whose life was being played out "in the fast lane" to rest was harder than getting a kid to volunteer to go to sleep early. Now these high-powered individuals are catching on. When they start to feel "out of it" they restructure their lives to be able to rest without the battle they used to put up. Why? Because it works!

In a speech before the American Natural Hygiene Society in New York in 1950, Dr. Herbert Shelton addressed this issue. He was aware of it then, way before others had realized what the situation was, and we know now how much worse the situation is today:

> All forms of overwork, over-indulgence and overdoing are causes of enervation. In civilized life today we live our lives on the basis of dissipation rather than on one of conservation. . . . We turn the night into day and seem to have a psychopathic dread of going to bed. For such reasons we . . . form great streams into and out of the offices of doctors of various kinds, into and out of the hospitals, and into premature graves. We build more and bigger hospitals, equipped with all the latest gadgets, and staff them with the best trained men in the world, but we never remedy the great and increasing amount of illness among us for the simple reason that we spend our day building more and more trouble. . . . Only by a cessation of the habits of living that produce and maintain enervation can the sick man become well again. What is needed most of all is not more institutions for the care of the sick, not more and better doctors, not health "insurance" and a program of "socialized" medicine, but a normal mode of life—one that conserves the precious energy of life and does not dissipate it.

In order for the level of health to improve in the United States, some things are going to have to change, and we are going to have to force the changes for our own good. You have to be your own health reformer. First change: When you are in need of rest, you *deserve* rest, and you *must* rest for as long as you need to do so. Cut out *every* noncritical activity and allow your body to rebuild as necessary to run properly. The more you rest, the faster you'll feel better. Your body will tell you how long that is.

Now that we have worked that out (and I hope I have made some headway in impressing on you that you have a right to rest, that it only makes sense for you to do so), make sure when you are resting that there is plenty of fresh air circulating in the room. We've already learned that one of the ways in which the body rids itself of toxins is through respiration. We breathe toxins out with every breath. If the room is stuffy and closed, guess what! We breathe them back in again and detoxification takes longer.

Pure water is the next important remedy during detoxification. Drink it as often as you feel the need. Remember the issue Harvey raised in the chapter on water. Most of what we drink only adds to the toxins in our bodies. Try, if it is available, *especially during a detoxification crisis*, to drink only distilled water.

All activity of the body takes energy, and eating, which forces the body to digest food, takes the most energy of all. When you are detoxifying, eat lightly, and if you are not hungry, listen to your body and don't force food on it. No matter what the uninformed may tell you about needing to eat to "keep up your strength," remember that **FOOD TAKES ENERGY BEFORE IT BECOMES A SOURCE OF ENERGY.** We have stored in our bodies enough nutrients to live for weeks without food, so going light for a few days certainly cannot hurt! If you are enervated, you have the need to *build* energy, not *use* it. If you are hungry —and only if you are hungry—depend on foods that drain the least amount of energy because they require little or no digestion. You know what those foods are: fresh fruit juices, fresh vegetable juices, and fresh fruits and vegetables. If you are sleeping, lying down and inactive, you are giving your body a physical and mental rest. Drinking water and eating only fresh fruits and vegetables will provide a physiological rest to a great extent. By following this simple regimen, energy will be built quickly and real hunger and the desire for activity will return soon.

One of the most important factors to be aware of during a detoxification crisis is the relationship factor. When you are out of energy, you may wish to be alone, and that is fine if that is how you feel. What is to be avoided is relating to others in an emotionally draining way. First of all, you know what is going on, but many around you may not understand. You have overdone it in some way, you have spent your energy, you are toxic because your body is enervated, and now you are recouping and detoxifying. Those with less up-to-date viewpoints may hear you sneeze or see you lying down and think you are "sick." They may ask you to get up and get help, when all you need is rest. Some people can become very pushy about health. Ask them to allow you the freedom to do what you know is best for you. You need no "harbingers of doom" around you telling you that if you don't do something, see someone, or take something for your fatigue and cleansing symptoms, you are going to be a statistic within the week.* One of the most important practices of the Asklepian priests of ancient Greece was to keep the spirits of those who entered the temples high. Morale was a big issue there. Faith in the healing process of the body was paramount.

Since positive thinking supports the healing process, I find it most curious that modern medical practitioners deal such low blows to the morale of the ill. Frequently we hear about people who are quite sick actually being told how long they have to live or that they have no chance to survive, and even the well are given statistics on how many will be sick in the future. Now, how can anyone know for sure what will happen in the future? How can anyone in this vast world of choices and variables tell us that we have *no chance*? History is full of stories about people who pulled off the unexpected when they were told they didn't have a chance. How can anyone have the audacity to tell us how long we have to live? You know the effect it has on someone in a weakened state to be told arbitrarily when death will arrive. Usually it only weakens them further. This negative approach has been challenged time and again by advocates of positive thinking. After all, what we think greatly affects how we feel, and if we are told by someone in a supposed position of authority to think we are going to die or are going to get sick, how will we feel? Not well! Not confident! Not hopeful! Not in control! Many people defy this thinking and prove the doomsayers wrong, but many also succumb when they might have had a chance.

Please, when you are detoxifying, don't let people bring you down. Make it a point to surround yourself with loving, supportive people. If someone dear to you has no understanding of your condition, invite that person to stay out of it. This is not the time for you to have to defend yourself. Trust your body's intelligence. It is far greater than your own or your friend's. You have overdone

---

*By all means, if you yourself feel a sense of alarm, contact a health professional whom you trust.

it and your body is regrouping. Let it. It will take care of everything that needs to be done. It is a natural, biological process that is taking place. Although this is new thinking for most of us, remember that it is really very *old* thinking, an instinctive response that we have disconnected from and are now returning to. We have been on the planet for millions of years; we survived and populated the globe during that time, undergoing tremendous physical tests and passing them. We were strong—we had to be—and all healing was a biological process. It had to be because we were without the 3000-year-old body of technology we now look to for health care . . . and yet, we made it, folks! So we once knew quite a bit, and we could know quite a bit again.

When I say that it is important to avoid emotional drain during detoxification and to surround yourself with loving, supportive people, I do not wish to imply that the loving go to the point of sexual interaction. Next to digestion, sexual activity is the greatest energy usurper. If your energy is depleted, please abstain. If you aren't feeling all that great, how can it be an enjoyable experience anyway? Making love is one of the most beautiful, creative, artistic experiences two people can share. A runny nose can definitely put a crimp on it.

Another of the elements that is also important to skip when you are detoxifying is exercise. *Exercise takes energy.* It does not contribute to the building of an energy supply. Rest! You will have plenty of energy for exercise when the crisis passes, and when you do start exercising again, be moderate. Overexercising is enervating. While detoxifying, a light bouncing on the rebounder to help clear the lymph system can be the exception, *if* you feel up to it.

People frequently ask how long a detoxification crisis lasts. There is no way of knowing. Your body is at work. When the work is completed the crisis will be over. Asking how long it takes is like asking how much time is needed for hair or fingernails to grow. For each person there are different variables. How enervated are you? How much did you overdo it? Having been involved in detoxification work for over a decade, I can tell you that I have seen absolutely everything! I have seen three-hour detoxes, six-hour detoxes, one-, two-, three-, or four-day detoxes, ten-day detoxes, and everything in between.

I'm talking to you now from the perspective of my own detoxification experience, from witnessing detoxification in Harvey and in my children, and from interaction with friends, students, clients, seminar attendees, and people who have attended our four-week detoxification workshops. In addition we have had thousands of calls and letters over the years from people seeking advice on detoxification.

When you first begin to realize the cause-and-effect factor that is behind detoxification, you will have a tremendous sense of your power to be well and remain well, *knowing* how to care for yourself if you begin to get sick. If in the beginning your body has detoxification crises as you learn to live a more intelligent life-style, you may notice that the crises have a particular set of symptoms. Some people get sore throats. A sore throat is a very healthful symptom—it is your body closing the door on food. The body is saying with pain, "More food will not be useful right now, my dear. I have more than I can deal with already." With a sore throat, you should definitely stop eating anything but juices and the lightest of fruits and vegetables until it goes away and the body once again clears the entry to the alimentary canal.

Other symptoms of detoxification include headaches, coughs, stomachaches, diarrhea, skin eruptions, and clogged sinuses. Emotional reactions such as irritability and depression are also frequently the result of enervation and symptoms of detoxification.* Whatever your particular experiences with detoxification are, you will come to understand that what you feel is the only way your body has to tell you to take it easy and lighten up. If year after year you ignore the signals of your body and, instead of resting and eating less, you go right on with your life and knock out the symptoms with a drug rather than dealing with the *cause*, your depleted energy, ultimately your body will speak to you in much stronger terms than just the sniffles or a cough. Allowing the biological process of detoxification to complete itself naturally whenever necessary is like smart investing or saving for the future. Drugging yourself so that you can continue to do what caused the symptoms in the first place is like spending more than you have earned. In the first instance, your future is secure; you have built health by listening to your body. In the second, your future does not look so great. Sooner or later, overspending of any commodity,

---

*We can only hope that if one of those show biz TV doctors decides to read these *possible* symptoms on national television, he or she will have the honesty and integrity *not* to read them out of context.

be it money or your energy, catches up with you and you must pay the price. The greater the debt, the more you pay.

Here is the most important point to remember: **YOUR BODY HAS THE INTELLIGENCE TO RESTORE ITSELF TO HEALTH.** *Only* it can do so! The magnificent power and wisdom that constructed you from a fertilized ovum *still remains with you*. Not only is it capable of restoring you to health, it is the only real power capable of doing so. **WHEN YOUR BODY GOES INTO A HEALING CRISIS—WHEN IT INITIATES ACTIONS TO DETOXIFY ITSELF—DON'T INTERFERE!** Leave it alone and it will do the job for you. It is totally self-sufficient if its simple biological needs are met from the outside. Rest, sleep, eat little, drink water, *smile*! Your body is the master of its domain!*

We are a society that has overspent in many ways for a long time. We are being given a chance to see how costly overspending can be when it comes to our health, since in spite of all the hospitals, doctors, medical plans, and insurance policies we have, our enervating life-style causes us to lead the world in the degenerative diseases. And as more hospitals are built, we have more disease, not less. An understanding of enervation and detoxification and their cause and effect relationship gives us a mighty tool to use in dealing with lesser symptoms appropriately, so that they do not ultimately lead to the graver health crises so prevalent in our society.

On the following pages you will find a list of recipes that are provided in the cookbook section for dishes that are appropriate eating during detoxification. They are classified from lightest to heaviest. When you feel unwell, *please eat as little as possible. Stay to the light side.* As your energy is restored, you can begin gradually to move to the heavier recipes. For some people salads, particularly those with heavier dressings, are not at all enticing

---

*Occasionally, symptoms of the body's cleansing efforts will include a fever or diarrhea. These two activities, *instigated by the body*, have long been misunderstood and therefore frequently feared unnecessarily. A mild fever or simple diarrhea lasting two or three days is uncomfortable to be sure, but not life threatening. If, however, either should persist longer than three days, or you feel personal concern, I would then seek out a professional opinion to verify that what you are experiencing is merely a temporary, therapeutic function of your body in its effort to be healthier.

during a detox. If you are one of those, the blended salad is for you. Have clear vegetable soups or steamed vegetables.

If salads do seem attractive to you while you are detoxifying, have them, because for most people, *only* living food during detoxification brings the best results. For others, whose digestive tracts are somewhat deficient in vitality, living food *initially* carries with it a bit too much cellulose. In these cases, a mixture of living food with steamed vegetables or vegetable soups works best. You will be able to sense what your body needs. The climate will also help determine your choices. In warm weather, living food will be more appropriate. In colder weather, a mixture of living food and warm, cooked soups and vegetables may feel best.

The most important principle to keep in mind is that the purpose of making changes in your food intake at all is to work *with* the body, freeing up energy to allow your body to carry out its healing efforts. The *less* you eat that taxes your digestive tract, the *more* energy your body will have to do its repair work. So **IF YOU ARE DETOXIFYING, PLEASE, REST YOUR WHOLE BODY, INCLUDING YOUR DIGESTIVE TRACT.**

Certainly, ample attention has been given to the importance of having a steady stream of energy throughout your body. All cleansing and detoxifying, all activity, mental and physical—every function of your body—is totally dependent upon this continuous flow of energy. For this reason I think it important to discuss the benefits of chiropractic adjustments. All energy in your body emanates from the nervous system, originating in your brain and spinal cord. Nerves come off of the spinal column and transport energy to every area of your body. Frequently, however, the spine can get out of alignment, and this not only causes discomfort in the back but, more seriously, it interferes with the flow of energy through the nerves. Organs that are waiting for energy to conduct a cleansing or healing are deprived of energy, and problems develop or become worse. Chiropractic adjustments realign the spine and normalize the flow of energy. Having your spine checked to see if it is in need of an alignment is a very simple and painless process. To get the name of a reputable chiropractor, you can contact the local chapter of the state Chiropractic Association in your city.

Professional massage is also another tool you can use to hasten the improvement in your health. When the body is enervated, the lymph system, our "sewage treatment plant," gets bogged down and the body becomes "swampy." Extra mucous is secreted by the body to sponge and clean out toxic material. Anti-histamines work against this elimination by drying things up. Wrong! The point is to move the waste material through, not stop it up! Certain massage therapies such as Swedish and lymphatic massage and reflexology will facilitate the lymphatic drainage. Aside from the important therapeutic value of these treatments, they feel great! Take advantage of them in sickness and in health.

Accupressure, based on the ancient Chinese study of the meridiens, which are like a map of our wellness system, will also help during detoxification, particularly if lighter touches to stimulate the nervous and circulatory systems are used. Deep accupressure should not be used during detoxification because it can be painful and enervating. Accupuncture, the 5000-year-old Chinese healing technique, can be used to repair shorts in electrical energy so healing can continue. Attacked vociferously until recently by medical science, this ancient healing art is now being accorded the respect it justifiably deserves.

RECIPES FOR DETOXIFICATION

ALL FRESH FRUIT AND VEGETABLE JUICES:

Tangerine
Strawberry-Apple
Orange
Grapefruit
Orange-Pineapple
Pineapple-Strawberry
Cherry-Grape

Watermelon-Cantaloupe
Tropical Ambrosia
Honeyloupe
Apple-Celery
Summer Vegemato
Carrot
Carrot-Celery-Tomato

SMOOTHIES

Orange Freeze
Persimmon Smoothie
Melon Smoothie
Watermelon Smoothie

Cantaloupe Smoothie
Honeydew Smoothie
Almond Sunrise

ALL FRUIT

FRUIT SALADS, SAUCES, TREATS, PLATTERS

Fruit for Life Salad with
Banana-Peach Sauce
Sliced Bananas, Strawberries,
and Kiwi
Mango MelonBerry Salad
with Honeyloupe Sherbet
Peach-Melon Bowl with
Cashew-Apricot Sauce

Sliced Apples in Cinnamon
and Figs with Grapes
Sliced Pineapple, Papaya, and
Banana
Sliced Oranges, Persimmons,
and Pears
Coconut-Apple Granola

VEGETABLE SALADS AND DRESSINGS

Sliced Tomato, Avocado, and
Cucumber
French Butter Lettuce Salad
Soft Lettuce Tacos with
Avocado and Fresh Herb
Dressing

Greens and Shredded
Vegetables with Grapefruit
Juice Dressing
Mixed Vegetable Salad with
Nori
Fit for Life Sprout Salad
Blended Salad

VEGETABLE SOUPS

Chinese Corn Soup
Cream of Romaine and
Cucumber Soup (creamless
version)
Miso Soup and Vegetables

Clear Broth and Vegetables
Country Carrot Soup
Green Soup with Fresh Herbs
Avocado Soup

ALL STEAMED VEGETABLES
(with or without lemon, butter, or olive oil)

STEAMED AND BAKED VEGETABLES

Braised Green Beans and
Gravy
Sweet and Sour Red Cabbage
Sweet Carrots *au Naturel*
Minute Asparagus
Easy Cauliflower Italiano

Steamed Potatoes and
Vegetables in Olive Oil
Mashed Potatoes
Plain Steamed Potatoes

DETOXIFICATION MENUS

If you are detoxifying, the idea is to concentrate on foods that will nourish your body without robbing it of its vital healing energy. The following examples of three possible detoxification eating plans are based on recipes that you will find in the **Living Health** recipe section. (NOTE: If fruit meals in the morning leave you feeling bloated, you can have the fruit with some raw celery and fresh lettuce leaves—but not iceburg lettuce.)

DAY ONE

An all-juice day will free up the maximum amount of energy for healing and repair. Stay in bed, rest, sleep, and *sip* eight to ten ounces of fresh juice *every two hours*, starting at 8 A.M. and continuing until 8 P.M. As long as the juices are fresh, you can choose whichever you prefer and you *can* substitute 8 ounces of water for two or three of the juice "meals" if desired. It is a good idea to stay with fruit juices in the morning and vegetable juices in the afternoon then have fruit juice again before bed. You don't have to have this much variety in one day. This is just to stimulate you to try some new juice combinations and flavors.

8 A.M. —Cantaloupe Smoothie
10 A.M. —Orange Juice
12 noon—Apple-Celery Juice
2 P.M. —Carrot Juice
4 P.M. —Vegetable Juice Cocktail
6 P.M. —Honeydew Smoothie
8 P.M. —Apple-Banana Smoothie

DAY TWO

A *living food* day will allow detoxification to proceed without draining a great deal of your energy toward digestion, unless you eat too frequently.

BREAKFAST Melon Smoothie of your choice, or plate of sliced cantaloupe, honeydew, and watermelon (or whatever fruits are available in your area) with lettuce

LUNCH   Blended Salad, sliced tomatoes, one-half avocado
             or peeled, sliced cucumber (if desired)

DINNER   A platter of sliced oranges, pears, persimmons, and
             bananas or fruits that are fresh in your area, with
             lettuce and celery.

DAY THREE

BREAKFAST   Fresh orange juice; plate of apples, figs, and grapes

LUNCH   Greens and Shredded Vegetables with Grapefruit
             Juice Dressing, sliced tomatoes

DINNER   Clear Broth with Vegetables, steamed broccoli, car-
             rots, spinach and cauliflower*

*A day of *living food* with a warm soup and vegetables in the evening is
most comfortable for some people when they are detoxifying. If you desire
a warm meal at lunch, have the soup then. It is good for the body to keep
variety to a minimum during detoxification, so have the same soup for
lunch and dinner.

CHAPTER 18
Questions Frequently Asked

HARVEY:

I work night shifts and have to sleep most of the daytime. How do I work this program into my schedule?

Although the body cycles are most efficient in those people on a "regular" schedule, if your night shift is worked on a *very consistent* basis, the cycles will accommodate themselves to your lifestyle. If your schedule fluctuates (one week regular, one week night shift), it will not be as easy to establish a routine. However, the single most important habit you can develop for the best results is to **CONSUME ONLY FRESH FRUIT AND FRESH FRUIT JUICE FOR THE FIRST FOUR OR FIVE HOURS AFTER YOU AWAKEN.** This is critical.

I am feeling better, but I would still like to lose more weight than I have so far on the program.

Be aware that your body works on priorities. When it deems it necessary to drop more weight, it will. More often than not the body will drop some weight, plateau while repair work is done internally, then return to the task of dropping more weight, *if necessary*. Let your body decide what weight it wants to be. It knows. You don't. Your only obligation is to feed yourself *correctly* and the body will do the rest. A good way to facilitate weight loss and "kick" your body off the plateau is to emphasize the living food days included in the menu section.

I have been losing weight and feeling too thin. Will I gain some weight back?

Practically everyone, no matter how thin, has some *waste* that needs to be removed from the body. If you lose weight and you do not want to lose more, realize that you have lost *waste* and **YOUR BODY WILL GO TO THE WEIGHT THAT IT WANTS TO BE** and remain there. In your case, you should emphasize complex carbohydrates in your diet. With correct eating *and exercise* (especially light weight-lifting), you will put on *healthy* weight.

Are there hot drinks to replace coffee?

Herbal teas are quite good, and there are many delicious flavors to choose from. They do not contain caffeine and are far superior to your run-of-the-mill commercial teas. Celestial Seasonings has a wide variety of delicious, caffeine-free teas. Also, hot water with the juice of a lemon squeezed into it is quite tasty and satisfies the desire for something hot in the morning. (The lemon will not ferment as it contains no sugar.)

What sweeteners are best?

I do not know of any sweetener that does not have something objectionable about it. Just pick one and use it moderately. I would use honey or maple syrup (raw) before aspartame or fructose or some other processed product. Also, some stores are carrying granulated date sugar and granulated maple sugar, neither of which are put through the refinement processes of other commercial sugars. These are very delicious, and you should give them a try if you can find them.

Occasionally when I eat fruit, even on an empty stomach as suggested, I feel bloated. Is there anything I can do about this?

The reason for occasional bloating after eating fruit is that fruit assists the body in cleansing toxic wastes from the lining of the stomach. When this waste is stirred up it ferments the fruit and causes the bloating. Eventually this toxic residue will be totally cleansed from the stomach and the bloating will not occur. But that's in the long term. However, there *is* something you can do now. The remedy may come as a shocker considering how frequently we caution against eating anything with fruit. But, as with all other "rules," there is an exception here and this is it: Eating celery stalks and/or lettuce leaves (any variety) together with your fruit buffers the interaction between the toxic residue and the fruit. These highly alkaline vegetables neutralize the acid in the stomach and prevent the bloating. This works! Hygienists have been doing this for a very long time. Some people, even after they have cleansed their stomachs and can eat fruit alone with no bloating, continue to eat celery and lettuce with their fruit simply because they like it.

I suffer from Candida, so how can I eat fruit?

This is not a subject that is easily covered in one short paragraph. However, one aspect of Candida is particularly important to understand: If you have the Candida yeast organism in your body, and almost everyone has, then be careful of fruit or anything else that can *ferment* in the body. **THE ONLY WAY FRUIT CAN AGGRAVATE A CANDIDA INFECTION IS IF IT IS EATEN INCORRECTLY.** When fresh fruit is eaten *alone* and on an *empty* stomach, *it will not ferment!* This is the key. When you eat cooked fruit or eat fruit with other foods, it spoils and ferments in the stomach. The Candida yeast proliferates on fermentable foods—carbohydrates. By consuming only *fresh* fruit when the stomach is *entirely* empty, there is no possibility of fermentation from bacteria or yeast. Also, it is exceedingly important for those with Candida to be very strict with food combining. All carbohydrates will ferment if eaten with proteins or if cooked. If you properly combine your foods, eat *fresh* fruit correctly, and avoid fermented foods (alcohol, vinegar, miso, yogurt), your Candida problem will become a thing of the past.

What about tofu?

This ancient food which originated in China over one thousand years ago has recently attracted our attention. It is an easily digestible protein which can play an important role in your diet as you begin to decrease your intake of animal protein. Tofu is made from soy milk, the liquid resulting when soaked and ground soy beans have been gently boiled for a short time. In high quality tofu preparation, the milk is then solidified with nigari (concentrate remaining when sea salt is extracted from sea water) or calcium sulfate (from gypsum). Tofu is rich in amino acids and calcium, containing more calcium by weight than dairy milk. It is also rich in iron, magnesium, phosphorous, potassium and sodium, essential B vitamins, choline and vitamin E. Unlike other proteins, it is alkaline, rather than acid. Because of this alkalinity and because it contains no crude soybean fiber, tofu combines well with starches, especially brown rice and other grains and whole grain breads. Watch for lots of new tofu recipes in the upcoming cookbook, THE FIT FOR LIFE KITCHEN.

Why are we allowed to include butter and oils in the **Fit for Life** *and* **Living Health** *programs?*

First of all, we need fat in our diets. It is one of the food groups necessary to the human body. Without fat our bodies do not thrive. In both programs, we are encouraging people to cut down on animal products, especially on meat and dairy. In so doing they are greatly decreasing the harmful animal fats that contribute so much to heart disease. The fact that we are asking people to increase their intake of vegetables, potatoes, and whole grains is one of the reasons we encourage a moderate use of butter. We are a society with a demanding palate. There are few people out there who would stay for very long on a high-vegetable regimen that did not include butter. And since so much animal fat is eliminated by cutting down on meat and dairy, the small amount of butter will not be harmful. The increase in high-water-content fruits and vegetables will help wash it through.

Notice that we are saying butter, *not margarine*. Margarine is very harmful and, contrary to advertising, it clogs the arteries. We call it "plastic fat." Use butter. Always go for the *real* rather than the synthetic.

The vegetable oils we recommend are the unrefined, cold-pressed varieties, not the hydrogenated oils, which are far too processed for your body to deal with them. Particularly recommended is olive oil, which has been reported by the University of Texas Health Science Center to actually *lower* blood cholesterol. People in Greece and southern Italy, who consume a lot of olive oil, have much lower blood cholesterol levels and a much lower rate of heart disease than people elsewhere in Europe and the United States.* Not many Americans would enjoy a salad without dressing, so use oils in moderation, and emphasize cold-pressed extra-virgin olive oils. In sautéeing, use a combination of safflower oil and butter, or use straight safflower oil.

Please explain exactly why butter is better than margarine.

Ah, yes! It's like wondering which is better, silk or polyester? Juice from a real piece of fruit or Gatorade? A diamond or a rhinestone? There's no comparison between the *real* and the *fake* in anything.

During World War II butter was real hard to come by, so a synthetic substitute, margarine, was created to take its place. Margarine is made by turning "pure liquid polyunsaturated oil" into a solid bar of grease. How is the liquid turned to solid? It is hydrogenated—hydrogen gas is bubbled through the oil until it solidifies. It can be made hard as a block of cement if enough hydrogen is used.

Margarine is touted as having less fat, being lower in calories, and providing some protection against heart disease. The truth is that butter and margarine have the *same* amount of calories and contain just as much fat, but margarine *will contribute to* the very problems commercials imply it will prevent, particularly heart disease! The manufacturers of margarine have often had to be constrained from making misleading statements. Although they have toned down somewhat, they are still very adept at giving the

*Tufts University Diet and Nutrition Letter, May 3, 1986.

impression that margarine prevents heart disease. It prevents heart disease about as much as a knife wound prevents bleeding.

Here's the lie. The word *polyunsaturated* is tossed around like it is heaven's answer to cholesterol in the blood. Not only do 999 people out of a 1000 have no idea what *polyunsaturated* actually means, **WHEN A POLYUNSATURATED FAT IS HYDRO-GENATED, IT IS CONVERTED TO A TOTALLY SATU-RATED FAT.** In fact, this type of fat causes an extremely high rise in cholesterol, and deaths from heart disease *and* cancer are highest among consumers of this type of fat, although you won't be hearing this in the advertisements. It's true that butter is an animal fat, but in moderate amounts it can be handled much more easily than hydrogenated oil. In the words of Dr. David Reuben, "In the process of making liquid corn oil, safflower oil, and all the other 'polyunsaturated' oils into margarine, they are transformed into plain ordinary 'saturated' oils. That has to be one of the greatest unexposed scandals in history. By hardening the vegetable oils, margarine sellers are offering you the very *saturated* fats they claim to be helping you to avoid. That's not too exciting, is it? It means, of course, that you are paying for polyunsaturates and getting all of the advantages of lard except for the lower price." Know what absolutely blows my mind? *Doctors* actually *recommend* margarine as a *healthy* substitute for butter! That's embarrassing. You just can't be more misinformed than that.

If you would like a terrific overview of this subject, there is a booklet by John H. Tobe called *Margarine*. This is what Mr. Tobe has to say about margarine: "[It is] a chemical compound that will not melt when you squeeze or rub it against your fingers. . . . What do you expect your bloodstream to do with these plastic particles? They feel and look exactly like flakes of celluloid, and that is exactly what you are putting in your body and your bloodstream every time you eat a food that contains hydrogenated fat." Wouldn't you rather have a little *real* butter on your food? Please do, instead of using a glop of congealed grease. Eating in accordance with the **Fit for Life** principles so drastically reduces animal fats that the modest amount of butter you consume will cause you *no* problems. The same cannot be said of plastic fat.

I love to eat popcorn and would like to know if this is okay.

Popcorn is a starch and should be treated as such. Try not to eat it with a protein in the stomach. Air-popped corn is best, without salt. A little melted butter, *not* margarine, is okay. Dr. Walker points out that the corn kernel, once popped, is very difficult to digest, so whenever we have popcorn we have either cucumber or celery with it. Sounds a little odd, but it tastes delicious. More importantly, the high water content of these vegetables assists greatly in facilitating the digestion of the popcorn and its movement through the body. Try it. You'll be very pleasantly surprised.

What about vinegar?

Vinegar is fermented and will suspend all salivary digestion. That goes for all vinegar: apple, wine or cider, and balsamic. Vinegar is vinegar and simply is not a food. It will not digest and will interfere with the digestion of other foods. Substitute lemon, tomato, or grapefruit juice whenever vinegar is called for.

I am diabetic and would like to know if this program could be something I can follow.

Of all the health situations that demand care and attention when altering diet, diabetes is the one with which one must be the most careful. **ABSOLUTELY NO DIETARY CHANGES SHOULD BE MADE WITHOUT THE KNOWLEDGE OF YOUR DOCTOR IF YOU ARE DIABETIC.** We have worked with many diabetics who have been successful in totally eliminating the need for insulin, and we have worked with others who have experienced no improvement whatsoever. It is essential that whatever changes you make are made under the supervision of your doctor. Whether you are one who will be successful or not is yet to be determined and will depend on your personal makeup and effort.

From the latest research observations it is clear that the fructose in fruit can assist a diabetic situation. Obviously, the fruit *must be eaten correctly*, which means alone on an empty stomach. Here is what to do:

Inform your doctor that you wish to try eating according to the principles you have learned and ask him or her to monitor your progress closely. As you start to implement the new eating life-style, *slowly* decrease the amount of insulin required. In a very short period of time, it will become clear to your doctor whether or not you can continue lowering your insulin. More than 50 percent of the patients with diabetes that we have worked with have shown marked improvement and have been able at least to lessen the amount of insulin necessary. We have several case histories of people we have worked with personally who have been able to either drastically reduce their insulin requirements or discontinue it altogether.

Let me tell you about Mr. Joe Gandolfo, who resides in Lakeland, Florida. Mr. Gandolfo, who is 50 years old, is an extremely successful businessman with a very active life-style. He has written five bestselling books on business and selling and is head of a major corporation. In 1982 he was diagnosed as having diabetes and went on insulin. The average number of units he required was between 15 and 20 a day, although he once was at 35 units. Because of his active life he deplored having to deal with the insulin, the needles and regular injections. But his efforts to get off of insulin all ended in failure. After reading **Fit for Life** about two and a half years ago, Mr. Gandolfo fashioned for himself a hygienic diet suited for his particular life-style and he has been able to reduce his insulin intake down to seven units. His physician recently told him that with requirements that low he might just as well go off of it entirely.

Interestingly, Mr. Gandolfo attributes much of his success in overcoming diabetes to celery. Why? Two reasons. First, celery, as has been amply stated, is highly alkaline. Since diabetes is aggravated in an acid environment, the more alkaline foods eaten the more chance there is of lessening the symptoms of the disease. Secondly, and this will come as a surprise to most, the green leaves of celery contain a valuable ingredient of insulin. Immediately after starting to eat celery every day and drinking celery juice (made with the leaves) Mr. Gandolfo was able to decrease his insulin intake. In fact he started to feel *worse* when he took his seven units, which in part prompted his physician to suggest his discontinuing it altogether.

I don't want to imply that celery can magically overcome diabetes. There are other variables including diet, exercise, mental attitude, etc. And I know there will be those to say the whole idea is ridiculous. They just better not say it in front of Mr. Gandolfo unless they want an earful. Please don't think that because you are on insulin that it is a life sentence. There are things you can do. Once again, this must be absolutely clear: **ANY CHANGES IN YOUR DIET IF YOU ARE DIABETIC MUST BE MADE UNDER THE SUPERVISION OF YOUR DOCTOR.**

When would be the best time to take brewer's yeast?

The best time to consume brewer's yeast is right after the sun turns to ice. We poor Americans are hopelessly gullible. We are constantly having *wastes* stuck down our throats, and more often than not we are convinced to pay for the privilege! Because of the gargantuan amount of food that is processed in this country, a tremendous amount of waste by-products are generated. These wastes are usually exceedingly difficult to dispose of, but then they are routinely labeled as "healthy" and *sold* to people who have been convinced that health can be purchased in neatly packaged tins.

Look at whey, the putrid, yellow-green by-product of cheese production. Only about 10 percent of the milk used to make cheese actually ends up as cheese. The rest of the unlovely liquid separates out as vile-smelling, vile-tasting whey. In the late 1970s there was a frantic search for ways to dispose of it. Before dairy consumption doubled, from 1960 to 1978, it was simply trucked to hog farms and fed to pigs, but that became too expensive. Strict federal and state regulations prohibit dumping raw whey down sewers. Whey is 100 to 200 times stronger a pollutant than residential sewage, and most municipal sewerage plants cannot treat it adequately. Disposal in streams is out because whey depletes waterways of oxygen, thus rendering them incapable of supporting marine life. Disposal on unused land or gravel pits is often unsuitable because of seepage into water supplies. Many cheese factories simply used to dump the stuff surreptitiously and illegally. An article in the *Los Angeles Times* (December 4, 1978) announced, "The solution hit upon by both industry and government is to apply high technology and sophisticated marketing techniques and feed the stuff to humans."

Right! Of course! Where else would they get rid of it? There may be strict regulations prohibiting whey from being dumped into the sewers, but there is nothing prohibiting them from dumping it into your food. Don't you just feel like throwing your arms around the food processors in this country and giving them a big kiss? They're in heaven. They get whey better than free—they are *paid* one cent a gallon to haul it away. The factories producing the whey are more than happy to pay a penny a gallon to have it hauled off so they don't have a waste problem to deal with. Now, start reading some labels and you'll see whey listed in a mind-boggling array of products —soup mixes, cocoa, pancake batter, Twinkies, margarine, packaged mashed potatoes, spaghetti sauces, salad dressings, baby foods, breads, etc., etc. Ovaltine has more whey than *any* other ingredient except sugar. Whey looks like pus and smells like vomit. It does not belong in your food.

The same goes for molasses, which is the by-product of the refining of sugar, sold for its "health-giving" qualities. Ha! It used to be trucked off and fed to cows, until it became apparent that people would pay a lot more for it than the cattle farmers.

Brewer's yeast is the by-product of beer production. The beer brewers didn't know what to do with their offal either, so the most dependable solution of all was used—call it a "health food" and dump it down the throats of the gullible population. Such a nice, easy, *profitable* answer to such a nasty, smelly problem.

I was once at a seminar where the subject of brewer's yeast was raised. A girl sitting directly in front of me said, "Ugh, brewer's yeast. I have some every morning, but it stinks up my whole kitchen when I take the top off the can." I tapped her on the shoulder and asked, "If it stinks up your kitchen, what do you suppose it's doing in your intestines?" She got the kind of perplexed look on her face of someone who has just been asked to spell *chrysanthemum*.

Whether the product is whey or molasses or brewer's yeast or fluoride or radioactive wastes, *we must not allow big business to use our bodies to solve their toxic waste problems.*

You mentioned Gatorade in a negative way. I thought it was a healthy thirst quencher.

Of course you thought that. It is exactly what the food processors pay the advertisers to get you to think. The truth is, dish water is probably a better drink. Gatorade is nothing but water and a bunch of chemicals—water, sucrose (refined sugar), glucose (more refined sugar), salt, sodium citrate (more salt), and yellow dyes number 5 and 6. Sounds like something used to remove paint from a wall. By law these drinks must say on the label how much actual fruit juice they contain. On the label of Gatorade, in print so small you need an extra set of eyes to see it, it states, "Contains no fruit juice." A fruit drink with no fruit. The food processors are taking P. T. Barnum's comment "There's a sucker born every minute" a little too seriously. Look, we can't keep falling for these things. If we're not careful, they're going to start feeding us radioactive waste while telling us how good it is for us. Whoops! I almost forgot. They already are.

What if I can't find all the products you recommend?

When we mention an unusual product, in the recipe section, we usually also note an alternative that is easier to find. When you cannot find the items recommended, substitute what you *can* find. For example, there are many varieties of seasonings that can be used for the broths and soups. At your *natural food* store, you may find vegetable bouillon cubes, powdered vegetable broths, liquid vegetable seasonings. (Do not use just any commercial product!) Use whatever is available to you. There are also food product catalogs that specialize in hard-to-find items. Three that you can take advantage of are put out by:

> Walnut Acres
> Walnut Acres Road
> Penns Creek, PA 17862

> Timber Crest Farms
> 4791 Dry Creek Road
> Healdsburg, CA 95448

> Pittman and Davis
> Box 2227
> Harlingen, TX 78551

You haven't mentioned eggs in any detail. Are they an exception to what you state about animal products?

They are not an exception, nor are they a valuable food. In chapter 14 we showed you how detrimental and disease-producing animal products are. Eggs are an animal product, being the embryo of a chicken. Also, remember what *all* health professionals are recommending that we eat—less fat and cholesterol and more fiber. Eggs are *very* high in fat and cholesterol and contain essentially *no* fiber. In fact, ounce for ounce, eggs contain eight times more cholesterol than beef! The egg industry, of course, denies all of the negatives about eggs in much the same way the tobacco industry defends itself, but don't fall for either's attempt to protect their profits at the expense of your health. Dr. John McDougall points to only six studies in medical literature that show that eggs don't dramatically affect blood cholesterol levels. Of these, three were funded by the American Egg Board, one by the Missouri Egg Merchandising Council, one by the Egg Program of the California Department of Agriculture (the sixth is not identified). As Dr. McDougall states, "The egg industry provides a timely example of how money can buy scientific nutritional information that can be detrimental to your health."

Here's a nice little example of how "credentialed" authorities are utilized to sway public opinion. In 1980 the National Academy of Sciences' Food and Nutrition Board came out with a controversial report suggesting that Americans needn't worry about fat and cholesterol in their diets, which would be akin to suggesting that you needn't worry about frostbite at the top of Mt. Everest. Two of the members of that board were Dr. David Kritchevsky and Dr. Robert Olson. Dr. Kritchevsky has received funding from the American Egg Board, the National Dairy Council and the National Livestock and Meat Board. Dr. Olson has been a consultant for the American Egg Board and the National Dairy Council. Hey! Pass me the air freshener!

If you wish to eat eggs, there are a couple of factors to bear in mind. First, it is really important to make an effort to get eggs that have not been tortured into existence. Fully 95 percent of egg-laying hens are maintained in production plants using a production line method that *has* to produce a poor quality product. The abuse these unfortunate animals endure is beyond belief. I'm not going to go into it extensively because it is too sickening to describe. Suffice it to say that the birds are crammed by the thousands into suffocatingly cramped cages—five fully grown hens in each twenty-inch by twenty-four-inch cage. (Some producers stuff four hens in twelve- by twelve-inch cages!) They can't spread their wings or even turn around. The wire flooring frequently tears open their feet. They are debeaked at one week and again at three to five months to prevent the pecking and cannibalism inevitably brought on by these grossly overcrowded conditions. Fluorescent bulbs provide seventeen hours of artificial daylight to stimulate laying. The birds are fed arsenic (some of which ends up in the eggs) to kill parasites and stimulate growth. And that's only part of this horror story. Indeed, there have been books on the subject that are absolutely frightening to read. One of the best is *Animal Factories* by Jim Mason and Peter Singer.

If you want eggs, at least do the best you can to acquire eggs that have been laid by hens in a more natural environment—birds that have been allowed to walk around in the outdoors. If more people demand eggs produced in a more natural environment, the industry will be forced to become more humane.

Secondly, eggs, being a very concentrated protein, should be eaten in proper combinations to minimize the negative effects. The traditional way of eating eggs with toast or potatoes is very harmful. It's best for eggs not to be eaten with other protein foods either, because two highly concentrated proteins are exceedingly difficult to digest simultaneously. Have eggs with slices of tomato and cucumbers, add eggs to salads, or have vegetable omelettes. This is the best way to consume your eggs. Do try to cut back and have as few as possible.

I am so confused about the nutrients issue—iron, zinc, riboflavin, B vitamins, and what seems like hundreds more. Where do we get them all?

Let's see if we can simplify this for you. The entire nutrient issue has been made so confusing with contradictory information that it is no wonder people are frustrated and bewildered when it comes to "where do I get what?" There is a *$3 billion* a year industry out there telling us that without their little bottles of expensive pills, we can't survive. I just wonder how we managed to make it for millions of years without them. Notwithstanding the never-ending onslaught of frightening propaganda designed to keep you a slave to the meat and dairy industries and pharmaceutical companies, who all profit directly from your fear and confusion, the entire nutrient issue is quite a simple one. Unfortunately, some people have been so totally scared and misguided that no amount of commonsense reasoning or even factual data will ever rescue them from the grip of these multibillion-dollar industries. The truth is frequently so profoundly simple, so manifestly conspicuous, so glaringly obvious that, strange as it seems, *it's missed!* Such is the case here. The simple truth is this: **WHATEVER NUTRIENTS THE BODY NEEDS THAT IT DOES NOT ITSELF PRODUCE CAN BE OBTAINED FROM THE PLANT KINGDOM.** In other words, if you can't get them from fruit, vegetables, nuts, seeds, sprouts, and whole grains, *you don't need them!* Those telling you otherwise are either in dire need of some courses in biology and physiology or they are seeking clear passage into your wallet. If you regularly partake of a well-rounded variety of the foods that fit your biological adaptation, you can no more have a nutrient deficiency than you can sprout wings and fly. Everything else you hear is propaganda and patently untrue. **NUTRIENTS COME FROM THE GARDENS AND THE ORCHARDS, NOT FROM PHARMACEUTICAL LABORATORIES OR DEAD ANIMALS!**

The pill pushers are quick to say that all soil is deficient. It's not nearly as deficient as their ability to recognize the truth. First of all, if a seed does not receive the elements it needs from the soil, *it won't grow!* Secondly, plants acquire nutrients in greater quantities from the sun, air, and water than from the soil. *Plants obtain only about 1 percent of their nutrients from the soil.*

The nutrient issue could easily take up the entirety of this book. Arguments for and arguments against the simple truths expressed above could go on forever. Use your common sense. What other species of animal is having difficulties in this area? None! Because they partake of the foods that fit their biological adaptations. If you will eat fruits, vegetables, nuts, seeds, sprouts, and whole grains, you will receive *all* that you need without constantly having to fret over long lists of possible deficiencies.

The greatest exposé I have ever read on this subject is to be found in the first seventy pages of Dr. David Reuben's book *Everything You Ever Wanted to Know about Nutrition*. Read those pages and you will never again look at this subject in the same way.

Is there any way of finding out where to locate health-oriented magazines and newsletters?

There sure is. In fact, there is a booklet entitled *Guide to Health Oriented Periodicals*, which is put out every year. You can receive this pamphlet by writing to:

> Sprouting Publications
> P.O. Box 62
> Ashland, OR 97520

There are several periodicals we very highly recommend you subscribe to. They will keep you up to date with what is *really* happening in the world of health. They will supply you with information that you simply can't find in your run-of-the-mill publications.

> *Healthful Living*
> 6600-D Burleson Road
> Box 17128
> Austin, TX 78760

This publication is from the American College of Health Science, and it is pure Natural Hygiene. It is brimming over with a wide variety of pertinent information that affects your health.

> *Health Science*
> Drawer B
> Box 30630
> Tampa, FL 33630

This is the official journal of the American Natural Hygiene Society in the United States. Treat yourself to this enormously informative and thought-provoking periodical.

> *The Hygienist*
> Shalimar
> Frinton-on-Sea
> Essex, United Kingdom

This is the oldest Natural Hygiene publication available anywhere. It is now in its twenty-seventh year of publication. It is edited by a brilliant doctor named Keki Sidhwa.

Health Freedom News
212 W. Foothill Blvd.
Monrovia, CA 91016

This publication is put out by the National Health Federation. The Federation fights for *your* freedom and keeps you on top of what is going on in Washington that affects your health. If not for the efforts of the Federation's president, Maureen Kennedy Salaman, we would probably be living in a "health dictatorship" in this country by now.

If you enjoy freedom, you should familiarize yourself with the National Health Federation. One drawback: Because this organization is open and honest enough to present *all* points of view, you have to contend with the monthly drivel of William C. Douglass, who is one of the medical advisers. Listen to him and you will find yourself consuming more animal products than a family of lions. This mustn't discourage you, however. This magazine is one of the best periodicals you could possibly read, in spite of William Douglass.

Nutrition Health Review
171 Madison Ave.
New York, NY 10016

This is a consumer medical journal, *packed* with a very wide range of information affecting your health that you won't read in your local newspaper.

Nutrition Action
1501 16th St., N.W.
Washington, DC 20036

This periodical is published by the Center for Science in the Public Interest (CSPI). The folks at CSPI work to bring to your attention the latest "tricks" by the food processors and others who present a danger to your health. Their efforts in Washington have held in check some of the more outrageous advertising claims and attempts to sneak into the marketplace products not worthy of entrance to your body. Unfortunately, their official nutritionist, Bonnie Liebman, although light-years ahead of many dietitians and nutritionists on some issues, is still stuck in the dark ages with many of her ideas, which are right out of a high school Home Economics class from the early 1950s. Don't let this discourage you, however. Just be aware of it.

I've been told that having a hysterectomy forces weight on the body that can't come off. Is that accurate?

The issue of surgery having an effect on weight is a very important one. Basically there are three surgeries that make weight loss more difficult: hysterectomies, removal of the thyroid, and removal of the appendix. However, there are measures that can be taken to minimize the negative effects of these. Over the years we have worked with many people who have had one of these three surgeries, and with very good results. It's interesting how we came to realize the effect these surgeries were having on weight loss. Whenever we see someone privately or conduct workshops with many people at once, we always take an in-depth case history of everyone. After compiling these records for seven or eight years, it was easy to recognize certain common denominators among individuals. No one has a 100 percent success rate in helping people lose weight. Although our success rate was very high—over 90 percent—in the 10 percent of those who either couldn't lose weight or had a very hard time of it, invariably we found they had had one of the three surgeries mentioned.

Generally speaking, the removal of *any* organ of the body will have some negative ramifications. After all, Mother Nature did not accidentally supply us with superfluous organs, despite what some surgeons will claim. *What we have we need.* Consider this: There is not one organ in the body that is not routinely removed unless its removal would cause instantaneous death. About the only ones safe from the scalpel are the brain, heart and liver. Even one kidney or one lung will be removed. The indiscriminate removal of organs as a means of fighting symptoms, as opposed to removing causes, is too ignorant for words.

In the case of hysterectomies, there are two contributing factors. First, the uterus is used by the female body to eliminate waste once a month to create as clean an environment as possible in case the ovum is fertilized. When this channel of elimination is lost, body wastes tend to build in the body. Second, the ovaries secrete a hormone that assists in breaking down fat in the body. When the ovaries are lost it becomes quite difficult to lose weight. In addition, when the ovaries are lost, almost without exception individuals start to suffer with thyroid problems. Why? Because the thyroid gland also helps to break down fat in the body. When the ovaries are lost, the thyroid has to do what it was doing *plus* what the ovaries were doing. Many of you right now, I'm sure, are saying something like, "Hey, that's right. After my hysterectomy I had to go on thyroid medication." Now you know why.

Those who have lost both the ovaries *and* the thyroid are in an unenviable position indeed. Not that you can't improve your situation. You can. But in all honesty, it takes a very dedicated effort. More than anyone else, you need to be extremely strict in following the principles laid out in this book. For those of you who have had a hysterectomy, lost your thyroid, or both and subsequently ballooned up (which, unfortunately, happens all too frequently) and now can't seem to lose weight even *with* following the principles, there is an emergency measure you can take. We have seen this work many times, but be forewarned that it is extremely rigid and only recommended in this particular instance.

Here's how it works. As you may already know, the brain only burns one substance for fuel—sugar in the form of glucose, which it gets from sugars and starches. When an insufficient amount of glucose is available in the blood due to a lack of sugar and starch consumption, the infinite wisdom of the body takes over, and through the remarkable process of gluconeogenesis the body breaks down fat and transforms it into sugar. Perhaps in the past you have heard of lettuce, celery, spinach, and other raw vegetables being classified as "zero-calorie foods." Many fad diets that rely on calorie counting usually allow the free consumption of these foods because the body actually uses up more calories to break them down than they bring into the body. If you are in the position of having had one of these surgeries and you can't get the weight back off that you put on, you can do it by eating *exclusively* these "zero-calorie foods." In other words, you eat *only* raw vegetables.

Eat raw vegetable meals at regular intervals, approximately three hours apart. It may sound strange to hear that you must *not* eat any fruit whatsoever, considering the importance we place on fruit, but if you eat fruit and supply your body with sugar, there will be no need for the body to go to the fat and break it down. The idea is to *force* the body to use its stored fat. As the fat is broken down and used, you lose weight. When the desired amount of weight is lost, start adhering to the **Fit for Life** eating principles, and that will maintain your weight loss so you don't put the weight back on. We have seen this work on many occasions, but remember: *It is an emergency measure and only suggested because once there has been surgery there are no more norms*. Also, it is very definitely *not* suggested that you jump straight into raw vegetables from a standard diet. If you have not cleansed your body somewhat by following the principles over a period of time, you can become very uncomfortable. You must build up to this very strict and rigid regimen. Please remember: *The zero-calorie diet is an emergency measure that you should employ carefully*.

The appendix is a small appendage (thus the name) that protrudes from the colon where it connects to the small intestine. The appendix is a lymph organ that detoxifies poisons in the colon. Losing the appendix is a severe blow. This is why people who have had appendectomies frequently complain of becoming bloated and/or constipated. For those who have lost their appendix, it is crucial to take whatever steps possible to keep the colon clean. It is dangerous not to! Allowing your colon to become clogged when the mechanism designed to keep it clean has been lost only invites trouble. The way to see to it that the colon is kept clean and flushed of its waste is to rely heavily on high-water-content foods and minimize the amount of more concentrated foods. Obviously, when more concentrated foods *are* eaten, they must be properly combined. Quite frankly, dealing with a lost appendix is considerably easier than dealing with the loss of the thyroid gland or a hysterectomy, but you do have to stay on top of it.

While on the subject of the appendix I must share with you the story of Dr. Alec Burton. Over thirty years ago Dr. Burton, who was in his third year of medical school, suffered a severe appendicitis attack. He was told by his physician that his *only* course of action was an appendectomy. Fortunately for him, he was in communication with a naturopathic practitioner who convinced

Dr. Burton not to allow his appendix to be removed, but rather to use a more natural approach which would allow his body to correct the situation. After a short seven-day fast and an improvement in his eating habits, the problem was indeed overcome and in Dr. Burton's words, "That was over thirty years ago and I still have my appendix."

So impressed by his recovery through natural measures was this young medical student that he discontinued his medical training in favor of a natural hygienic approach. He earned his doctorate in osteopathy and chiropractic and he is today one of the most brilliant, articulate, and well-respected natural hygienists in the world. For the last sixteen years, he has been director of a clinic in Sydney, Australia, where people from all over the world go for the opportunity to be under his care. He is a great humanitarian and his record is one of fantastic success in treating a wide range of ailments. If you would like to communicate with Dr. Burton, you can contact him at his clinic:

> Arcadia Health Center
> 31 Cobah Road
> Arcadia, New South Wales
> 2159-Australia
> phone: (02) 653-1115.

Realizing the importance of detoxifying, are there places where one can go for supervised help—a little "hand-holding" to oversee the process?

Yes, there are. The following are centers in the United States with practitioners well versed in hygienic principles who can support and supervise your efforts to gain control over your health.

CENTER FOR
  CONSERVATIVE
  THERAPY
4310 Lichau Road
Penngrove, CA 94951
Dr. Alan Goldhamer, Director
(707) 792-2325

SCOTT'S HEALTH
  RETREAT
P.O. Box 8919
Cleveland, OH 44136
Dr. David J. Scott, Director
(216) 238-6930

HYGEIA HEALTH
  RETREAT
439 E. Main St.
Yorktown, TX 78164
Dr. Ralph Cinque, Director
(512) 564-3670

PAWLING HEALTH
  MANOR
P.O. Box 401
Hyde Park, NY 12538
Joy Gross, Director
(914) 889-4141

REGENCY HEALTH
  RESORTS
2000 S. Ocean Ave.
Hallandale, FL 33009
Dr. Gregory Haag, Director
(305) 454-2220

ESSER'S HYGIENIC REST
  RANCH
P.O. Box 6229
Lakeworth, FL 33466
Dr. William Esser, Director
(305) 965-4360

SHANGRI-LA HEALTH
  RESORT
P.O. Box 2328
Bonita Springs, FL 33923
Frances Cheatham, Director
(813) 992-3811

HAWAIIAN FITNESS
  HOLIDAY
P.O. Box 1287
Koloa, Hawaii 96756
Dr. Grady Deal
(808) 332-9244

If there are questions you have that have not been answered in this book or in this particular chapter, please don't hesitate to write to us and we will answer them in our newsletter. (The address is on page 443.)

CHAPTER 19
Two Weeks of Living Health

HARVEY AND MARILYN:

Now the elements of health are familiar to you. But familiarity doesn't necessarily guarantee practical application. We know that frequently people very much want to adopt new behavior, but for many reasons they just can't. This chapter will help you bring these elements into your life-style in a sensible way. Remember, the elements of health discussed in this book are not mere words on a page that you read and then intellectualize about. **THEY CAN TRULY HELP YOU FEEL BETTER IF YOU WILL USE THEM AND INCORPORATE THEM INTO YOUR LIFE-STYLE.**

On the following pages we will outline the **health-style** we recommend. It is an easy-to-follow two-week program that will enable you to begin to weave the elements of health into your daily routine. These elements are actually *your biological needs*. In order to become a person who is totally confident about his or her health, you must fulfill your biological needs. When you deprive your body of what it needs, you create the environment for disease. On the other hand, it is amazingly easy to give your body what it requires, because Mother Nature provides you with all the raw materials. Just take advantage of them and you're on your way!

As we have already said, often, even given all we know about what we need, we still don't always do what is best for us. We intend to, but we just keep slipping. The desire is there, but we have *many* desires, and often the willpower to fulfill one particular desire is weak.

We have taken this into consideration in designing the program so that it will be *easy* for you to incorporate the elements of health into your life-style regularly, no matter what conflicting desires you may be experiencing. Part of our strategy in creating this program for you is to help you work into your life, in the most comfortable way, new behavior that will increase your willpower so that very soon you will be able to do what is best for your health without conflict among all the diverse and demanding desires that make up your personality.

You are not unique in your tendency to feel a tug-of-war of opposing forces within yourself. The human personality is a battleground. The mind taps into all of them and, like a director, chases its wants and needs here and there, pushing this one out, giving that one a larger share of attention. Meanwhile, a very quiet, *instinctive* inner voice that we all possess *knows* what is right, but very often it simply can't make itself heard above the raucous whirring of the mind as it runs this way and that, pulling the body after it, reacting to whichever desire is making itself most strongly felt at a particular moment. Once you realize what is going on, you can overcome the flip-flop mechanisms of the mind. You can observe what it does but allow your stronger inner voice to prevail. You can go about your business, instinctively doing what will benefit your health the most.

We know you wish to live healthfully—otherwise you wouldn't be reading this book. Within you are forces that wish to control your health totally, doing whatever will bring an improvement in the way you feel and supply a new found confidence that *you* are in charge. We also understand that there are other desires within you that are not so interested in your health. They want to watch television and eat or sleep instead of exercise. They want coffee and doughnuts or bagels instead of fruit in the morning. They want to party all the time and disregard how your body feels. They want to yell and scream and make a mess of your relationships, so that later on you feel terrible. The **Living Health** life-style will help you bring those desires into balance. It will enable you to be aware of all of your desires but not sit in judgment on any of them. It will help you to intuitively take the right action in spite of them, because **THE RIGHT ACTION FEELS THE BEST**.

The **Living Health** life-style we recommend is designed to help you *feel good*. There is no better feeling than the feeling that comes when you really begin to take care of yourself. Everything you do from that point on is better, too, because when you feel better, the world is a better place. Joy begins to build inside of you, and it radiates out to the world. This life-style is intended to nourish that joy.

The two-week **Living Health** program consists of two categories of activities. One category includes activities that we suggest you do every day. These are called the "Dailies," and they are so helpful that we encourage you to take advantage of them six days a week. The second category consists of "Weeklies," the activities we recommend that you start doing once a week. (Once a week is the *minimum*.) As you progress, you can increase the frequency of these weekly activities to whatever feels comfortable.

The **Living Health** life-style should be followed six days—not that the seventh day should be *un*healthy. It is, however, a day of rest. It is a day to spend in whatever fashion you wish to spend it. You may skip the Dailies on your day of rest, or you may include them. That is your choice. The seventh day is your "breather." It is your day to structure any way you wish.

THE DAILIES

These are the activities that you will want to do *every day* as you begin to practice the **Living Health** life-style. Implementing each "daily" for two consecutive weeks will definitely make a noticeable difference in how you feel.

1. Sleep with the window open at night. If you live in a cold climate, open it just an inch or so and add an extra blanket or two to your bed. How will this benefit you? Remember, when you sleep you exhale toxins and carbon dioxide from your lungs. In a closed room you re-inhale the toxins and the carbon dioxide, which is also poisonous. The fresh air circulating through the open window will allow you to *detoxify*, not *retoxify*, while you sleep. You will wake up in the morning fresh and invigorated. If you are worried about leaving the window open for security reasons, you can purchase window stops at your hardware store. These are easy to install and make it impossible to raise an open window more than an inch or two when they are in use.

2. Stretch your body for one minute before retiring and one minute upon awakening in the morning. Just stretch gently, comfortably—to the sides, to the floor. (Bend your knees as you come up!) Stand on your toes and try to reach the ceiling. Stretching your body is like ironing the wrinkles out of a shirt before you wear it. It just makes you *feel* better. You'll sleep more restfully and soundly, and you'll spring into action faster in the morning.

3. Do six abdominal or alternate nostril breaths before retiring, when you awaken, or sometime during the day. Before retiring is a good time. You will sleep more soundly. If you have a particularly hectic day, six alternate nostril breaths sometime during the day will even things out. The day may remain hectic, but *you* will be more relaxed.

4. Drink a glass of water when you awaken in the morning. Drink an additional glass five to ten minutes before each meal. This minimum amount of water will prevent dehydration in your body. We need to respond to thirst. Sometimes we get too busy to do so. Many people are, in fact, dehydrated. Dehydration manifests as lethargy and muscle weakness.

Water has many functions in your body. It is an energy conductor. A glassful before you eat will help you control your appetite and will also supply you with necessary fluid so that you won't be thirsty *after* you eat. A glass of water first thing in the morning will help wash out any food debris that may be clinging to your stomach lining and digestive tract.

5. Take a twenty-minute walk every day. Take it in the morning, in the evening, or during your lunch break—but *take it!* Walk briskly to get your heart really pumping. The heart is the most important muscle of your body. You *must* exercise it every day. Be kind to it and it will be kind to you. Remember, heart disease is the number one killer in this country.

Your daily walk will bring you many unsuspected benefits. People who walk daily rarely suffer from constipation. Their skin has a better color because of increased circulation. Their eyes are clearer. They think and feel better because they have taken the time to oxygenate their blood with fresh air. Walking during your lunch break will help you get out of the office and into the sun and fresh air. Your afternoon will be more pleasant.

Many people we know keep rebounders at the office for rainy days. Twenty minutes on the rebounder in the office will do for your heart and circulation what twenty minutes of walking will do—except, or course, for the fresh air and sunshine benefits that come from being outside.

If you are elderly and cannot go out regularly on your own or if you live where the climate is very severe, you should also consider investing in a rebounder. They are *not* expensive and they are well worth the investment. Doing even the gentle health bounce we recommend for the elderly (see page 161) will help strengthen your heart, pump the lymph system, and prevent constipation.

6. Observe the Fit for Life eating principles. Eat only fruit in the morning and properly combine your midday and evening meals.

7. Take five minutes or more to focus on the inner you every day. This is a very important "daily." A *minimum* of five minutes in a quiet place, by yourself, sitting comfortably with eyes closed and your attention focused on "what lies within" you, will strengthen you and keep you more aware of your identity, your needs, and your goals. Take five minutes in the morning, after you stretch or at some other *regular* time during the day to focus your attention away from the outside world and on your inner world. While you sit, you will have the opportunity to observe your mind running tapes of all your conflicting desires. Just objectively watch all these desires come and go. Breathe in love, breathe out negativity. You will be stronger and less at their mercy as a result, and that means able to focus in on actions that will most benefit your health. **NOTHING YOU DO WILL KEEP YOU MORE DEVOTED TO YOUR NEW "HEALTH-STYLE" THAN THE QUIET, FOCUSED TIME YOU SPEND WITH YOURSELF.**

THE WEEKLIES

These are the health-producing activities that, if done *at least* once a week from now on, will bring you great rewards. Ideally, some or all of them should be done more frequently, but when you begin, just make sure to do them once a week—and be proud of yourself that you are making so many positive changes so quickly.

1. Yoga. The yoga routine given in this book (see pages 166–181) is designed to keep you flexible and young. It is a basic routine, not extreme in any way, and it will strengthen and release toxins from your entire body. Many people who practice the yoga routine once a week enjoy it so much and are aware of so much benefit that over time they find themselves turning this ''weekly'' into a ''daily.'' Remember, the routine is to be done *gently*. You are not supposed to push yourself to the point of pain!

2. Be in bed by nine. This investment in your energy once a week will have remarkable payoffs. You will awaken more refreshed than on days when you stay up later. Remember, the hours you sleep before midnight are the most valuable. When you sleep your body regenerates its nerve energy, and with abundant energy it carries out all its processes more effectively. That means *you feel better*. Our ancestors went to sleep every night when darkness fell. Rest and sleep are gifts to us from nature. Why not take advantage of them? Once a week! You deserve it!

3. Have a living food day. Once a week eat three living food meals. (If your digestive tract is impaired or severely devitalized and raw vegetable salads present a digestive problem, lightly steam your vegetable meal or simmer all the vegetables in a broth— however, *only if you must!* The vitality you will receive from this day is diminished when the food is cooked. Some people are able to rely on the Blended Salad—see page 378—rather than steam the vegetables.

Your living food day should consist of juice in the morning, a fruit or vegetable salad meal at lunch, and a fruit or vegetable salad meal in the early evening. This is also a good day to have nut milks, an almond milk shake, ''smoothies,'' or fruit ices if the weather is warm. If the weather is cold, have peppermint tea. Some people misunderstand the nature of a living (raw) vegetable meal. They will try to eat lots of raw, fibrous vegetables like cauliflower and broccoli. I have not found that to be the most comfortable way to do it. Rely on salad vegetables like lettuce (all varieties), sprouts, cucumbers, tomatoes, carrots, celery, bell peppers, jicama and avocados. Small amounts of other raw vegetables can be added, if you like, but they should not predominate in the salad. The more watery vegetables you use, the more digestible the salad will be.

The living food day will give you an opportunity to really get into some of the living food recipes in the recipe section that follows. Avocado Gazpacho (see page 407), thick and creamy, garnished with fresh minced vegetables, is a meal in itself! You can try the Strawberry-Almond Milk Shake (see page 438), the Blended Salad (see page 378), a fresh vegetable soup, delectable new juice ideas, creamy "smoothies," and fruit and vegetables galore. These may well inspire you to create some of your own living food recipes, which I hope you will share with us! One of the best living food cookbooks is *Light Eating for Survival* by Marcia Acciardo (Omangod Press, P.O. Box 64, Woodstock Valley, CT 06282).

On living food days your body will accelerate and maximize cleansing. You will be lighter, more glowing, and happier in the days that follow. You will also become more conscious of your eating the rest of the week because you won't wish to fritter away the benefits of your living food day.

4. Take a long, hot bath (once a week or as often as you can). This may sound so basic that it amuses you. But we tend to rush so much these days that many people routinely take only a quick shower. Of course, a daily shower will keep you clean, but it will do nothing to moderate the stresses of modern living the way a bath will. Dim the lights, light a candle, put on some music, fill your tub with lots of hot water, and *soak*! Before you get into the tub, you can use a soft skin brush all over your body to remove the dead cells on the surface of your skin. Use a natural loofah sponge once you have soaked for a while to remove the dead cells that remain. Your skin will feel wonderful, and body elimination will proceed faster through the skin because the pores are not clogged with dead cells. Make sure when you *do* take your relaxing bath that you have allowed enough time to enjoy it—at least twelve minutes!

The therapy you will receive from hot baths is invaluable beyond your wildest dreams. Recent research on hot bath therapy by Dr. Kevin Michael, a highly credentialed and skilled chiropractor in Studio City, California, reveals that this age-old relaxation technique has always been used to prevent disease in highly developed societies where stress is the order of the day. In his words, "A large portion of the human brain is dedicated to SURVIVAL. Its systems are divided into two basic halves. There is a TRANQUIL side which is contemplative, creative, tends to see the overall picture and prepares our bodies to take advantage of the abundance which life has to offer. It quietly oversees the functions of digesting our food, absorbing nutrients, eliminating wastes, healing wounds, making babies and in general maintaining the health necessary to pursue all other life goals.

"The opposite half of the survival system is almost totally devoted to ALARM. It prepares our bodies to cope with immediate physical dangers and emergencies. Much of its work is accomplished by causing an aggitation in the nerves of our body (like cocking the trigger on a gun) and moving as much as 60% of the blood from within our intestines out to the muscles, priming them for action, thereby greatly reducing and at times actually stopping digestion, absorption and elimination.

"The continual stresses of modern society tend to push the ALARM side into our driver's seat and keep it there. Help, however, is not far away.

"The simple act of allowing ourselves time for a soothing bath can dramatically change this picture. The action of hot water as it envelopes our bodies, pulls the trigger on our nerves and heats the blood within our muscles. Together they signal our body to regain its balance and move blood back into our intestines, allowing our TRANQUIL side to once more take control of the wheel."

5. Walk in the woods or the park. Once a week, take a walk in nature. It is such a grounding, stabilizing, uplifting activity. All week long, we find ourselves under pressure from the constraints of our man-made world. A walk among the trees and plants, where it is peaceful, can erase the tension modern living causes. Trees and plants give off fresh, clean oxygen, which we need, especially after a week of confinement where we work. Since we are a species that first lived in nature, whenever we return to it even briefly, we get a peaceful feeling, because nature is where we are *naturally* intended to be.

6. Do something nice for someone without expecting anything in return. A loving act, unsolicited and unconditional, will brighten another's life and come back to you as love. The act can be as small or large a gesture as your spirit moves you to make. We have become a "me"-oriented society, and we sometimes forget that " 'tis better to give than to receive." What you give comes back to you anyway in the form of loving and positive vibrations. The best way to get love is to give it!

Once in a while, give in some way to the elderly. People who should be honored for the wisdom and experience of their years have become the forgotten, shoved aside castoffs of our modern society. Up to quite recent times, people lived with or close to their parents throughout their lives. It is part of our nature to do so. When we don't there is a void that no amount of friends can fill. With some effort, we can change the way the elderly are treated in our society. And we should—before we get old!

Imagine how many lives would be lightened and brightened if once a week *millions* of us showed someone forgotten that *we care*!

7. Spend time with friends or family in a festive, happy setting. We are *social* beings. We need the input and support of others around us. The ancients did not live in a solitary way, and neither should we. Come together with those you care about once a week—to eat, laugh, talk, and generally enjoy life and each other. This is an important activity for all of us, especially since families who in years past would get together regularly are now scattered all over the country. Children thrive on the social interaction of family and friends. If you have lost this great gift of nature, reclaim it. It will do you a world of good!

Any one of these Dailies or Weeklies, taken alone, may not appear to be all that significant. But when all are forged together into a "health-style," the result is remarkably powerful. When all of the elements of health are used in concert with one another, the ensuing benefits are enormously magnified. In the same way, a quarterback on a football team may be highly talented, but the true extent of his abilities cannot be demonstrated until he has the supporting interaction of all the rest of his teammates. Only when the team members work together and in harmony with one another are they able to perform at full potential and win.

There is no way to fully describe to you the exhilaration and peace of mind awaiting you when your body has the benefit of the simultaneous interaction of all the elements of health. This heightened state of being cannot be described any more easily than can the fragrance of a rose. To *experience* it is the only way to appreciate its true value. Your life is transformed—physically, emotionally, spiritually, and psychologically. Please don't take our word for this. Try it for two weeks. Then you will understand what we are trying to put in words for you. You will have given yourself the opportunity to know *firsthand* the joy that is intended to permeate human existence. You will experience the vast difference in your life when your body is fully supplied with what nature intends it to receive.

As we have said before, the mere fact that you are reading this book is an indication that you are interested in your health. Have you been searching for a long time for answers that made sense to you? Have you felt confused by "academic" explanations that tended to contradict each other and weren't bringing good results to anyone around you? Have you been frustrated by a lack of power over your health and the resulting feeling of helplessness that it created? We wonder if you are willing to give Mother Nature a chance to work in your life. **YOU CAN DO IT!** And if you do, years from now, you will look back on this day, and *you will bless it!*

THE
LIVING
HEALTH
COOKBOOK

INTRODUCTION

MARILYN:

The most important aspect of new information lies in its versatility. How valuable is it, after all, if we cannot integrate its practical features into our lives? Of course, not everything we learn can be used to the letter. There is always the situation of the real versus the ideal. For example, you know that the freshest air is ideally what you want to breathe, but sometimes you have no choice, so you do the best you can. Since distilled water is really the purest water available, you make an effort to get it *when you can*. Perhaps you can purchase a home water distiller or, if there are water delivery companies in your area, perhaps you can take advantage of them. With all the other elements of health—rest and sleep, exercise, sunshine, positive emotional influences—you do the best you can whenever you can. The area where you actually can have a great amount of choice, the area where you can really take control and notice a definite change in your life-style because of the new information you have received, is in the area of food.

In **Fit for Life** I focused on the preparation of well-combined, balanced meals. That was my greatest emphasis, because that was the most important new information to integrate into a practical, workable life-style. **Fit for Life** is only fourteen months old, as of the writing of this book, and in just a short fourteen months, there is a new consciousness in the area of food preparation *in general* that is *really exciting*. This is the greater, more widespread demand for light, quickly prepared, simple and elegant, *fresh* food meals. Combined with the more time-consuming, homespun, country kitchen quality of healthful food preparation (calling for thick, hearty soups, hot whole-grain breads and muffins, pastries, and creamy sauces) are simple, easy, and quickly prepared dishes that are light and extremely satisfying at the same time. This was a trend started by the Nouvelle Cuisine approach, which for many people was excessive in its sparsity. The positive and lasting effect of Nouvelle Cuisine seems to be the food preparation techniques it employs. They leave the food fresh and wonderful due to its own nature and not because of all that has been done *to* it.

Food combining and an emphasis on fresh, unadulterated foods and fruits and vegetables are the backbone of any cuisine that purports to support efficient digestion and good health, because food combining ensures a correct relationship with the physiology of the body, and fresh fruits and vegetables are our biological foods.

In the following recipe section, you will find many new, properly combined dishes and menus. In addition, the new emphasis on freshness, which has been so exciting over the past year, will really make itself felt in the recipes presented. Sweet and refreshing juice combinations, simply prepared fresh vegetables, lightly dressed, crisp salads, and delicate and discerning accents on pasta, potatoes, chicken, and fish are all emphasized.

You will find some new entries in the baking department. There are even some fresh frozen treats and goodies for those with a passion for sweets. I think the most fulfilling aspect of compiling these recipes for those who are interested in truly *living health* has been the continued variety, change in mood, "something for everyone" quality that seems to predominate in the evolution of this cuisine. Although this is nutritious home cooking that definitely maintains a certain gourmet standard, it is also very grounded rather than esoteric, economical rather than expensive, and developed with sophisticated and worldly as well as relaxed and casual family life-styles in mind.

You will notice that in spite of all the new information contained in this book on the effects of animal products, I have nonetheless included a few recipes containing chicken and fish. It is not our desire to impose vegetarianism on our readers. We wish merely to point out its potential benefits, especially during detoxification, and to allow the process to unfold in the life of each reader if it is appropriate. Even when one has become a vegetarian, the craving for flesh food will come up periodically; after a few days of feeling less and less satisfied by even the most tempting vegetarian meal, one simply should listen to one's body and satisfy the craving. With the exception of a sugar craving, which is a harmful addiction, other cravings are your body telling you of its needs, and you should not ignore them if they persist. Whenever you do eat flesh food, try to eat only a few ounces, as they do in Asian countries. Otherwise you will notice a significant drop in your energy and a less "shiny" feeling.

In this "**Living Health Cookbook**" we are presenting some sample *living food* days. I know Harvey has already discussed the benefits of living food in depth, but I want to take the opportunity to add some practical information based on our personal experience. The idea of eating only living food may not be attractive to those who have never tried it, but I really encourage you to give yourself the chance to know what it is like and to feed your body *nothing* but living food now and then, especially in warm weather, *if the idea appeals to you!*

We personally know many, many people who flourish on living foods a great deal of the time. From my own experience, the benefits of eating only living foods from time to time are immeasurable—they are that great, especially in warm weather! If you are feeling sluggish or enervated after having "overdone it," your energy level is restored almost immediately. If you have minor aches or pains, they tend to clear up. If you feel you have a little extra weight on your body, it washes right out. If your nails are weak, they strengthen. Your hair shines, your skin glows. Your eyes get very, very clear and white.

Living food will help alleviate a toxic condition in one person and enhance and improve the healthy state of another. You may notice:

● The special mellow, even feeling of a body free from food stimulants and depressants

● That you experience an extraordinarily peaceful, calm, sound sleep at night

● An increased ability to focus, concentrate, and work long hours without fatigue

● A total absence of stress

I think the most extraordinary consequence of eating living food, which takes people *completely* by surprise, is the almost total absence of hunger once you have "made it" through the first day. The first day poses the greatest challenge because your body craves what it is used to and psychologically you feel you may not be satisfied. Obviously, that is a misconception. With living food your body will be receiving an abundance of live, buzzing-with-energy nutrients. Of course you will be nourished! More than from the greatest cooked food banquet. The pure living essence of the food will be incorporated directly into healthy cell structure with a minimal expenditure of body energy and an abundance of energy conserved that would normally be required to break down the cooked foods. When you are on your second day of only living foods, you will be able to verify how your appetite decreases. You will hardly be hungry. This is because your appestat is satisfied and turned off due to the nutritious nature of your food.

Two mistakes many people make when they experiment with uncooked food are either to feel that they must eat all the time or to not eat enough. The best way to incorporate living food into a life-style is to eat small meals at more frequent, regular intervals with definite rest periods in between—rest for the digestive tract. Because you are eating only living food, do not take the license to eat all the time. For example, you can start the day with fresh juice around 8:00 A.M. At 10:00 you might have some melon, staying with light fruit early in the day. At noon, you might have a fruit salad and some more juice, or a plate of sliced tomatoes and cucumbers. Around 2:00 to 3:00, you would have bananas, a smoothie, or some raw nuts. At dinner time, a salad and some sliced avocado or guacamole and salad with raw vegetables. Before bed, you might have some more fruit, a shake, or some juice.

If you wish to have your vegetable salad at midday rather than dinner, you can. If you are interested in dropping weight, you will emphasize vegetables that burn calories stored in your body during digestion. If you wish to maintain your weight, you will eat lots of fruit, vegetables, and an avocado or nuts each day. This living food approach, coupled with weight lifting and aerobic exercise can be effective for people who wish to gain weight. Professor T. C. Fry, the dean of the American College of Health Science, went from 128 pounds after a serious automobile accident to 163 pounds on a living food life-style coupled with weight-lifting.

Remember that cancer cells thrive on cooked food and refuse to grow on living foods. Try living food days one at a time, or lump two or three of them together. A living food interlude, coupled with exercise and rest, will enhance, restore, and rejuvenate—and you deserve all three!

Fourteen Days
of Living Health Menus

In the following menus, I have included several ideas for entertaining, since that is a question that has come up quite frequently since the publication of **Fit for Life**. You will find menus for an outdoor "Vegetable Barbecue," a buffet dinner party, a more formal sit-down dinner, and several brunches. In addition, there are plenty of family menus, foods for kids, and two sample total living food days. Remember, as in **Fit for Life**, these menus are merely suggestions, examples of how to plan and enjoy properly combined high-energy meals. Feel free to substitute according to your preferences.

All starred items are appropriate foods to eat during detoxification (see Detox List, page 316). Cross-references are provided to dishes for which recipes appear in this book.

DAY ONE—"PASTA IN THE WOK"

BREAKFAST Fresh Tangerine Juice* (see page 367)
      Sliced Peaches and Cantaloupe with Blueberries*

LUNCH   Tomburgers (see page 408) with Coleslaw *or*
      Steamed Potatoes and Vegetables in Olive Oil
      (see page 417)

DINNER   Pasta in the Wok (see page 429)
      Herbed Buttermilk Biscuits (see page 432)
      Grilled Shiitake Mushrooms (see page 401)
      French Butter Lettuce Salad* (see page 387)

DAY TWO—"MASHED POTATOES AND GRAVY"

BREAKFAST   Fresh Strawberry-Apple Juice* (see page 367)
Sliced Melon*

LUNCH   Cauliflower Salad on Whole-Grain Toast (see page 409), topped with Fresh Tomato or Cucumber Slices

DINNER   Chinese Corn Soup* (see page 402)
Creamy Mashed Potatoes (see page 415)
Braised Green Beans* (see page 400)
Summer Greens with Fresh Herb Dressing* (see page 382)

DAY THREE—"FLOUNDER IN LEMON DILL"

BREAKFAST   Fresh Orange Juice* *or*
Persimmon Smoothie* (see page 373)
Fruit

LUNCH   Avocado-Tomato Sandwich on Whole-Grain Bread
Cream of Romaine and Cucumber Soup* (see page 403)

DINNER   Sole, Flounder, or Orange Roughy in Lemon-Dill Sauce (see page 434)
Crispy Broccoli with Garlic, Butter Lettuce, Arugula and Spinach in Seven-Herb Dressing*

DAY FOUR—"VEGETABLE BARBECUE"

BRUNCH   Tropical Ambrosia* (see page 371)
Fruit for Life Salad (see page 375) with Banana-Peach Sauce* (see page 377)
Blue Ribbon Bran Muffins with Butter (see page 431)
Peppermint-Camomile-Rose Hips Tea*

AFTERNOON   Chilled Cucumber Soup (see page 403)
BARBECUE   Barbecued Vegetable Kebabs (see page 398)
              Pasta with Butter and Fresh Herbs (see page 428)
              Sweet and Sour Red Cabbage* (see page 397)
              Limestone and Lamb's Lettuce Salad* (see page 379)

DAY FIVE—"QUINOA!" OR "MESQUITE-GRILLED SWORDFISH BEVERLY HILLS"

BREAKFAST   Pineapple-Orange Juice* (see page 367)
              Sliced Bananas, Strawberries, and Kiwi*

LUNCH   Mexicali Goodwich (see page 410)
              Clear Broth with Vegetables (see page 407)

DINNER   Millet (page 419) or Quinoa (see page 418) with
                 Burnt Onion and Tarragon Gravy (see page 416) *or*
              Mesquite-Grilled Swordfish Beverly Hills (see page 435)
              Beverly Barney's Italian Zucchini (see page 396)
              Romaine Lettuce and Cucumbers with Seven-Herb Dressing* (see page 390)

DAY SIX—"PILAF OF BROCCOLI AND BASMATI"

BREAKFAST   Pineapple-Orange-Strawberry Juice* (see page 367)
              Fruit of Choice

LUNCH   Miso Soup and Vegetables* (see page 405)
              Whole-Grain Toast with Butter

DINNER   Summer Vegemato Juice* (see page 369)
              Easy Broccoli Pilaf (see page 419)
              Sweet Carrots *au Naturel** (see page 396)
              Caesar Salad (see page 382)

DAY SEVEN—"LIVING FOOD DAY"

BREAKFAST Cherry-Grape Juice* (see page 368)
Watermelon and Honeydew Balls*

LUNCH Mango-MelonBerry Salad with Honeyloupe
Sherbet* (see page 374)
Coconut-Apple Granola* (see page 375)

DINNER Soft Lettuce Tacos with Avocado Dressing* (see
page 380) *or* Lisa's Salad with Nori* (see page
381)

EVENING SNACK Banana Shake Divine (see page 439)

DAY EIGHT—"LEMON DILL CHICKEN"

BREAKFAST Melon Smoothie* (see page 372)
Grapes and Figs*

LUNCH Sprout Salad Sunset Plaza (see page 380)

DINNER Lemon-Dill Chicken (see page 436)
Minute Asparagus* (see page 395)
Easy Limestone Lettuce Salad with Basil-Garlic
Dressing* (see page 379)
Grilled Shiitake Mushrooms (see page 401)

DAY NINE—"BUFFET DINNER"

BRUNCH Banana Milk* (see page 370)
Strawberry-Mint Soup* (see page 376)
French Toast with Maple Syrup (see page 430)

AFTERNOON SNACK Carrot-Celery Juice*

BUFFET Potato Burek (see page 420)

DINNER Dolmas (see page 421)
      Linguine with Pesto and Broccoli (see page 427)
      Stuffed Mushrooms Francesca (see page 394)
      Easy Cauliflower Italiano* (see page 395)
      Sweet Carrots *au Naturel** (see page 396)
      Mixed Greens with Tarragon Cream Dressing
       (see page 390)

DAY TEN—"PASTA IN MUSHROOM SAUCE"

BREAKFAST Fresh Orange Juice *or*
       Orange Freeze (see page 371)

LUNCH   L.A. Goodwich (see page 412) *or*
       Avotilla (see page 410)
       Clear Broth with Vegetables* (see page 407)

DINNER   Pasta in Mushroom Sauce with Garlic, Oil, and
       Parsley (see page 426)
       Butter Lettuce Salad with Regent of Fiji French
       Dressing (see page 391)
       Chinese Zucchini (see page 393)

DAY ELEVEN—"LIVING FOOD DAY"

BREAKFAST P.J.'s Honeyloupe Juice* (see page 369)
       Sliced Kiwis and Pears*

LUNCH   Peach-Melon Flower Bowl (see page 374) with
       Cashew-Apricot Sauce* (see page 376) *or*
       Platter of sliced Avocado, Tomato, and
       Cucumber*

AFTERNOON Juice or Fruit
SNACK

DINNER   Fresh Grapefruit Juice
       Fit for Life Sprout Salad* (see page 378)

EVENING   Juice
SNACK   Bananas
          Rainbow Cream* (see page 439) *or*
          Carob Shake (see page 439)

DAY TWELVE—"SOUP AND SCONES"

BREAKFAST   Fresh Apple Juice*
            Sliced Apples in Cinnamon*

LUNCH   Broiled Potato Slices (see page 416)
            Hearts of Lettuce in Thousand Island Dressing
               (see page 391)

DINNER   Green Soup with Fresh Herbs* (see page 404)
            Onion Scones and Butter (see page 433)
            Summer Greens with Fresh Herb Dressing (see
               page 385)

DAY THIRTEEN—"SIT-DOWN DINNER PARTY"

BREAKFAST   Fresh Strawberry-Apple Juice* (see page 367)
            Sliced Pineapple and Papaya*

LUNCH   Avotillas (see page 410) or Cuke-a-Tillas (see
               page 409) *and*
            Chinese Corn Soup (see page 402) *or*
            Summer Greek Salad with Seven-Herb Dressing
               (see page 382)

DINNER   Mango-MelonBerry Salad with Honeyloupe
               Sherbet* (see page 374)
            Country Carrot Soup* (see page 403)
            Roast Potatoes Bonne Femme (see page 417)
            Grilled Shiitake Mushrooms (see page 401)
            Braised Courgettes* (see page 392)
            Glazed Baby Beets* (see page 393)
            Whole-Wheat Garlic Triangles

Limestone and Lamb's Lettuce Salad (see page 384)

DAY FOURTEEN—"PASTA WITH FRESH TOMATO SAUCE"

BREAKFAST Watermelon-Cantaloupe Juice* (see page 368)
Sliced Oranges and Kiwi*

LUNCH Steamed Potatoes and Vegetables in Olive Oil* (see page 417)
Country Carrot Soup* (see page 403)

DINNER Hot or Chilled Cream of Romaine and Cucumber Soup (see page 403)
Pasta with Fresh Tomato Sauce (see page 425) *or*
Warm Chicken and Broccoli Salad (see page 435) with Regent of Fiji French Dressing (see page 391)
Limestone Lettuce with Avocado and Fresh Herb Dressing (see page 387)

Juices and Smoothies

There is a marvelous world of juices to discover. The juice concept has gone far beyond the days of just good old orange or apple juice. Thanks to all the affordable home juicers that are now available, people can create an unlimited variety of juice blends that are filling, nourishing, full of energy, and delicious! Juicing can become a very rewarding pastime, especially during the warm weather when many fruits are in season. Fresh juices help to cleanse the body of accumulated waste. They provide excellent nourishment without requiring *any* energy expenditure by the body. They are very helpful during detoxification since they afford a continuous energy supply to the bloodstream while allowing the body to use *all* of its available energy simultaneously for cleansing and repair. *Remember to drink juices slowly*. Mix them with the saliva in your mouth before you swallow them.

The following are some of our favorite juice combinations. (Smoothies are simply juices made with ice or frozen fruit or juice mixes that include pureed banana.) In order to make them, you will need a Champion juicer or one of the many other juicers that are available for home use. We find the Champion to be the handiest and easiest to use, because it does not require the cumbersome process of emptying accumulated pulp from the inside of the machine. The Champion dispenses juice from one opening and expels unusable pulp from another. It is simple to clean and will make an unlimited amount of juice. It is easy to assemble, durable, and best of all, it makes delicious, smooth juices as well as delectable frozen fruit creams.

Kids love juices. Use them as a base and blend in frozen fruit for smoothies, shakes, and slushes. Freeze juices in plastic pop containers as a healthy alternative to commercial pops, which frequently contain no juice at all and always contain sugar and other chemicals.

The following are just a few suggestions. There is really no end to the possible combinations of juices, and you can vary the amounts of fruits in any blend according to taste. Many people do not like to combine melon juices with other juices. I have actually done so quite successfully from time to time, for example, in Tropical Ambrosia (see page 371).

If you serve some of these innovative juices to guests when you are entertaining, be prepared for some very enthusiastic reactions.

TANGERINE JUICE

You can juice the tangerines on a regular citrus juicer, or you can peel them and put them through the Champion for a frothier, thicker juice. (The same can be done with oranges and grapefruit.)

STRAWBERRY-APPLE JUICE

Run a mixture of strawberries and cored apples through the Champion, or make the apple juice first and then combine it in a blender with fresh or frozen whole strawberries.

PINEAPPLE-ORANGE JUICE

1 fresh pineapple
1 large orange

Peel a fresh pineapple and cut into long spears. Peel an orange. Run both fruits through the Champion for a thick and frothy creation.

PINEAPPLE-ORANGE-STRAWBERRY JUICE

Follow the directions above, adding fresh strawberries, or combine pineapple-orange juice in blender with frozen strawberries.

CHERRY-GRAPE JUICE

This is a very sweet blend of pitted cherries and Red Flame grapes. Run both through the Champion. You will not believe the result!

GRAPE-APPLE JUICE

Use seedless grapes for juicing. (Seeds make the juice a little bitter.) Adding grapes to apple juice will sweeten it if the apples you have used are tart.

WATERMELON JUICE

This is a classic, thirst-quenching juice that should not be missed during watermelon season. No need to remove seeds from the watermelon. Just cut it in chunks from the rind and pass it through the Champion.

How to pick a watermelon

The trick of thumping a melon and listening for a hollow sound does not always guarantee a ripe melon. Other indications of ripeness are rounded and well-filled-out ends. The melon should be very heavy for its size and feel firm. The skin should be slightly dull, not waxy or shiny. The bottom should be a pale, creamy yellow.

If the melon is cut, the job is easier. Look for firm, juicy, bright red flesh with dark brown or black seeds. Avoid melons with whitish streaks or white seeds.

WATERMELON-CANTALOUPE JUICE

The addition of cantaloupe will sweeten and thicken watermelon juice. Peel and seed the cantaloupe and run it through the Champion with the watermelon. Great for entertaining!

APPLE-CELERY JUICE

6–8 quartered, cored apples
1 stalk celery

This may sound unorthodox, but this is a very refreshing juice combination. The first time I had it was at the Hygeia Health Retreat in Yorktown, Texas. It is served on the day a fast is broken.

P.J.'S HONEYLOUPE JUICE

A fourteen-year-old friend shared this recipe for his favorite juice with me.

2 cups honeydew chunks
2 cups cantaloupe chunks

Run melon chunks through juicer. *Yields 1–2 servings.*

SUMMER VEGEMATO JUICE

This is a terrific juice to have on hand in the summer, when tomatoes are abundant. We make large pitchers of it twice a week. It has a good refrigerator shelf life of two to three days, but remember, the best benefits from fresh juice are there for you immediately after the juice is prepared. Still, when tomatoes are in season this is a great juice to have cold in the refrigerator. Its high alkalinity will neutralize acids in your body.

4–6 medium, ripe tomatoes
 14 medium carrots
  2 stalks celery
  2 red bell peppers
  1 green bell pepper
  1 tiny beet
  1 small handful parsley
  1 small pickling cuke

Quarter tomatoes. Wash carrots and trim ends. Do not peel them. Wash and trim ends of celery. Quarter peppers and remove seeds. Thoroughly wash beet. Rinse parsley. Peel cucumber.

Run all the vegetables through juicer. A squeeze of lemon may be added for a tangier flavor. Shake before serving. *Yields 1 quart.*

BANANA MILK

In 1979, Dr. Philip Welsh, a retired eighty-seven-year-old dentist turned health advocate, told me about almond milk while we both selected produce at a local natural food store. In 1983, I once again ran into Dr. Welsh at the same store, carefully selecting for himself some beautifully spotted, unsprayed bananas from Mexico, and I thanked him for the almond milk recipe, telling him what a difference it had made in my life and in the lives of the people I was counseling. "I'm telling everyone about it," I said.

Dr. Welsh winked his amazingly clear and sparkling ninety-one-year-old eyes and answered with a big smile, "Now tell them about banana milk!"

I have since shared this recipe with many young mothers, who have reported back to me that their children love it. Banana milk is a complete protein, containing all the eight essential amino acids in as live a form as we can hope to obtain them. It's delicious and nourishing, no matter how old you are.

  1 **large banana**
1–2 **cups water**

Place banana and water in a blender. Blend until smooth. Add additional water if a thinner milk is desired. This is an ideal "baby bottle" food. *Yields 1½ to 2½ cups.*

ALMOND SURPRISE

1½ **cups Almond Milk (see page 438)**
1½ **cups fresh orange juice**
  1 **orange, peeled and seeded**

Combine all the ingredients in a blender and blend several minutes until smooth. Strain. *Serves 2.*

TROPICAL AMBROSIA

*The preparation of this ambrosia requires a Champion, Acme,
Ultramatic, or one of the many other juicers capable of extracting
the juice from any fruit or vegetable. The enjoyment of this juice
is well worth the investment you will be making in the juicer. You
can also come up with your own version of ambrosia. When you
find that you have a large quantity of fruit that is ripening too
quickly, that is a good time to make ambrosia.*

    4 cups watermelon chunks
    2 cups cantaloupe chunks
  6–8 oranges
    2 cups pineapple cubes
 1½ cups apricot halves
    1 cup plum halves
    2 cups Red Flame grapes
    1 banana

Run all the fruit but the oranges and the banana through the juicer.
Juice oranges on orange juicer. Place orange juice and banana in
blender and liquefy. Combine melon blend and orange-banana
blend in a large jar with a tight-fitting lid. Shake well. Refrigerate.
Ambrosia may be used as a punch for parties. Place it in a punch
bowl and add several trays of watermelon juice ice cubes. You
may also add several sprigs of fresh mint. *Yields 8 to 10 cups,
depending on the juiciness of the fruit.*

ORANGE FREEZE

 1½ cups fresh orange juice
    2 frozen bananas
  4–6 soft dates, seeds removed
 ½–1 cup crushed ice

Combine juice and dates in blender and blend until smooth. Add
ice and bananas. Blend until thick and creamy. Serve immediately.
Serves 2.

MELON SMOOTHIE

This smoothie can be made with all fresh melon, some fresh and some frozen, or all frozen. If you use only frozen, it will be a Melon Slush.

1 cup fresh or frozen watermelon
1 cup fresh or frozen cantaloupe, honeydew, Persian, or Crenshaw melon

Place melon in blender and blend until smooth. *Yields 2¼ cups.*

WATERMELON SMOOTHIE

  2 cups watermelon
3–4 ice cubes (optional and not recommended during detoxification)

Place watermelon (and ice cubes, if desired) in blender—it's not necessary to remove seeds. Blend for several minutes until thick pink frothy juice forms. Strain. *Serves 1.*

HONEYDEW SMOOTHIE

  2 cups honeydew melon
3–4 ice cubes (optional and not recommended during detoxification)

Place honeydew (and ice cubes, if desired) in a blender. Blend several minutes until a creamy juice has formed. *Serves 1.*

CANTALOUPE SMOOTHIE

  2 cups cantaloupe
3–4 ice cubes (optional and not recommended during detoxification)

Place cantaloupe (and ice cubes, if desired) in a blender. Blend several minutes until a creamy juice has formed. *Serves 1*.

PERSIMMON SMOOTHIE

2 cups fresh orange juice
2 medium persimmons, very ripe
6–8 ice cubes
3–4 soft dates, pits removed

Blend dates and orange juice in a blender until smooth. Add ice and persimmons and blend until frothy. This smoothie can be frozen in individual pop holders for great pops. *Makes 3 individual smoothies or 6 to 8 pops*.

Fruit Salads and Sauces

PEACH-MELON FLOWER BOWLS

 2 peaches, cut in 8 slices each
½ cantaloupe or Persian melon, cut in 1-inch balls
¼ honeydew, cut in ½-inch balls
    Several red seedless and Thompson seedless grapes,
    halved lengthwise
    Several fresh mint leaves

Using 2 fruit plates or shallow fruit bowls, arrange the peach slices in a ring around the edges of the bowls. Combine the melon balls and mound them in the center of the ring. Place the grape halves at appropriate places in the form of flowers. Garnish the "grape flowers" with mint leaves. This makes a lovely first course. *Serves 2.*

MANGO-MELONBERRY SALAD WITH HONEYLOUPE SHERBET

 6 ½-inch slices honeydew, cut in bite-sized pieces
36 cantaloupe balls
 2 peaches, cut in 12 slices each
12 strawberries, stemmed and halved lengthwise
 1 large or 2 small mangoes, peeled and cut in thin slices
 2 Bartlett pears, peeled and cut in 12 slices
 2 cups frozen honeydew chunks
 2 cups frozen cantaloupe chunks

On 6 pretty plates, divide fresh fruit in equal portions. Run frozen melon through Champion juicer using blank instead of juicing screen. Top fruit arrangements with one scoop of honeydew ice and one scoop of cantaloupe ice. You are not going to believe this delightful eating experience! Serve for lunch or as a first course for a dinner party while your guests chat and you put the finishing touches on the rest of the meal. You will find that they will be chatting about what they are eating! I usually tell people that this is their dessert and they get to eat it first! *Serves 6.*

FRUIT FOR LIFE SALAD

  ½ **Persian melon, cut in balls**
  ¼ **honeydew melon, cut in balls**
1½ **cup Red Flame grapes**
  1 **cup blueberries**
  ½ **papaya, peeled, seeded, and cubed**
  1 **mango, peeled and cubed**
  ½ **cup soaked raisins or currants**

Cut all fruit and toss together in a glass bowl or place in layers of alternating colors in parfait glasses. Top with Cashew-Apricot or Banana-Peach Sauce (see page 377), or Rainbow Cream (see page 439). *Serves 3 to 4.*

COCONUT-APPLE GRANOLA

This delightful, grainless granola is light and sweet and can be a perfect breakfast for kids who "want something more." Make it in the food processor or use electric or hand grinders.

  1 **large Delicious apple, peeled and cored**
  1 **large handful fresh coconut chunks**
  1 **tablespoon currants**
  ¼ **cup fresh almonds**
  2 **teaspoons maple syrup**
  ½ **teaspoon cinnamon**
2–4 **tablespoons fresh apple juice**

Run the apple, the coconut, and the currants through the fine grater of a food processor. Run about half the almonds through the slicer blade of the food processor, and grind the rest to meal in a nut grinder or blender. Add the maple syrup and cinnamon and mix well. Add apple juice to taste. *Serves 2*.

STRAWBERRY-MINT SOUP

This is a wonderful light lunch with Coconut-Apple Granola, or it makes a beautiful first course at a dinner party.

2 pints fresh strawberries
2 tablespoons maple syrup
18 fresh mint leaves, washed and patted dry
¼ cup fresh orange juice
2 pints frozen strawberries
2 tablespoons grated coconut (optional)

Reserve 4 large fresh strawberries. Place remaining fresh strawberries in blender with maple syrup, 10 mint leaves, and fresh orange juice. Blend until completely smooth. Refrigerate until cold.

Thinly slice remaining fresh strawberries. Refrigerate until serving time.

Run frozen strawberries through Champion juicer (using blank), or process with metal blade until thick sherbet forms.

To serve, ladle strawberry-mint soup into 4 broad, shallow bowls. Place a scoop of strawberry sherbet in center. Garnish with strawberry slices and mint leaves. Sprinkle with coconut, if desired. *Serves 4*.

CASHEW-APRICOT SAUCE

¾ cup watermelon, watermelon-cantaloupe, or orange juice
¼ cup (scant) cashews
4 frozen or fresh apricots
2 teaspoons maple syrup
Fresh ground nutmeg to taste (optional)

Blend cashews in juice until completely smooth. Add apricots and syrup and continue blending. Add nutmeg.* Blend until thoroughly combined and smooth. Serve with fruit salad of your choice or Fruit for Life Salad. *Serves 4*.

BANANA-PEACH SAUCE

1 **ripe banana, fresh or frozen**
¼ **cup raisin water (from soaked raisins) or fresh orange juice**
1 **fresh or frozen peach**
 Dash of nutmeg
 Dash of cardamom

Place all the ingredients in a blender or food processor and blend until smooth. If both banana and peach are frozen, you may need to add ¼ cup extra liquid. Serve over fruit salad of your choice or Fruit for Life Salad. *Serves 4*.

Vegetable Salads and Dressings

BLENDED SALAD

2 medium tomatoes
3 inches hothouse cucumber, unpeeled, or 3 inches regular
   cucumber, peeled
   Small red or green bell pepper
   Large stalk celery
5 or 6 leaves Romaine lettuce

Place tomatoes in blender and liquefy. Add cucumber and bell pepper and liquefy. Add lettuce leaves, pushing them down with stalk of celery. Blend 1 to 2 minutes to liquefy entire salad. This makes an incredible lunch with a half large avocado per person. *Serves 2.*

FIT FOR LIFE SPROUT SALAD

Sprouts are more and more available and they make wonderful change-of-pace salads. Some that you can look for are alfalfa, buckwheat, sunflower, mung or azuki bean, brown or red lentil, pea, wheatberry, soybean, or garbanzo bean. Alfalfa, buckwheat, sunflower, mung bean, and lentil are the most easily digested. Alfalfa sprouts are very common, and red clover, a similar sprout with a larger leaf, is also more and more available. Fenugreek and radish are quite spicy and a matter of personal taste.

2 cups buckwheat sprouts, broken in half
2 cups sunflower seed sprouts, broken in half
1 cup mung bean sprouts
½ cup red lentil sprouts
½ cup azuki bean sprouts
1–2 cups alfalfa sprouts
1 large tomato, coarsely chopped
1 7-inch section hothouse cucumber, peeled and cubed

DRESSING

1 large avocado
⅓ cup water
1 teaspoon fresh lemon juice
¼ teaspoon cumin
Seasoned salt or salt-free seasoning to taste

Place all the sprouts in a medium salad bowl and toss them well so they are mixed. Mash the avocado by hand or process until smooth, adding water, lemon juice, and seasonings. Pour the dressing over the sprouts. Add the cucumber and the tomato and toss well. Roll in toasted nori, sushi style, if desired. *Serves 2 to 3.*

EASY LIMESTONE LETTUCE SALAD WITH BASIL-GARLIC DRESSING

Limestone lettuce is a crunchy, lighter alternative to butter or Boston lettuce—slightly more expensive, but delicious.

3 tablespoons olive oil
1½ tablespoons fresh lemon juice
1 small clove garlic, crushed
½ teaspoon Dijon mustard
¼ teaspoon salt
1 head limestone lettuce
1 tablespoon almonaise (see p. 388) or mayonnaise
Fresh ground pepper to taste
1 tablespoon fresh basil, minced

In salad bowl, whip together oil, lemon juice, garlic, mustard, and salt. Add limestone lettuce broken gently in bite-sized pieces and almonaise or mayonnaise. Add pepper and fresh basil and toss again to combine. *Serves 2 to 3*.

SPROUT SALAD SUNSET PLAZA

½ medium avocado
1 tablespoon mayonnaise
1 teaspoon Dijon mustard
1 teaspoon fresh lemon juice
   Seasoned salt or salt-free seasoning to taste (Trocomare)
3 tablespoons water
3 cups buckwheat sprouts
2 cups sunflower sprouts
1 cup alfalfa sprouts
2 whole-wheat chapatis or tortillas (Garden of Eatin')

In a large salad bowl, mash the avocado with a fork or potato masher. Incorporate the mayonnaise and mustard. Beat in the lemon juice, seasoned salt and the water until a thick creamy dressing has formed.

Gently break the buckwheat and sunflower sprouts in half and add them to dressing. Separate the alfalfa sprouts and add them. On a dry, hot skillet, heat the chapatis or tortillas one at a time until they are soft and pliable. Break them into the salad. Toss *very* well until the sprouts break down just a bit and the chapatis are coated with dressing. You won't believe how good this is. *Serves 2*.

SOFT LETTUCE TACOS WITH AVOCADO DRESSING

Your choice of fresh vegetables (tomatoes, bell peppers, carrots, cucumbers, celery, zucchini, jicama)
Several leaves of iceberg or butter lettuce, washed and dried
Avocado slices
Alfalfa sprouts

Clean and peel all the vegetables. Chop them finely by hand or in a food processor. Place a slice of avocado in center of lettuce leaf. Top with chopped vegetables and alfalfa sprouts and drizzle Avocado Dressing with Fresh Herbs (see page 387) over the top. *Serves 1.*

LISA'S SALAD WITH NORI

My teenage daughter Lisa invented this salad one day when she was craving sushi. She said it totally satisfied the craving because of the nori it contained. Now that nori is commonly eaten as a result of the popularity of sushi, people may be ready to begin experimenting with it in salads. It is a delicious salad ingredient.

  2 **cups red leaf or butter lettuce**
  2 **cups iceberg lettuce**
  ½ **cup red lentil sprouts (or brown, if red are not available)**
  1 **cup bean sprouts**
  1½ **cups sunflower sprouts, cut in half**
  2 **cups buckwheat sprouts, cut in half**
  2 **large tomatoes, diced**
  1 **medium large avocado, cubed**
  2 **sheets toasted nori (pressed seaweed, available in natural food stores or in Oriental section of your market)**
  ¼ **cup olive oil**
  2 **tablespoons fresh lemon juice**
     Seasoned salt or salt-free seasoning to taste
  1 **teaspoon ground celery seed (optional)**

In a large salad bowl, break the lettuce into small pieces. Add the red lentil sprouts, the bean sprouts, and sunflower and buckwheat sprouts. Add the diced tomatoes and cubed avocado. Break the nori in ½-inch pieces and add to salad. Beat together olive oil, lemon juice, and seasonings and pour over salad. Toss very well. Season to taste. *Serves 2 on a living food day as a complete lunch or dinner.*

SUMMER GREEK SALAD WITH SEVEN-HERB DRESSING

    1 cup red leaf lettuce
    1 cup iceberg lettuce
    1 cup butter lettuce
    1 cup spinach
    1 medium tomato, chopped
    ⅓ cup green or black olives (Capello's or Greek olives)
    ½ cup chopped cucumber
    1 large handful buckwheat or alfalfa sprouts
    1 tablespoon minced celery
    ¼ cup carrot, cut in fine, long slivers with zester or grated
    ¼ cup red pepper strips
    ¼ cup yellow squash, cut in fine, long slivers with zester or
       grated
    ¼ cup zucchini, cut in fine, long slivers with zester or
       grated
    ½ cup Seven-Herb Dressing (see page 390)
    ¾ cup crumbled fresh feta cheese (or substitute same
       amount grated Jack cheese)

Combine all vegetable ingredients in medium salad bowl. Add
dressing and cheese and toss gently but well. *Makes 1 or 2 servings*.

CAESAR SALAD

This is the Fit for Life *Caesar Salad with an almonaise addition.
The almonaise (see page 388) makes it quite special.*

   *Remember the food-combining principle here. If you are adding
the parmesan cheese, you must omit the croutons. If you are using
almonaise, you may include croutons. You may omit both the
cheese and the almonaise, and the salad will still be delicious.*

    1 **clove garlic**
    3 **tablespoons olive oil**
       Dash of Robbie's Worcestershire Sauce (optional)
1–2 **tablespoons fresh lemon juice**
    1 **teaspoon Dijon mustard**
    1 **sheet nori (pressed seaweed, available in natural food stores or in Oriental section of your market—optional)**
   ¼ **teaspoon sea salt**
   ¼ **teaspoon Spike or salt-free seasoning**
    1 **small head romaine lettuce, washed and rolled in a towel to dry**
    2 **tablespoons Parmesan cheese (omit croutons below) or 2 tablespoons almonaise (croutons may be included)**
½–1 **cup Garlic Croutons (see below)**
      Fresh ground pepper to taste

Place garlic in a large salad bowl and crush with a fork. Add the oil and stir briskly with a fork or whisk. Add the Worcestershire, lemon juice, and mustard, stirring briskly. Remove the garlic pieces and discard. Holding nori in your hand, toast it over hot burner (gas or electric) for 1–2 seconds on each side, until it turns from black to green. Crumble into pieces and mix into dressing. Add sea salt and Spike and mix briskly.

Break washed and dried romaine into bite-sized pieces, discarding the heaviest part of the stalk. Add to bowl and toss thoroughly. Add parmesan cheese or almonaise and croutons. Add fresh ground pepper to taste. Toss thoroughly. *Serves 2–3.*

GARLIC CROUTONS

These are easy to make and far superior to the packaged variety!

1 **slice whole-grain bread**
2 **teaspoons butter or olive oil**
1 **clove garlic, crushed or cut in 2–3 segments**

Cut bread in ½-inch cubes. Heat butter or oil in small skillet. Add crushed garlic or garlic segments. Sauté over medium heat to flavor the butter. Remove the larger garlic segments. Add bread cubes and sauté, turning frequently, until crisp. Add cubes to salad, soup, or vegetable dishes. *Serves 2*.

LIMESTONE AND LAMB'S LETTUCE SALAD

This light and flavorful salad of the tenderest of greens is a perfect accompaniment to any festive dinner menu. The lamb's lettuce, or "mache," is a small-leafed green with a mild flavor that has a truly elegant effect in a salad. Limestone lettuce, although similar to butter or Boston lettuce, but of much finer texture, is also more costly but well worth the price. The light Dijon dressing comple-·ments rather than distracts from other flavors you may wish to feature.

   2 **heads limestone lettuce**
   4 **ounces lamb's lettuce**
  ¼ **cup plus 2 tablespoons extra-virgin olive oil**
   1 **small clove garlic, halved**
   2 **teaspoons lemon juice (fresh)**
  ¼ **teaspoon seasoned salt or salt-free seasoning to taste (Trocomare)**
   1 **teaspoon fresh savory, minced**
¼–½ **teaspoon Dijon mustard**

Throughout the preparation, take care to handle the delicate greens as gently as possible, because it takes very little abuse for them to wilt. Wash the greens gently and place them in bowl of cold water in the refrigerator to crisp them until you are ready to prepare the salad. Place the cut clove of garlic in the olive oil and set aside. Drain the lettuce and, using a lettuce centrifuge, dry it in small batches. Break the lettuce gently into a large bowl, removing the tiny root portion at the base of the lamb's lettuce clusters so the leaves separate.

    Add the fresh lemon juice, seasoned salt, fresh savory, and Dijon mustard to the garlic and oil mixture. Whip with a fork to combine, and then remove and discard the garlic. Pour over the greens. Toss gently and thoroughly. *Serves 4*.

SUMMER GREENS WITH FRESH HERB DRESSING

This is a lovely entertaining salad, which is why the recipe has been written with larger amounts than usual. This type of green salad particularly complements a rich entrée such as Mushroom Cream Crêpes or Vegetable Pie.

1 small Belgian endive
1 large or 2 small heads butter lettuce
1 small head red leaf lettuce (or several leaves)
1 small head curly endive (or several leaves)
1 bunch arugula
2 cups lamb's lettuce/mache (optional)
1 bunch enoki mushrooms

Dressing

2 tablespoons fresh oregano, minced
1 tablespoon fresh basil, minced
1 tablespoon fresh thyme, minced
⅓ cup olive oil
½ teaspoon sea salt
  Juice of 1 small lime
  Fresh ground pepper to taste
1 scant teaspoon Dijon mustard or Dijon-tarragon mustard

Cut bottom from Belgian endive and soak in salt water until ready to use. Break butter lettuce and red leaf lettuce into bite-sized pieces, discarding heavy ribs. Break curly endive into slightly smaller pieces, discarding heavy ribs. Remove arugula leaves from stems. Leave mache leaves whole, removing roots. Cut away and discard roots from enoki. Slice Belgian endive in thin lengthwise strips. Combine lettuces, mache, arugula, curly endive, enoki, and Belgian endive in large salad bowl. Add minced oregano, basil, and thyme and toss well. Add olive oil and sea salt and toss again. Add lime juice, pepper, and Dijon and toss thoroughly. *Serves 8.*

GREENS AND SHREDDED VEGETABLES

This is an excellent light salad for one and especially good when you are detoxifying, because it contains no free oils. (A free oil is any bottled oil that has been extracted from another food—i.e., olive, safflower, peanut, corn, etc.) Three no-oil dressing alternatives are provided here.

6 leaves red leaf lettuce
6 leaves butter or salad bowl lettuce
1 tomato, coarsely chopped
¼ cup sliced celery
½ medium avocado, peeled and cubed (optional)
1 medium carrot, finely shredded (¾ cup)
1 chunk jicama, peeled and finely shredded (¾ cup)

Break the lettuce into bite-sized pieces. Add the tomato, celery, and the avocado. Finely shred the carrot and jicama, using a hand grater or the fine shredding blade of a food processor. Add to salad. Season with one of the no-oil dressings below.

Grapefruit Juice Dressing

Lemon juice is an obvious no-oil dressing, but have you ever tried *grapefruit* juice on your salad? It is absolutely delicious! Because there is a relatively small amount of sugar in the grapefruit juice, there is no food combining problem. Simply add ¼ cup of freshly squeezed grapefruit juice to the above salad and toss well.

Carrot Juice Dressing

Fresh carrot juice by itself makes a great dressing. Or you can use it as a base and blend it with small amounts of other vegetables like avocado, tomato, cucumber, celery, or spinach.

Blended Vegetable Dressing

 1 small tomato
 ½ stalk celery
 ¼ bell pepper (red or green)

Blend vegetables together until pureed and smooth. Pour over above salad. Toss well.

FRENCH BUTTER LETTUCE SALAD

This is an easy salad that can be used as a standard with almost any meal.

 1 head butter lettuce, broken in bite-sized pieces
 2 tablespoons olive oil
 ¼ teaspoon sea salt
   Fresh ground pepper to taste
 1 small clove garlic, crushed
 1 tablespoon fresh lemon juice

Break the lettuce into a large bowl. Add the olive oil and the salt and toss well. Add the pepper, garlic, and lemon juice. Toss well. *Serves 2 to 3.*

AVOCADO DRESSING WITH FRESH HERBS

 1 medium avocado
 ½ cup water
 2 tablespoons olive, safflower, or grape seed oil
 1 teaspoon fresh savory leaves
 2 medium fresh basil leaves
   Seasoned salt or salt-free seasoning to taste (Trocomare)
 1 tablespoon fresh lemon juice

In food processor or blender, place avocado and water and process until smooth. Stop motor and push down all avocado chunks from sides of container with spatula. Add oil, herbs, seasoned salt, and lemon juice. (Dried herbs may be substituted, using ¼ teaspoon of each.) Process to incorporate all ingredients until dressing is creamy with little green flecks of herbs. Serve over cold, crisp summer greens such as limestone, red leaf, and lamb's lettuce. This light and flavorful dressing may also be used as a dip. *Yields enough for 1 large salad, approximately ¾ cup.*

DIAMOND'S ALMONAISE

This incredible mayonnaise substitute is a truly new eating experience. Made from a base of thick almond cream, it is lighter and less oily than its egg counterpart. You can verify this when you wash your blender after making the almonaise. It will be much easier to clean than when used to make regular mayonnaise.

As in the making of all mayonnaises, certain basics apply in this procedure. First of all, all the ingredients must be at room temperature. Secondly, it is necessary to carefully observe the indicated amounts. And last, oil should be added in a thin, fine stream and very slowly.

Most people find the flavor and consistency of almonaise to be somewhat of a cross between mayonnaise and cream cheese. It will truly enhance your sandwiches and salads, can be used as a dip for vegetables and even in some pasta dishes, and you will find the result to be excellent in terms of flavor and digestibility. This versatile spread, however you use it, is well worth the effort. If you are too busy to make it during the week, make a blenderful on Sunday to last the week.

To blanch almonds, simply place them in a skillet of boiling water for one minute. The skins will loosen and easily pop off. I used to give Harvey the blanched almonds to pop out of their skins while he was watching the weekend sports. Children also make good assistants for this chore, since they find peeling the nuts to be somewhat of a game. Almonds can also be blanched in advance and stored in the refrigerator in water for a day or two, but remember to bring them to room temperature before you use them.

Since all mayonnaises are a food-combining compromise when used with starches, it is worth having the choice of this lighter, more digestible variety over the traditional egg mayonnaises. If you occasionally have a "failure" when preparing the almonaise, don't worry about it. Sometimes too much moisture in the atmosphere interferes with the emulsification process.

½ cup blanched almonds
½ cup purified or distilled water
1 small sliver garlic (approximately ⅛ teaspoon)
½ teaspoon sea salt (optional)
½ teaspoon Spike or salt-free seasoning
2–3 tablespoons fresh lemon juice
    Dash of cayenne (optional)
    Fresh ground pepper to taste
2–3 cups safflower oil

Place blanched almonds and purified water in blender and blend on high speed until a thick cream forms. If the blender refuses to turn, add 1 to 2 tablespoons water until blade moves freely. Add garlic, sea salt, lemon juice, and pepper. Blend briefly. Remove center plug from top of blender and, while blender is on high, slowly drizzle oil into almond cream mixture. Blade will turn more and more freely as you blend. When mixture refuses to accept any more oil, the oil will begin to sit in a bubble on top of the almonaise. At this point, remove the lid and continue to add oil in a thin stream, beating shallowly with a spoon so that you do not hit the moving blade. This will force more oil into the mixture and guarantee a thicker product. Final consistency should be between that of mayonnaise and whipped cream cheese. Store in a covered glass container in the refrigerator. Almonaise keeps for at least a week (if it isn't used up by then!). *Yields 3 to 4 cups.*

SEVEN-HERB DRESSING

This is a great dressing to prepare in large quantities and keep on hand in your refrigerator. The flavors blend the longer the dressing sits. Mix all ingredients directly in a large jar with a tight lid. Refrigerate until use.

1 clove garlic, minced or crushed
5 tablespoons olive oil
2 tablespoons fresh lemon or lime juice
½ teaspoon dried chervil
½ teaspoon basil
½ teaspoon dried thyme
½ teaspoon dried oregano
½ teaspoon savory
¼ teaspoon coriander
⅛ teaspoon sage
½ teaspoon sea salt, seasoned salt, or salt-free seasoning
1 teaspoon mustard
1 tablespoon mayonnaise or almonaise (see page 388)

TARRAGON CREAM DRESSING

¼ cup avocado oil or olive oil
2 tablespoons heavy cream
1 tablespoon minced fresh tarragon or 1 teaspoon dried
1 clove garlic, crushed
¼ teaspoon sea salt
1½–2 tablespoons lemon juice
Fresh ground pepper to taste

Combine all the ingredients in a measuring cup. Beat well with a fork until thick and creamy. *Yields enough for 4 limestone lettuce salads.*

REGENT OF FIJI FRENCH DRESSING

*During a stopover in Fiji after our 1986 tour of Australia to
promote* **Fit for Life**, *we really enjoyed the incredible food at the
fabulous Regent Hotel in that South Pacific paradise. Thomas
Brossmer, the executive chef at the Regent of Fiji, prepared wonderful, properly combined meals for us and was also happy to
share this unusual and delicious salad dressing recipe with me so
that I could share it with you. It pays to make a large quantity of
this dressing so that you can have it on hand for several days.*

  4 **cups vegetable broth, preferably from 2 Hugli**
    Vegetable Bouillon Cubes
  2 **onions, chopped**
  2 **cups mayonnaise or almonaise (see page 388)**
1–2 **tablespoons Dijon mustard**
    Fresh ground white pepper to taste
    Sea salt to taste (optional)
  1 **tablespoon fresh lemon juice or to taste**

Bring the vegetable bouillon to a boil. Add the chopped onions.
Boil for 40 minutes. Cool and strain.

   Put mayonnaise or almonaise in large bowl. Add cooled liquid
slowly, whisking until mayonnaise has dissolved. Add mustard,
pepper, sea salt, and lemon juice to taste. Store in closed container
in refrigerator. *Yields 3 cups.*

THOUSAND ISLAND DRESSING

½ **cup mayonnaise or almonaise (see page 388)**
½ **cup sour cream**
 1 **small dill pickle, finely grated**
   Scant tablespoon fresh lemon juice
¼ **teaspoon dried basil**
   Spike, Herbamare, or salt-free seasoning to taste

Combine all the ingredients in the order given. Mix thoroughly.
Enough for 2 large salads.

Vegetable Dishes

BRAISED COURGETTES

This is such an easy and marvelous vegetable dish. If you can find the tiny zucchini with their blossoms intact, use them. They have a wonderful flavor and the blossoms have a fabulous consistency. When the baby zucchini are unavailable, use small whole zucchini as a substitute and braise them for twice the time with double the braising liquid. Or you may substitute Belgian endive, baby bok choy, or fennel.

  1 pound baby zucchini with blossoms
  1 tablespoon butter
  1 tablespoon olive oil
  1 tablespoon minced onions
  ½ vegetable bouillon cube or 1 heaping teaspoon powdered
    vegetable broth
  ¾ cup water
  1 tablespoon fresh sage leaves or ⅛ teaspoon dried sage

Trim the stem end of the zucchini. Melt the butter and heat the oil in a heavy skillet with lid. (The skillet must be heavy or the water will cook off too fast. The Fogacci skillet is the best I have ever used for braising.) Add the minced onion and the baby zucchini. Sauté the zucchini over medium heat to seal in the juices, turning with tongs as you sauté. Dissolve the vegetable bouillon or broth in the water. Add the sage. Add to the skillet. Bring to a boil. Cover and braise over medium low heat for 15 minutes to an hour or until the vegetables test tender when pierced with a sharp knife and the liquid is reduced to a thick glaze. Serve as part of a vegetable plate with glazed baby beets, baked dumpling squash and artichokes, accompanied by a bibb lettuce and arugula salad with French dressing and hot buttered monkey bread. *Serves 3.*

GLAZED BABY BEETS

These are easy to make and they look very special on a vegetable plate. If baby beets are not available, substitute one bunch regular beets.

2 bunches baby beets, with greens and ends removed
 Water to cover
1 tablespoon honey, maple syrup, or maple sugar

Wash beets well. Place in small saucepan with lid. Add water to cover and bring to a boil. Cover and reduce heat to medium low. If beets are cooked at too high a heat, the water will spatter all over the stove. Simmer for 20 minutes or until the beets are tender when pierced deeply with a sharp knife. Remove from water and peel off skins. At this point, if you are using regular-sized beets, you can cube, slice, or julienne them. Return beets to beet water. Add sweetener. Bring to a boil and simmer until water is reduced to a thick, sweet glaze. *Serves 6.*

CHINESE ZUCCHINI

1 large clove garlic, crushed
2 tablespoons safflower oil
½ cup vegetable broth
2 teaspoons mirin (Japanese sweetener made from rice) or
 1 teaspoon honey
2 tablespoons light soy sauce
1 teaspoon roasted sesame oil
1 tablespoon cornstarch dissolved in ¼ cup water
6 medium zucchini, sliced in ¼-inch diagonals

Heat wok over high heat for several minutes. While the wok is heating, prepare the other ingredients and have everything ready at your fingertips. Wok cooking is quick and there is no time to start slicing or measuring once the process has begun.

Crush the garlic and place it in a small bowl with the first tablespoon of safflower oil. Combine the vegetable broth, mirin, soy sauce, and sesame oil. Combine the cornstarch with ¼ cup cold water.

Place second tablespoon of safflower oil in the heated wok. Swirl the wok to coat the sides. Add the garlic and oil combination and immediately add the zucchini. Toss the zucchini in the hot oil, blending it with the garlic so the garlic does not brown, sprinkling it with a few teaspoons of broth if it begins to scorch. Continue tossing until zucchini is bright green and just tender. Add the broth mixture. Toss well. Add the cornstarch mixture. Toss as sauce thickens.

This dish mixes very well with Japanese rice vermicelli. Simply mix the cooked vermicelli directly into the wok, adding another ½ cup of vegetable broth. *Serves 3 to 4.*

STUFFED MUSHROOMS FRANCESCA

My beloved mother, Frances, has shared so many wonderful, easy recipes with me. This is one I thought you would really enjoy.

12 large mushroom caps, stems reserved
 1 small onion, finely chopped
 ½ cup parsley, finely minced
 ¼ cup (scant) bell pepper, minced (optional)
 2 tablespoons butter
 1 teaspoon lemon juice
 ⅓ cup fine whole-wheat bread crumbs
 ¼ teaspoon oregano
 ¼ teaspoon basil
 ¼ teaspoon coriander

Wash and dry mushrooms. Mince stems. Heat 1 tablespoon butter in medium skillet. Add onion, parsley, and bell pepper, and sauté until soft. Add lemon juice, bread crumbs, and herbs. Mix well. Stuff into caps. Dot with remaining tablespoon butter. Bake in buttered Pyrex baking dish at 375° for 20 minutes. *Yields 12 stuffed mushroom caps.*

EASY CAULIFLOWER ITALIANO

This simple method of preparing and seasoning cauliflower can be used for practically any vegetable. You can substitute sliced potatoes for a delicious warm salad or string beans, zucchini, celery, peas, bok choy, or snow peas. The possibilities are endless. After a day on living food, a warm bowl of simple vegetables Italiano is absolutely satisfying, and so easy to prepare that even a child can put this together.

1 **medium cauliflower, quartered, cored, and cut in 1-inch florets**
1 **tablespoon olive oil**
2 **teaspoons fresh lemon juice**
  Dash of sea salt (optional)
  Fresh ground pepper to taste

Place the cauliflower in a vegetable steamer over boiling water. Steam covered for 7 to 10 minutes or until the cauliflower tests very tender when pierced with the tip of a sharp knife. Place florets in large bowl and coarsely chop. Add olive oil, lemon juice, and salt and pepper and toss well. *Serves 1 to 2 as a main course or 3 to 4 as a side dish.*

MENU TIP: After a day on fruit and salad, Easy Cauliflower Italiano makes a terrifically satisfying one-dish meal; a vegetable fruit platter makes a nice accompaniment.

MINUTE ASPARAGUS

2 **pounds asparagus**
4 **tablespoons butter**
1 **large clove garlic, minced (approximately 1 teaspoon)**
1 **tablespoon fresh lemon juice**
1 **tablespoon reduced-sodium soy sauce**
  Fresh ground pepper to taste

Roll cut asparagus in 1-inch diagonals or slice them thin in ¼-inch slices. Blanche for 1 minute in boiling water. Drain and shock under cold water. Melt butter in wok or skillet. Add garlic and stir-fry, taking care that the butter does not brown. Add asparagus and stir-fry briefly. Add lemon juice and soy sauce. Toss gently. Season with pepper. *Serves 4 to 6.*

SWEET CARROTS AU NATUREL

1 pound carrots (approximately 6–7 medium carrots), peeled
2–3 tablespoons sweet butter
1 teaspoon basil
 Sea salt and fresh ground pepper to taste
2 tablespoons maple syrup

Cut carrots in ¼-inch rounds, 2-inch by ¼-inch strips, or you may cut them into fine julienne strips for a more elegant effect. Place carrots in heavy earthenware casserole with cover. Dot with butter, sprinkle with basil and salt and pepper, and drizzle with maple syrup. Bake covered at 375°, stirring occasionally, for 1 hour or until carrots are tender. *Serves 8.*

BEVERLY BARNEY'S ITALIAN ZUCCHINI

Beverly Barney of Phoenix, Arizona, was kind enough to write and share some of her newly developed, properly combined recipes with me after she started the **Fit for Life** *program. Her accompanying note read: "I had fun developing some of my recipes to fit the* **Fit for Life** *program. I feel 10 years younger!" Since I spend so much of my time working to develop all the new recipes that are constantly needed, it is really great when people on the program feel inspired to share some of their own innovations with me. This is an easy side dish for a large group.*

3 **pounds zucchini, scrubbed**
¼ **cup (or a bit more) safflower oil**
1 **cup freshly chopped parsley**
1 **cup freshly chopped basil**
2 **cloves garlic, minced or crushed**
   Fresh ground white pepper to taste

Trim ends from zucchini and cut into julienne strips. Heat oil in a large skillet. Add zucchini and remaining ingredients and sauté until crispy-tender, adding additional oil as needed. *Serves 6 to 8.*

SWEET AND SOUR RED CABBAGE

1 **small red cabbage, shredded (approximately 10 cups)**
3 **tablespoons butter**
½ **cup thinly sliced red or white onion**
3 **tablespoons honey**
3 **tablespoons fresh lemon juice**
½ **teaspoon sea salt**
   Fresh ground pepper to taste

Shred cabbage and soak it in cold water for 10 minutes. Heat butter in heavy enamel, flameproof casserole with lid. Add onion and sauté until soft. Lift cabbage from water, keeping it moist, and transfer it to casserole. Cover and simmer 10 minutes over medium heat. Mix together the honey, lemon juice, and salt. Pour over the cabbage and mix well. Cover and simmer over very low heat for 1 hour, adding small amounts of boiling water if cabbage becomes dry. If water has not been absorbed when cabbage is done, uncover and cook it gently until it is absorbed. Season with pepper and additional salt or salt-free seasoning, if desired. *Serves 4.*

SUGGESTED MENU:
   Chilled Cucumber Soup (see page 403)
   Lisa's Salad with Nori (see page 381)
   Beverly Barney's Italian Zucchini (see page 396)
   Creamy Mashed Potatoes and Gravy (see page 415)
   Sweet and Sour Red Cabbage (above)

BARBECUED VEGETABLE KEBABS

These lovely barbecued brochettes of vegetables can be used as hors d'oeuvres, appetizers at a buffet, or as part of a sit-down dinner. They have a tangy marinade that can be used after barbecuing as a sauce. Thread them either on short, individual skewers as appetizers or on longer skewers for entrées. Any assortment of vegetables you prefer will work. The longer the vegetables are marinated, the better their flavor will be.

Marinade

¼ cup olive oil
¼ cup safflower or avocado oil
1 teaspoon roasted sesame oil
2 tablespoons fresh lemon juice
2 tablespoons tamari sauce
2 teaspoons Worcestershire sauce (preferably Robbie's)
1 large clove garlic, crushed
2 teaspoons dried oregano or 2 tablespoons fresh, finely chopped
2 teaspoons dried savory or 2 tablespoons fresh, finely chopped
½ teaspoon dried rosemary or 1 tablespoon fresh rosemary
2 teaspoons dried basil or 2 tablespoons fresh, finely chopped
Fresh ground pepper to taste

Vegetables

6 medium Japanese eggplant, peeled and cut in 1-inch slices
12 tiny new potatoes, presteamed for 15 minutes or until just tender
1 sweet red pepper, cut in 1½-inch sections
1 sweet yellow or green pepper, cut in 1½-inch sections
12 mushrooms, halved
12 artichoke hearts
4 small zucchini, cut in ¾-inch sections (or you may use the baby summer squash)

If you can get the Japanese eggplant, they are preferable, as they are less bitter than regular eggplant. If using regular eggplant, cut it in cubes after peeling, salt it, and let it sit for ½ hour to remove bitterness. Rinse and pat dry. If you cannot find the tiny new potatoes, use the smallest you can find and halve or quarter them after steaming.

Mix the marinade. Cut all the vegetables in the desired sizes. Place in a large, shallow dish and pour marinade over vegetables. Mix well, making sure all vegetables are coated with marinade. Cover and refrigerate for several hours. Stir the vegetables two or three times while they are marinating. Arrange the vegetables on skewers. You can arrange an assortment of vegetables on each skewer for appetizers or, if the barbecued vegetables are the entrée, you can put each type of vegetable on its own skewer to ensure proper cooking. For example, potatoes and zucchini take longer than eggplant and mushrooms. If you are grilling each vegetable on its own skewer, place the finished vegetables in a pretty bowl or platter from which guests can help themselves, rather than leaving them on the skewers. Grill the vegetables 15–25 minutes over medium coals, turning frequently. Baste frequently with the marinade. Pour remaining marinade over the vegetables after they have been placed in the bowl or serve as a dipping sauce. Serve with chow mein udon with garlic butter (available in Asian food section of your supermarket) and a summer green salad with Dijon dressing. Sour cream and chives can be passed as an additional dip for the grilled potatoes. *Serves 4 to 8.*

CRISPY BROCCOLI WITH GARLIC

   2 **bunches broccoli**
   2 **tablespoons safflower oil**
2–3 **large cloves garlic, according to taste**
  ½ **cup vegetable broth**
   2 **tablespoons light soy sauce**
   1 **tablespoon dark soy sauce (low sodium)**
   2 **teaspoons mirin (Japanese sweetener made from rice)**
     or 1 teaspoon honey
   1 **teaspoon roasted sesame oil**
   2 **tablespoons cornstarch dissolved in ⅓ cup water with 1**
     teaspoon safflower oil

Trim heavy stalks from broccoli and reserve for another use. Using florets and about 2 inches of remaining broccoli stems, cut lengthwise in ½-inch-thick lengths. Place in vegetable steamer over boiling water for 3 minutes. Turn out on cookie sheet to cool.

Preheat wok over high heat. Prepare sauce ingredients: Crush garlic into small bowl, and add 1 tablespoon safflower oil. Combine broth, soy sauces, mirin, and sesame oil in a separate bowl. Set both bowls close to the wok so they will be easily available during wok preparations. Combine cornstarch and water and 1 teaspoon safflower oil. Set near wok.

Heat remaining 1 tablespoon safflower oil in wok. Turn wok to coat sides. Add garlic-and-oil mixture and immediately add broccoli and begin tossing. Toss immediately so that garlic on bottom of wok does not burn. Toss for several minutes until all broccoli has been well coated with the oil. Add soy sauce mixture and cornstarch thickener and toss well until broccoli is coated with thick, light brown sauce. This combines well with chow mein udon in basil butter and head lettuce and avocado vinaigrette. *Serves 4.*

BRAISED GREEN BEANS

This wonderful preparation for green beans is very quick and easy. Combined with mashed potatoes and using the sauce from the green beans as a gravy, you will have an absolutely delicious main course that takes less than 40 minutes to prepare. It is a real hit with kids, too! When you are buying your green beans, hand pick those that are young and slender. The older, thicker ones are usually very stringy. Use a heavy, covered skillet for braising (see Braised Courgettes, page 392).

- 1 tablespoon powdered vegetable broth (Bernard Jensen's salt-free is great) or 1 vegetable bouillon cube
- 2 cups water
- 2 tablespoons butter
- ½ tablespoon olive oil
- 1 teaspoon minced shallot
- 1 pound tender green beans, ends trimmed and halved
  Several fresh sage leaves or ¼ teaspoon dried sage
- ⅛ teaspoon dried thyme or 1 teaspoon fresh thyme leaves
- 1 tablespoon fresh oregano leaves or ⅛ teaspoon dried oregano

Dissolve the vegetable broth in the water. Melt the butter and heat the oil in the skillet. Add the minced shallot and sauté briefly over medium heat, allowing shallot to soften but not to crisp. Add the beans and sauté, turning frequently until they are well sealed.* Do not allow beans to brown. Add the braised liquid and sprinkle the beans with the herbs. Bring to a boil, cover and simmer 20 minutes over medium low heat until the green beans are tender and the liquid is reduced by approximately half. If you do not wish to use the liquid as a gravy for potatoes or noodles, remove the beans and boil the liquid until it is reduced again by half. Pour over the beans as a glaze. *Serves 3*.

GRILLED SHIITAKE MUSHROOMS

1 **package dried shiitake mushrooms**
   Water to cover
1 **tablespoon butter**
1 **teaspoon safflower or olive oil**

Soak dried shiitake for ½ hour in warm water to cover. Drain and remove stems with a sharp knife. If mushrooms are very large, you may wish to cut them in half. While you are trimming mushroom stems, preheat wok. (This dish may also be prepared in a heavy skillet.) Add butter and oil to heated wok. Immediately add shiitake and begin tossing them in the hot butter-oil mixture. Toss shiitake continuously until they are tender. This only takes 2 or 3 minutes. If you like the mushrooms a little bit crispy, allow them to sear for a minute or two longer. *Serves 3*.

*Sealing cooks in the natural juices of the vegetables.

Soups, Sandwiches, and Rolled-Up Yummies

CHINESE CORN SOUP

This easy corn soup can be whipped up in a few minutes. Kids love it. It is satisfying during detoxification.

 1 tablespoon safflower oil
 ¼ cup chopped green onions
 2 teaspoons Bernard Jensen's Natural Vegetable Seasoning
 2 teaspoons vegetable "chicken" broth
 4 cups water
 4 cups corn, fresh cut from cob or frozen
 ½ teaspoon sesame oil
 1 teaspoon light soy sauce
 1 teaspoon low-salt dark soy sauce
 ½ teaspoon mirin (Japanese sweetener made from rice)
 ¼ teaspoon (scant) Chinese Five Spices
 ⅛ teaspoon powdered ginger
 1 bunch green chard or bok choy greens, cut into 3-inch
   sections
 1 teaspoon (heaping) cornstarch or arrowroot, dissolved in
   2 tablespoons cold water (optional)

Heat wok over high heat for several minutes. Add safflower oil and immediately add green onions. Add seasoning, vegetable broth, and water. Cover and bring to boil.

Add corn, sesame oil, soy sauces, and mirin. Add Chinese Five Spices and powdered ginger. Return to a boil and add chard or bok choy greens. Simmer until greens wilt.

Stir in cornstarch-and-water thickener if desired. Allow to bubble and thicken. *Serves 4.*

CREAM OF ROMAINE AND CUCUMBER SOUP

Using the potato version, this is a good soup to incorporate into the third or fourth day of detoxification. The small amount of potato makes it filling but not too heavy. This is also a good soup for people who have difficulty digesting lettuce.

1 **large head romaine lettuce, thoroughly washed**
1 **large hot house cucumber (English) or 2 medium cucumbers, peeled**
1 **tablespoon butter**
2 **teaspoons olive oil**
1 **small red or white onion, coarsely chopped**
½ **cup celery, chopped**
7 **cups water**
1 **teaspoon Bernard Jensen's Natural Vegetable Seasoning**
1 **salt-free vegetable bouillon**
2 **medium potatoes, peeled and cubed, or 4 tablespoons heavy cream**

Coarsely chop romaine. Cut cucumber in ¼-inch slices. Heat butter and oil in soup kettle. Add onion, cucumber, and romaine and mix well. Add celery and continue stirring until vegetables begin to wilt slightly. Add water and vegetable seasoning and bouillon. Bring to a boil and add potato *or,* if you wish to serve this soup as part of a fish or chicken dinner, omit the potato and add cream later *as a final step.* Simmer soup for 30 minutes, liquefy in a food processor, blender, or Vita-Mix. If using cream, add it before reheating. Do *not* allow soup to return to a boil. *Serves 4 to 5 people.*

GREEN SOUP WITH FRESH HERBS

1 medium onion, coarsely chopped
1 bunch green onions, coarsely chopped
3 stalks celery, coarsely chopped
1 large carrot, coarsely chopped
2 tablespoons butter
1 10-ounce box frozen cut green beans or 2 cups fresh, cut in 1-inch segments
2 10-ounce boxes frozen Fordhook lima beans
3 tablespoons vegetable broth or vegetable chicken broth
½ teaspoon thyme
¼ teaspoon sage
13 cups water
1 10-ounce box frozen chopped spinach or ½ bunch fresh, coarsely chopped
2 medium zucchini, cut in ⅛-inch rounds
1 small head Chinese (Napa) cabbage, cut in fine shreds
1 tablespoon Bernard Jensen's Natural Vegetable Seasoning or 1 vegetable bouillon
2 tablespoons fresh basil, coarsely chopped
2 tablespoons fresh savory, coarsely chopped

This is a quick and easy soup to make and comes out fantastically well if the water is added in stages and a lot of stirring takes place during the short preparation time.

Using a food processor, coarsely chop the onion, green onions, celery, and carrot. Melt the butter in a large soup kettle and add the chopped vegetables. Sauté, stirring frequently for 2 or 3 minutes or until the vegetables turn a brighter color. Add the frozen green beans and the limas. Stir to combine. Add the vegetable broth, thyme, sage, and 6 cups of the water. Bring to a boil and stir in the frozen spinach, cut in cubes, or the fresh spinach and the zucchini. Cook, stirring frequently, for several minutes. Add the shredded Chinese cabbage and the remaining water. Bring to a boil. Add the vegetable seasoning or bouillon. Stir in the fresh basil and savory. Simmer, uncovered, for 5 minutes. Soup will be ready when limas are tender. The entire cooking time should not exceed 25 minutes. This is a large amount that keeps very well and can be frozen. Serve with vegetable fusilli, if desired. Accompany with whole-grain toast.

COUNTRY CARROT SOUP

This delicious soup can be served textured or blended to a smooth cream. With the help of a food processor, it is a breeze to prepare.

   1 **onion**
   2 **ribs celery**
   1 **tablespoon butter**
   6 **medium carrots**
   ½ **cup parsley**
      Water
1–2 **vegetable bouillon cubes**
      Herbamare or salt-free seasoning to taste

In a food processor, chop onion and celery. Melt butter in a medium soup kettle; add onion and celery and sauté. Meanwhile, coarsely grate carrots. Add to sautéing vegetables. Chop parsley and add to vegetable mixture, stirring to combine. Add water to cover vegetables by approximately ½ inch. Add vegetable cubes and Herbamare. Bring to a boil, cover, and simmer for 1 hour. For a richer soup stir in 2 tablespoons cream at end of cooking. Do *not* return to a boil. For a carrot cream soup, blend soup and add cream after blending. Serve hot or cold. *Serves 4 to 6.*

MISO AND VEGETABLES

Miso is a soybean paste that is used in Japanese and macrobiotic cooking as a base for soups. It is also made from brown rice or barley, but these are not as common. I used to buy miso only in health food stores, but now I find it in the Asian food section of my supermarkets. In soup it has a mellow flavor and does not require the addition of any other flavorings, especially since it already has a slightly salty quality.

6 **cups water**
2 **medium new potatoes, presteamed for 20 minutes**
2 **summer squash**
1 **medium yellow squash**
2 **small zucchini**
1 **large or 2 medium carrots, presteamed for 20 minutes**
1 **medium bok choy or ¼ cabbage**
1 **tablespoon white, yellow, or red miso**

Bring water to a boil. Peel potatoes and cut into bite-sized chunks. Cut squashes, zucchini, and carrots into bite-sized chunks. Coarsely chop bok choy (leaves only) or cabbage. Add with miso to boiling water. Stir to dissolve miso. Cover and simmer 10 minutes or until squashes are tender. *Serves 3.*

CHILLED CUCUMBER SOUP

This delicious, creamy cold soup is filling, as it contains cream and sour cream. It is a good first course when you are serving a predominantly vegetable meal. I like to serve it first when I am making Barbecued Vegetable Kebabs (see page 398) and a big salad.

     3 **large cucumbers, peeled, seeded, and thinly sliced**
    ½ **cup sliced scallions**
     3 **tablespoons butter**
   1½ **cups potatoes, peeled and cut in ½-inch cubes**
     6 **cups vegetable broth**
    ½ **teaspoon seasoned salt or salt-free seasoning to taste**
    ¼ **teaspoon dried tarragon or 1 teaspoon fresh tarragon, minced**
    ½ **teaspoon dried dill or 2 tablespoons fresh minced dill**
    ¼ **cup raw cream or heavy cream**
    ¼ **cup sour cream**
        Fresh ground white pepper to taste

Use the thin slicing blade of the food processor to slice cucumbers and scallions, or slice them thin by hand. Reserve 1 teaspoon of scallions and ½ cup of sliced cucumber as garnish for the soup.

Heat butter in soup kettle. Add scallions and sauté until soft and transparent. Add cukes and potatoes and sauté several minutes, stirring. Add broth, seasoned salt, tarragon, and dill. Cover and simmer 15 to 20 minutes or until potatoes are tender. Cool slightly and blend until smooth. Stir in cream and sour cream with whisk. Add pepper. Do *not* reheat. Refrigerate until cold. Serve cold with fresh cucumber and scallion garnish. A fresh mint leaf in each bowl adds a nice touch. *Serves 6.*

AVOCADO GAZPACHO

6 stalks celery
1 medium cucumber, peeled, or ½ hothouse cucumber, unpeeled
1 green bell pepper
1 large or 2 small avocados, peeled and seeded

Garnish

½ cup diced tomatoes
½ cup diced red pepper
½ cup diced peeled cucumber
½ cup diced celery
½ cup diced avocado

Put celery, cucumber, and bell pepper through a juicer. Place green juice in blender. Add avocado and blend until smooth. Chill. When ready to serve, pour avocado soup into large bowls and garnish with 2 heaping tablespoons each of minced vegetables and avocado. *Serves 3.*

CLEAR BROTH WITH VEGETABLES

This is a very easy-to-prepare soup when light eating is indicated or anytime that a hot, easy-to-digest vegetable soup is desired. Morga Salt-free Vegetable Cubes, Bernard Jensen's Natural Vegetable Seasoning, or Vogue Vegetable Bouillon are among the many excellent vegetable seasonings now available, and all will make adequate bases for this soup. Those who wish something heavier can serve the soup over hot couscous or any noodle or pasta. Kids love this clear, simple soup.

6 cups water
2 teaspoons Bernard Jensen's Natural Vegetable Seasoning
1 cube Morga Salt-free Vegetable Bouillon
6 small zucchini, cut in ⅛-inch slices
  Greens of one very large bok choy or 2 medium bok choy, shredded

Bring water to a boil. Add the powdered broth seasoning and bouillon. Add the zucchini and bok choy greens and simmer, covered, for 5–10 minutes or until vegetables are tender and bright green. *Serves 4.*

TOMBURGERS

These "burgers" are juicy and delicious! A real treat with soup and coleslaw!

> 1 **whole-wheat burger bun**
> 1 **1-inch slice tomato from large beefsteak tomato or several slices from smaller tomato**
> ½–1 **cup alfalfa sprouts or shredded lettuce**
> 1–2 **tablespoons mayonnaise or almonaise (see p. 359) or 2 teaspoons butter**
> 2 **slices dill pickle (optional)**
> 1 **slice red onion (optional) or 2 tablespoons barbecued onions (optional; see recipe under the New York Goodwich, p. 411)**
> **Spike or any salt-free seasoning**

Use burger bun fresh and soft or lightly toast it under a hot broiler for 2 minutes. Spread mayonnaise, almonaise, or butter on bun. Slice tomato and layer on bun with sprouts or lettuce. Sprinkle with Spike, if desired. For a "lustier" burger, add pickle and/or onion or barbecued onions.

CAULIFLOWER SANDWICH FILLING

This is a fabulous substitution for tuna or egg salad. It is absolutely delicious on toast. A real favorite!

1 small cauliflower, steamed until soft
2 teaspoons lemon juice
¼ teaspoon Spike
¼ teaspoon sea salt
½ teaspoon Parsley Patch Oriental Blend or ¼ teaspoon oregano
⅛ teaspoon dried mustard (optional)
¼–½ cup almonaise (see page 388) or mayonnaise

Mash the cauliflower. Add the remaining ingredients. Serve as a sandwich filling on whole-grain toast with sliced tomato and sprouts, as a stuffing for pita pockets with sprouts, shredded carrots, and lettuce and chopped tomato, or as a stuffing for artichokes or tomatoes. *Serves 3 to 4.*

CUKE-A-TILLAS

Cucumber spears
Corn tortillas
Mayonnaise, almonaise (see page 388), or butter
Alfalfa sprouts or shredded lettuce
Spike, Vegesal, or Parsley Patch Mexican Seasoning (salt-free)

Peel a cucumber and cut it into thin spears 5 or 6 inches in length. Heat one tortilla on hot, *dry* skillet, turning from one side to the other until it is soft but not crisp. Spread the hot tortilla with spread of your choice. Arrange a line of cucumber spears down center of tortilla. Top with sprouts or lettuce and seasoning. Roll tightly. *Serving suggestion: 2 to 3 Cuke-a-Tillas per person.*

NOTE: Mexican food buffs might want to drizzle a thin line of salsa alongside the cucumbers.

AVOTILLAS

2–3 **corn tortillas**
   **Mayonnaise, almonaise (see page 388), mustard, or
   butter**
½ **medium avocado, cut in 4–6 slices**
   Spike or any salt-free seasoning
   Alfalfa sprouts or shredded lettuce

Heat tortillas on hot *dry* skillet until they are soft but not crisp.
Apply spread of your choice. Place two slices of avocado down
the center. Sprinkle with Spike. Add a layer of alfalfa sprouts or
lettuce. Roll tightly. *Serves 1.*

NOTE: Almonaise is particularly good with Avotillas. Mexican food
buffs might want to add a line of salsa alongside the avocado.

MEXICALI GOODWICH (VEGERITO)

8 **cups chopped lettuce, combining red leaf and iceburg
   lettuce**
1 **cup alfalfa sprouts**
1 **cup chopped tomato**
3 **cups corn, steamed**
½ **cup broccoli, steamed and chopped**
3 **tablespoons Barbara's Barbecue Sauce**
3 **tablespoons mayonnaise or almonaise (see page 388)**
2 **tablespoons olive oil**
1 **tablespoon lemon juice**
8 **whole-wheat tortillas**

Combine all the vegetables. Toss well with the barbecue sauce,
mayonnaise, oil, and lemon juice. Heat tortillas; add salad stuffing.
Fold up one side to catch drips. Roll envelope style. *Yields 8
goodwiches.*

NEW YORK GOODWICH

Believe it or not, this conglomeration of vegetables results in an absolutely delectable "handwich"—something that can really become a great addiction! Seven hundred and fifty people devoured sixteen hundred of these at one of our seminars on the Queen Mary in Long Beach, California. It was a new experience, and they loved it!

- 1 **cup broccoli**
- ½ **cup cauliflower (optional)**
- 2 **tablespoons carrot, finely grated**
- 2 **tablespoons red cabbage, finely grated**
- 2 **tablespoons yellow squash, finely grated**
- ¼ **cup Barbecued Onions (see below) (optional)**
- 1 **whole-wheat tortilla, chapati, or pita**
- 1 **tablespoon mayonnaise**
- 3 **thin slivers dill pickle**
- ½ **cup lettuce, finely shredded**
- ½ **cup alfalfa sprouts**
- 2 **slices avocado (optional)**
   Dash of sea salt, Spike, or salt-free seasoning (optional)

Prepare the vegetables.

Cut broccoli into thin lengths, using only florets and upper portion of stalk. Break cauliflower into tiny florets. Place broccoli and cauliflower in vegetable steamer, covered, over boiling water for 5 minutes or until vegetables are tender when pierced with tip of sharp knife. Combine carrot, cabbage, and squash, and mix thoroughly.

Barbecued Onions for Goodwich:

- 2 **teaspoons safflower oil**
- 1 **small white onion, sliced**
- ½ **tablespoon Hain or Robbie's barbecue sauce**

Prepare the Barbecued Onions.

In small skillet, heat oil. Add onion, and sauté until it begins to soften. Add barbecue sauce, and continue sautéing, stirring frequently, until onion is thoroughly wilted. Makes enough for 3 or 4 Goodwiches. Leftover Barbecued Onions are delicious in any vegetable soup.

Assemble the Goodwich.

In hot *dry* skillet, heat tortilla or chapati, turning from one side to the other until soft but *not crisp*. Place on large sheet of plastic wrap. If using pita, heat in oven for a few minutes to soften it, and cut a sliver from top so pocket opens easily. Combine all other ingredients, mix well, and stuff into pocket.

Spread tortilla with mayonnaise. Add a line of broccoli down center. Crumble cauliflower and place a line of it on broccoli. Add a line of pickle, a line of grated vegetables, a line of Barbecued Onions. Top with lettuce, sprouts, and avocado. Sprinkle with Spike, if desired. Roll tortilla tightly, crepe-style, around vegetables. Wrap tightly in plastic wrap until ready to serve. This Goodwich will keep for 2–3 days in the refrigerator (if you hide it from your friends and family)! Cut it in half and push plastic wrap partially down, but leave one end closed to catch the drippy sauces. YUM! *Serves* 1.

THE L.A. GOODWICH

The New York Goodwich (see above) has lots of barbecued onions, "à la Sabrett." In Los Angeles we forgo the onions and add lots of avocado instead.

   1 whole-wheat tortilla
   1 tablespoon mayonnaise or almonaise (see page 388)
   2 teaspoons barbecue sauce (optional)
     Several thin florets of broccoli approximately 2 inches in length (¾ cup)
   ¼ medium avocado, sliced
   ½ cup alfalfa sprouts
     Several thin slices of dill pickle
     Handful of shredded lettuce
     Dash of Spike (optional)

Heat the tortilla on a hot dry skillet until it is just pliable. Spread the mayonnaise or almonaise over the entire tortilla. Add a line of barbecue sauce down the center of the tortilla. Layer the steamed broccoli on the line for the entire length of the tortilla, with florets facing each end. Layer the avocado slices, alfalfa sprouts, pickle, and lettuce on top of the broccoli. Add a dash of Spike, if desired. Roll tightly, burrito style. Wrap in plastic wrap and store in the refrigerator or eat immediately. This recipe serves 1, but usually a hungry person can eat more. These will keep several days tightly wrapped in the refrigerator, *if* they last that long.

Potatoes and Grains

COLD NEW POTATOES IN OLIVE OIL WITH FRESH OREGANO

This light version of an Alsatian potato salad is very digestible and pleasing to the palate on a day when you want something a little heavier but don't feel like eating breads or grains. Potatoes will always do the trick, and cold or room temperature potato dishes are a nice change of pace. This is a nice entry on a cold buffet of salads and chilled soups.

6 medium new potatoes, thoroughly washed
6 tablespoons extra virgin olive oil
1 tablespoon fresh lemon juice
   Seasoned salt or salt-free seasoning to taste
2 tablespoons fresh oregano leaves, minced
1 teaspoon Dijon mustard

Place the potatoes in a vegetable steamer over boiling water. Steam, covered, for 20 minutes to ½ hour or until the potatoes are tender when pierced with the tip of a sharp knife. Cool slightly and cut in ¼-inch slices. Mix together the olive oil and lemon juice. Pour over the warm potatoes. Sprinkle with seasoned salt and oregano, add mustard, and toss well. Serve warm, room temperature, or chilled. *Serves 3 to 4.*

CREAMY MASHED POTATOES

**8–10 small all-purpose, white, or russet potatoes, peeled
and cut into 2-inch cubes
1 stalk celery, including leaves
1 bay leaf
1 large clove garlic
4 tablespoons butter
¼ cup heavy cream
½ teaspoon sea salt or salt-free seasoning
½ teaspoon Spike
Fresh ground pepper to taste**

Peel potatoes, cube (there should be 8–10 cups), and place in large kettle. Add cold water to barely cover potatoes. Add celery, bay leaf, and garlic. Bring to a boil and simmer, covered, for 20 minutes to ½ hour or until the potatoes are tender. Remove from water with slotted spoon, reserving ⅓ cup of liquid for mashing. The remaining liquid can be used as a stock in gravies and soups. Discard celery, bay leaf, and garlic.

Melt the butter and add the cream. Heat until hot, but do not boil. Place potatoes in food processor or mash by hand, incorporating butter-cream mixture, salt, Spike, and pepper. Add small amount of boiling liquid from potatoes to achieve desired consistency. Whip thoroughly until desired smoothness is achieved. Serve with Braised Green Beans (see page 400) and Burnt Onion Gravy with Tarragon (see below). *Serves 5 to 6.*

NOTE: Mashed potatoes should be served immediately. They become stiff if they sit too long. Add any leftover mashed potatoes to soups.

Burnt Onion Gravy with Tarragon

    1 tablespoon safflower or grape seed oil
    1 large white onion, sliced
1½ cups water
    2 teaspoons Bernard Jensen's Natural Vegetable
      Seasoning or 1 cube Hugli Vegetable Bouillon
   ¼ teaspoon tarragon
   ⅛ teaspoon sage
     Dash of nutmeg
   ¼ teaspoon chervil

Heat oil in a large skillet. Add sliced onion and sauté, stirring frequently over high heat until onion begins to brown. Add water, vegetable seasoning, tarragon, sage, nutmeg, and chervil. Bring to a boil, lower to medium heat, and simmer until gravy is reduced to about ¾ of a cup. *Makes 2 servings.*

BROILED POTATO SLICES

These are a great treat for kids as an alternative to baked potatoes. They're real speedy to make.

2 large Idaho russets
3 tablespoons melted butter
  Spike, Herbamare, or salt-free seasoning to taste

Thoroughly scrub potatoes and cut them lengthwise in thin slices. Arrange in overlapping layers on a cookie sheet. Do not stack. Brush with melted butter. Sprinkle with Spike. Place in preheated oven to broil 15–20 minutes or until slices are crispy golden. Slices can be dipped in ketchup or Cappello's Barbecue Sauce before eating. *Serves 4.*

ROAST POTATOES BONNE FEMME (WITH ROSEMARY)

2 pounds tiny new potatoes
3 tablespoons butter
1 tablespoon olive oil
2 teaspoons fresh oregano leaves, minced
½ teaspoon fresh rosemary leaves, minced
  Seasoned salt or salt-free seasoning to taste
  Fresh ground pepper to taste

Wash the potatoes thoroughly and place them in a vegetable steamer over boiling water 20–25 minutes or until they are tender when pierced with the tip of a sharp knife. Cool slightly and cut the potatoes in half or, using a paring knife, cut a strip of the peel from around each potato, leaving an attractive round cap on both top and bottom. Toss the potatoes gently with the 2 tablespoons of the butter, cut in ⅓-inch cubes, the olive oil, half the minced oregano, half the minced rosemary, the seasoned salt, and the pepper. Place in a preheated 425° oven for 15 minutes. Stir well, lower heat to 300° and roast for an additional 20 minutes. Remove from oven and toss with the remaining butter and fresh herbs. Serve with Braised Courgettes (see page 392), Limestone and Lamb's Lettuce Salad (see page 384), and buttered corn on the cob. *Serves 4.*

STEAMED POTATOES AND VEGETABLES IN OLIVE OIL

This is a really nice light lunch or dinner, and it is an especially satisfying meal when you are coming to the end of detoxification. The olive oil is an aid in the elimination process, as are the soft steamed vegetables.

4 small or 2 large potatoes
2 medium carrots
2 medium zucchini
2 medium yellow squash
2 medium summer squash
5 tablespoons olive oil
  Salt-free seasoning or fresh ground sea salt to taste

Wash potatoes thoroughly and cut in quarters or sixths, depending on size of potato. Peel carrots and cut them in quarters. Place cut vegetables and *whole* zucchini and squash in top of large vegetable steamer over boiling water. Cover and steam 20 minutes or until zucchini and squash are very tender and potatoes and carrots are soft. Peel potatoes and cut in bite-sized pieces. Cut carrots and squash in bite-sized pieces. Arrange on platter and drizzle with olive oil. Add salt-free seasoning or sea salt, if desired. *Enough for 2 meals.*

QUINOA
(pronounced "keenwa")

Quinoa is a "new" grain available in natural food stores. It comes from the Andes mountain regions of South America and is an amazing food with ancient origins. Along with corn and potatoes it was one of the three staple foods of the Inca civilization. It was then—and still is—known with respect as the Mother Grain.

Quinoa is absolutely delicious! It contains more high-quality, usable protein than any other grain. It is high in the amino acids lysine, methionine, and cystine, which other grains are low in. It is a rich and balanced source of starch, sugar, oil, fiber, minerals, and vitamins. It is light (not sticky or heavy) and easy to digest. It is easy to prepare, quick and versatile. A little goes a long way. (One cup of quinoa expands five times, as opposed to brown rice, which expands only three times.) Quinoa is an excellent source of nutrition for children and nursing mothers. Try it! You'll love it!

1 cup quinoa
2 cups water
   Dash of salt (optional)

Rinse quinoa *thoroughly* in cold water to remove slightly bitter coating—place it in a very fine sieve and run water over it or place it in a bowl with water and work it gently with your hands. Strain and place in medium saucepan with water and salt. Bring to a boil, cover, and simmer until all water is absorbed (10–15 minutes). Grains will have turned from white to transparent. Season with butter and sea salt or salt-free seasoning to taste.
Serves 2 to 6.

MILLET

This is the ideal grain, because it is the only one that is not acid forming in the body.

 2 cups water
 1 cup millet
 1 tablespoon butter
 ¼ to ½ teaspoon salt

Bring water to a boil. Add millet, butter, and salt. Return to a boil, stirring frequently. Cover and simmer over medium-low heat for 15 minutes. Water should be absorbed and millet will be fluffy. Add butter to taste or serve with gravy. Millet, steamed vegetables, and salad is a perfect meal! *Serves 2 to 3.*

EASY BROCCOLI PILAF

 3 tablespoons safflower oil
 1 teaspoon mustard seed (optional)
 1 teaspoon coriander
 1 teaspoon turmeric
 ¼ teaspoon cinnamon (optional)
 2 bay leaves
 1 teaspoon garlic, minced
 ½ cup onion, minced
 1 bunch broccoli, cut into small florets, stems peeled and
   cut crosswise into ⅓-inch slices
 3 cups steamed rice (Basmati rice is preferable, but brown
   rice will work.)
   Juice of 1 small lemon (2–3 tablespoons)
 2 tablespoons chopped cilantro (optional)
 1 teaspoon sea salt

Heat the oil in a large skillet with lid. Add the cumin seed and the mustard seed and sizzle the seeds briefly. Stir in the coriander, turmeric, cinnamon, and the bay leaves. Add the garlic and onion and cook the mixture, stirring, until the onion is soft and beginning to brown. Add the broccoli and cook, stirring, for 5 minutes over medium heat. Add ⅓ cup water, cover, and steam the mixture over medium low heat for 5 minutes or until the broccoli is tender. Stir in the rice and cook, stirring frequently, until the mixture is hot. Stir in the lemon juice, cilantro, and the salt. Mix well. *Serves 5 to 6.*

POTATO BUREK

Burek are Yugoslavian in origin, remarkably easy to make and delicious. They make great hors d'oeuvres but should be served hot. They are an exciting accompaniment to a soup, salad, and bread meal and take star billing on any buffet table. (Before preparing burek, check "Working with Phyllo" on page 421.)

4 large russet potatoes, peeled and coarsely grated
1 small onion, finely minced
½ teaspoon sea salt
   Fresh ground pepper to taste
2 teaspoons safflower oil
1 package phyllo leaves
½ cup butter, melted

Place grated potatoes in collander and squeeze to press out moisture. Place in bowl and combine with onion. Season with salt and pepper. Add oil and mix thoroughly. Use immediately before potatoes begin to discolor.

Place one phyllo sheet with short side facing you. (Cover remaining phyllo with slightly damp towel to prevent drying.) Fold phyllo sheet one-third up from the bottom. Brush immediately with melted butter. Spread large handful of filling along folded edge, leaving 1-inch margins at bottom and along sides. Fold phyllo over filling and fold in sides. Roll until burek is completely rolled.

Place burek on lightly buttered cookie sheet, seam side down, and brush immediately with butter. Cut slashes in burek, 6 for hors d'oeuvres, 4 for dinner burek. When all burek are rolled, buttered and slashed, sprinkle sparingly with water or sparkling mineral water. Bake in 425° oven 20 to 25 minutes or until golden brown, brushing once more during baking with melted butter. Cut along slashes and serve hot. Makes approximately 10 burek rolls. Serve with green salad with garlic-oil dressing, buttered asparagus, buttered yellow beets. *Serves 6.*

WORKING WITH PHYLLO

Phyllo are of Greek origin. They are very thin leaves or sheets of pastry that can be used when a very light result is desired. Although people tend to avoid working with phyllo leaves, they are actually quite simple to handle once you have had a little experience with them. Don't try using them for the first time when you are expecting twelve people to dinner. Get used to working with them first on an informal occasion, so you will feel confident when the results are up for scrutiny. Here are a few little tricks to make your experience easier:

1. Since phyllo leaves have a way of drying out remarkably fast, cover them with a *slightly damp* dish towel as soon as you have laid them out flat. If the dish towel is too damp, the phyllo will become gluey and stick together.

2. As soon as you have separated the sheet you are planning to use from the stack, cover the stack. After laying the sheet out flat, brush it immediately with melted butter. It will dry out almost immediately and be difficult to work with if it is not brushed.

3. Be willing to sacrifice a few sheets if necessary. Batches of phyllo do not tend to be uniform. Sometimes they are torn or tear when separated. Don't worry, there are usually more sheets in a pound package than you will need for any one recipe.

DOLMAS (STUFFED GRAPE LEAVES)

These marvelous little goodies have a Middle Eastern origin. Recipes frequently call for pine nuts to be added to the filling, but this merely creates an additional food-combining problem and adds nothing to the flavor of the dolmas. The small amount of currants does not seem to create a digestive problem for most people, but if you wish to remain a purist, simply leave them out. I love to incorporate dolmas into a party buffet. They can be made two or three days in advance and stored in a tightly closed container in the refrigerator. Many Middle Eastern markets sell jars of grape leaves that contain absolutely no preservatives. Those commonly found in the supermarket contain an acid preservative. Fresh grape leaves can be steamed in a lightly salted lemon water solution containing a clove of garlic for 3 to 5 minutes or until they are tender. They make a fine substitute for the bottled version. If you are using the bottled grape leaves, remove them gently from the jar and rinse them under cold water to remove some of the salt. Drain on layers of paper towel in a collander.

    9   tablespoons olive oil
    1   small onion, minced
    1   teaspoon dried dill
    3   tablespoons dried currants
    1   teaspoon fresh ground nutmeg
    ¼   teaspoon cardamom
    2   cups steamed white basmati rice (see recipe next page),
        omitting salt since leaves are salty
    1   8-ounce jar grape leaves
        Juice of 1 lime (2–3 tablespoons)
        Water
        Several thin slices lemon
  2–3   bay leaves

Heat 5 tablespoons olive oil in a large skillet. Add the onion and sauté until it is transparent but not brown. (You may add a tablespoon of water to prevent browning.) Add the dill, currants, nutmeg, and cardamom. Remove from heat and pour into the steamed rice. Mix thoroughly.

Place 1 heaping teaspoon to 2 heaping tablespoons of the filling in the center of each grape leaf (depending on size of the leaf). Cut the protruding stem from the leaf, if there is one. Fold the sides of the leaves over the filling and roll gently from the bottom to the top. Arrange the dolmas in lines in an ovenproof baking dish. (Dolmas may be refrigerated overnight and baked the next day.)

Mix together the lime juice, the remaining olive oil, and water to equal one cup of liquid. Pour over the dolmas. Top with several slices of lemon and two or three bay leaves. Layer any remaining grape leaves over top. Cover loosely with aluminum foil. Bake at 350° for 45 minutes or until the liquid is almost completely absorbed. *Yields 28–36 dolmas.*

MENU SUGGESTION:
   Country Style Vegetable Pie*
   Sweet Carrots *au Naturel* (see page 396)
   Curried Cabbage**
   Caesar Salad (see page 382)
   Dolmas
   Fresh Basil Green Beans***
   Honey Cornbread****

BASMATI RICE

There are two varieties of basmati rice, white and brown. The white has a nutty flavor and lends itself very well to salads, stuffings, and such delicacies as stuffed cabbage and Dolmas (Stuffed Grape Leaves). The brown basmati is chewier and a little heavier than the white, but it is absolutely delicious as a main course with vegetables and salad.

White Basmati

   1 cup white basmati, washed and picked over for impurities
   2 cups water or vegetable broth
   1 teaspoon butter or oil
   ½ teaspoon salt (optional—do *not* add when you are making dolmas, since the grape leaves are usually cured in brine)

Place rice, water, butter or oil, and salt in a saucepan. Bring to a boil. Stir lightly, cover, and reduce heat to lowest setting. Simmer covered for 18 minutes. Remove cover and fluff with a fork. *Serves 2 to 3.*

*From *A New Way of Eating*, page 89
**From *Fit for Life*, page 163, 164
***From *Fit for Life*, page 154
****From *Fit for Life*, page 219

Brown Basmati

2 cups water or vegetable broth
1 cup brown basmati, washed and picked over for
   impurities
1 teaspoon butter or oil
½ teaspoon salt (optional)

Bring water to a boil. Add rice, butter, and salt. Bring to a boil
again and stir well. Reduce heat to low, cover and simmer 40 to
45 minutes or until all the water has been absorbed. Remove from
heat. Fluff with fork. Allow to sit 5 minutes before serving. *Serves
2 to 3*.

Pastas and Sauces

QUICK FRESH TOMATO SAUCE FOR PASTA

Since cooked tomatoes are so acid, fresh tomato sauces for pasta are the answer. This one is a winner tossed over brown rice udon or any pasta you prefer. Chopping the vegetables in a food processor makes this quick sauce even quicker.

2 tablespoons olive oil
1 small onion
1 medium clove garlic
1 small carrot
1 small rib celery
¼ cup fresh parsley
¼ cup fresh basil
1 vegetable bouillon
¼ cup water
6 medium, fresh tomatoes
   Seasoned salt or salt-free seasoning to taste (Herbamare)

Heat olive oil in a medium saucepan with lid. Coarse chop the onion and sauté in olive oil. Coarse chop the garlic and add to the onion. Sauté briefly. Fine chop the carrot and celery and add to sautéing vegetables. Stir well. Fine chop the parsley and basil and add to vegetables. Add bouillon and ¼ cup water. Cover and simmer over low heat for 15 minutes or until carrot and celery are tender. Cool to room temperature.

While vegetables are cooling, place tomatoes in boiling water for 30 seconds or until skins loosen. Peel tomatoes and coarsely chop them by hand in a bowl so that none of the juice is lost. (I avoid chopping peeled tomatoes in a food processor because they get too frothy and pale.) Stir the cooked vegetables into the chopped tomatoes. Add seasoned salt or salt-free seasoning to taste. *Serves 2 to 3 people.*

MUSHROOM SAUCE WITH GARLIC, OIL, AND PARSLEY

½ ounce dried Italian mushrooms
1 pound fresh mushrooms
½ cup olive oil
2 teaspoons minced garlic
3 tablespoons minced parsley
   Sea salt and fresh ground pepper to taste

Soak dried mushrooms in warm water to cover for ½ hour or until soft. Thinly slice fresh mushrooms—you should have about 6 cups. Strain soaked mushrooms, reserving all liquid, which you can strain again through cheesecloth or a very fine sieve. Chop soaked mushrooms until they are semi-fine. Combine liquid and chopped dried mushrooms in a small saucepan. Bring to a boil and simmer until all the liquid has evaporated. Heat olive oil. Sauté garlic in the oil. Add parsley and fresh mushrooms. Cook 1 minute. Add dried mushrooms, then add salt and pepper and cook until all mushroom liquid has evaporated. This yields enough sauce for 1 pound of Chinese lo mein, Japanese soba, or any fresh or dried pasta. *Serves 3.*

PESTO GENOVESE

Many pesto recipes call for the addition of parmesan or romano cheese, but I have found that if you balance the amounts of basil, pine nuts, and garlic, cheese is not at all necessary. The amount of pine nuts in this recipe is also not substantial. Food-combining purists can omit the pine nuts. For those who don't mind stretching the rules once in a while, pesto as a sauce is far superior to meat sauces or those containing cooked tomatoes or cheese. Pesto can also be used as a sauce for vegetables such as cauliflower, spaghetti squash, or sliced tomatoes. Avoid using too much. A little goes a long way!

  4 **medium cloves garlic**
  2 **cups fresh basil leaves, packed down**
  2 **heaping tablespoons pine nuts**
  ¼ **to ⅓ cup olive oil**

With motor running and using steel knife, drop garlic into food processor and process until minced. Place basil leaves and pine nuts in food processor. Process while adding olive oil in steady stream, but reserve 2 tablespoons of the olive oil. Store pesto in tightly covered jar. Pour remaining olive oil over pesto before storing. *Yields ¾ cup.*

TO USE PESTO: Prepare pasta of choice, reserving ¼ cup of pasta water, then toss pasta with 1 tablespoon butter. For a 12-ounce portion of pasta (enough for 2 or 3 people) place ⅜ cup of pesto in a small saucepan. Add ¼ cup pasta water. Heat but do not boil, stirring until sauce just begins to bubble. Pour over hot buttered pasta. Add salt and pepper to taste.

PESTO WITH CREAM

To make a pesto cream sauce, boil ½ cup cream per serving to reduce to ¼ cup. Stir 2 tablespoons pesto per serving into cream.

LINGUINE OR UDON WITH PESTO AND BROCCOLI

  1 **bunch of broccoli**
  1 **pound linguine or brown rice udon**
  ½ **cup pesto (see recipe above)**
  5 **tablespoons water**
  1 **tablespoon butter**
    Sea salt and fresh ground pepper to taste

Cut broccoli in very thin 2-inch-long florets. Cook linguine or udon according to package directions. While pasta is cooking, steam broccoli in vegetable steamer over boiling water for 4 minutes or until it is bright and crisp. Set aside. Drain pasta thoroughly when done. Toss immediately with the butter. Heat pesto gently with the 5 tablespoons water and pour over pasta. Add broccoli and seasonings and toss well. *Serves 4 to 6.*

PASTA WITH BUTTER AND FRESH HERBS

1 **pound jinenjo noodles, brown rice soba, chow mein udon, or any pasta of your choice**
2 **tablespoons butter**
2 **teaspoons olive oil**
 Salt-free seasoning or sea salt to taste
 Fresh ground pepper to taste
⅓ **cup fresh basil, oregano, or savory, minced**

Bring several quarts of water to boil in a large pasta kettle. Add pasta gradually so water continues to boil, and cook according to package directions. Drain and toss immediately with butter, olive oil, and seasonings. This is a wonderful accompaniment to salads, vegetables, soups, or barbecues. *Serves 4 to 6.*

PASTA IN THE WOK WITH ZUCCHINI AND BOK CHOY

8 ounces chow mein udon, brown rice soba, or any long
   pasta of your choice
2 medium zucchini
1 small carrot, peeled
6 baby bok choy or 1 medium bok choy
1 clove garlic (optional)
1 tablespoon safflower oil (plus 2 teaspoons if using garlic)
2 tablespoons light soy sauce
2 teaspoons Japanese mirin (Japanese sweetener made from
   rice) or 1 teaspoon honey
1 teaspoon roasted sesame oil
¼ cup water
1 teaspoon powdered vegetable broth

Cook pasta according to package directions for *al dente*. Drain,
rinse with cold water, and set aside. Using the thin julienning
blade of a food processor, julienne the zucchini and the carrot.
Using the entire baby bok choy or the upper half, including the
leaves, of a medium bok choy, cut the bok choy lengthwise in
thin slivers. Heat the wok. If you are using the garlic, mince or
crush it and mix it with 2 teaspoons safflower oil. Combine the
soy sauce, mirin, sesame oil, water and broth.

   Place 1 tablespoon of safflower oil in the heated wok. Add the
garlic, zucchini, carrot, and bok choy and toss in the hot oil
continuously, adding a little of the seasoning liquid if the vegetables begin to sear. When the vegetables are barely softened and
bright in color, add the pasta and continue tossing to combine the
pasta and vegetables. Add the seasoning liquid as you toss. This
is an excellent accompaniment to a big salad. *Serves 3*.

Muffins, Biscuits, and Scones

FRENCH TOAST WITH MAPLE SYRUP

This delicious version of an old favorite is much lighter and more digestible than the usual recipe because it has no egg. You can use cream or almond milk to moisten. Either yields a very successful result. This is a favorite for brunch or lunch for kids.

1 cup almond milk or ⅓ cup cream diluted with ⅓ cup water
¾ teaspoon cinnamon
¼ teaspoon nutmeg
4 slices flourless or whole-grain bread
3 tablespoons butter, plus butter for topping
  Maple syrup, warmed

Combine almond milk or diluted cream mixture with cinnamon and nutmeg. Cut the bread in half on the diagonal. Dip the bread in the liquid mixture. Melt the butter in a large skillet over medium heat. Add the moistened bread. Cook in the butter over low enough heat so that the butter does not brown. Bread should become golden and toasty. Place on heated platter. Top with bits of butter and warm maple syrup. *Serves 3.*

BLUE RIBBON BRAN MUFFINS

   3 **cups bran flakes, soaked in 1 cup boiling water**
   1 **cup honey or blackstrap molasses or ½ cup of each (best with ½ cup blackstrap molasses, ½ cup maple sugar)***
   2 **cups buttermilk****
   2 **eggs (optional)**
   ½ **cup sunflower or safflower oil**
   3 **cups whole-wheat flour or 1½ cups unbleached white flour and 1½ cups whole-wheat pastry flour for a lighter muffin**
 2½ **teaspoons baking soda**
   ½ **teaspoon sea salt (optional)**
   1 **cup presoaked raisins (optional)*****

Soak bran in boiling water. Combine honey, buttermilk, eggs, and oil. Add to bran. Combine flour and soda. Mix well. Add to bran mixture. Stir in presoaked raisins. Bake 25 minutes at 350°. These muffins are delicious served hot with butter, and they freeze beautifully. *Yields 18 bran muffins.*

*Maple sugar, available at natural food stores, may be substituted for honey or molasses.
**Water may be substituted for buttermilk. The resulting muffin, especially if you also omit the eggs, will be smaller and "grainier." If you are using buttermilk and raw buttermilk is available, by all means use it. Check the section in chapter 8 for a better understanding of the raw (natural) versus pasteurized (processed) dairy product controversy.
***Fresh or frozen blueberries may be substituted for raisins.

HERBED BUTTERMILK BISCUITS

This variation on a buttermilk biscuit recipe is absolutely fantastic. These herbed biscuits are a real winner when topped with creamed peas or other vegetables. Have all ingredients at room temperature before combining.

1¾ cups whole-wheat pastry flour
½ teaspoon salt
 2 teaspoons double acting baking powder
½ teaspoon baking soda
 5 tablespoons butter
¾ cups buttermilk
 1 teaspoon honey
 2 tablespoons bran flakes (optional, and if you are not
   using the flakes, cut buttermilk to ⅔ cup)
1½ teaspoons sage
 1 teaspoon rosemary
1½ teaspoons thyme

Preheat oven to 450°. Sift flour before measuring. Sift again with salt, baking powder, and baking soda. Cut in butter until mixture resembles coarse meal. Make a well in center and pour in buttermilk combined with honey. (Remember to reduce amount of buttermilk if not using bran.) Add bran, if desired, and herbs. Mix briskly with fork until dough forms into a ball. Turn out on floured board and knead 1½ minutes. Roll or pat into ½-inch thickness. Cut with 2–2½-inch biscuit cutter. Arrange close together on buttered cookie sheet. Bake 12–15 minutes at 450°. *Yields 16 biscuits*.

SUGGESTED MENU:
    Creamed Peas
    Carrot-Leek Bisque
    Herbed Buttermilk Biscuits
    Easy Limestone Lettuce Salad with Basil-Garlic Dressing (see
page 379)

ONION SCONES

>   2 cups whole-wheat pastry flour
>   2 teaspoons baking powder
>   2 teaspoons baking soda
>   ½ teaspoon sea salt
>   ¼ cup (½ stick) cold, sweet butter, cut into bits
>   1 teaspoon honey or maple sugar (optional)
>   ½ cup minced white onion
>   1 egg or egg replacer
> ⅔–1 cup heavy or raw cream, plus additional cream for
>   brushing

Sift whole-wheat pastry flour before measuring. Sift again with the baking powder, soda, and salt. Cut in the butter until the mixture is like coarse corn meal. Stir in the maple sugar and the onions. In a separate bowl, beat together the egg and ⅔ cup of the cream. Add honey if you are using it (but do not use both maple sugar and honey). Make a well in the center of the flour mixture and add the cream and egg mixture. Stir with a fork, adding more cream, if necessary, until the dough forms a sticky but workable dough. On a floured surface, knead the dough for 30 seconds and pat it gently into a rectangle ¾-inch thick. Cut out rounds with a 2¼-inch cutter or glass dipped in flour. Form the scraps into a ball, pat the dough into a ¾-inch rectangle, and cut out scones in the same way. Brush the tops of the scones with the remaining cream and bake in a preheated 400° oven for 12 to 15 minutes or until they are golden. These are light and delicious, an excellent accompaniment to soup and salad meals. *Makes about 12 scones.*

Fish and Chicken

FLOUNDER IN LEMON-DILL SAUCE

Any white fish fillet works well in this marvelous recipe. If orange roughy, an absolutely delectable fish, is available at your fish market, substitute it for the flounder.

3 tablespoons butter
1 tablespoon chopped fresh dill or ¼ teaspoon dried dill
1 tablespoon fresh lemon juice
¼ teaspoon seasoned salt, sea salt, or salt-free seasoning to taste
1 medium green onion, thinly sliced
1 pound fresh or frozen flounder fillets, cut in serving-sized pieces
   Lemon slices for garnish

Heat butter, dill, lemon juice, salt, and green onion in large skillet over medium-low heat. Stir occasionally. Add flounder to butter mixture in skillet; cover and cook 8–10 minutes, basting occasionally with butter mixture from skillet. Flounder will flake with a fork when ready. Arrange flounder in warm platter. Pour sauce over fish and garnish with lemon slices. *Serves 4.*

MESQUITE-GRILLED SWORDFISH BEVERLY HILLS

The fresh food cuisine coming out of Los Angeles these days is really innovative. L.A. chefs are setting the pace for fine and healthful gourmet food with their "California Cuisine."

6 tablespoons olive oil
2 cloves garlic, minced
2 tablespoons minced fresh parsley or 2 teaspoons dried
2 tablespoons minced fresh tarragon or 2 teaspoons dried
1 tablespoon minced fresh savory or 1 teaspoon dried
1 tablespoon minced fresh chervil or 1 teaspoon dried
2 teaspoons ground coriander
2 tablespoons fresh lemon or lime juice
1 large tomato, peeled, seeded, and coarsely chopped
   Salt-free seasoning or sea salt to taste
   Fresh ground pepper to taste
4 6-ounce skinned and boned swordfish, tuna, mackerel, or striped bass "steaks"

Combine 4 tablespoons olive oil, garlic, and herbs in food processor. Add lemon and tomato juice and process only for a few seconds. Add salt and pepper. Set aside.

Brush grill and both sides of fish with remaining olive oil. Grill fish 8–9 minutes per inch of thickness, turning once, basting with sauce as you start grilling and after turning.

Place a small ladle of sauce on four warm plates. Top with fish. Cover with remaining sauce. Serve with lightly steamed asparagus or string beans and salad. The fish is the main event. *Serves 4.*

WARM CHICKEN AND BROCCOLI SALAD

2 large whole chicken breasts
1 clove garlic
1 onion, peeled
   Handful of parsley
1½ to 2 cups vegetable stock
2 cups small broccoli florets
1 sprig fresh rosemary or a pinch of dried rosemary
½ cup Regent of Fiji French Dressing (see p. 391)

Cut chicken breasts in halves and place in medium saucepan. Add garlic, onion, parsley, and vegetable stock to barely cover chicken. Bring to a boil. Reduce heat and simmer, covered, over medium-low heat until chicken is tender, about 20 minutes.

While chicken is cooking, place broccoli in vegetable steamer over boiling water in which you have placed rosemary. Steam 5 minutes or until broccoli is just *al dente* and bright green.

Remove chicken from stock and cut into bite-sized pieces. Discard broth, which is too acid to be of use. Combine chicken and steamed broccoli. Add dressing and toss. Add fresh ground white pepper to taste. Serve warm or chilled. *Makes 4 servings.*

LEMON-DILL CHICKEN

This is basically the same recipe used for Flounder in Lemon-Dill Sauce (page 434), but the cooking time is approximately doubled.

 3 tablespoons butter
 1 tablespoon chopped fresh dill or ¾ teaspoon dried dill
 1 tablespoon fresh lemon juice
 ¼ teaspoon seasoned salt, sea salt, or salt-free seasoning to taste
 1 medium green onion, thinly sliced
 1 pound chicken breasts, skinned, boned, and cut in 4 pieces

Heat butter, dill, lemon juice, salt, and green onion in large skillet over medium-low heat. Stir occasionally. Add chicken to butter mixture in skillet, cover, and cook 10 minutes, basting occasionally with butter mixture in skillet. Turn chicken and cook, covered, 10 more minutes. Arrange in warm serving dish. Pour sauce over chicken. *Serves 4.*

Nut Milks, Shakes, and Frozen Goodies

NUT AND SEED MILKS

This is the basic nut and seed milk recipe. Almonds, sesame seeds, cashews or sunflower seeds will all work with this recipe. The milk keeps well for 24–48 hours in the refrigerator, although it is best consumed when freshly made. It will separate slightly when refrigerated, so shake well before using. If you wish the milk to be cold but do not have time to refrigerate it, substitute 3 or 4 ice cubes for ½ cup of water.

 ½ cup blanched almonds* or unhulled sesame seeds
 2 teaspoons maple syrup or raw honey (optional)
2–2½ cups water, depending on how concentrated you wish
 the milk to be

Line a strainer with several layers of moist cheesecloth. Place nuts or seeds in a blender. (You may soak them several hours or overnight first, but this is not required.) Add sweetener and 1 cup water. Blend until a smooth cream forms, using the highest setting on the blender. Add the remaining water and continue blending for several minutes. Strain well. If there is a great deal of pulp, you have not blended long enough. Remaining pulp can be blended again with additional water for more milk. *Yields 2 cups.*

*To blanch almonds, simply place them in a skillet of boiling water for 1 minute. The skins will loosen and pop right off.

DATE OR STRAWBERRY-ALMOND MILK SHAKE

1 cup Fresh Almond Milk (see below)
2 frozen bananas
6 pitted dates *or* 6 fresh or frozen strawberries

Place almond milk and fruit in blender. Blend until thick and creamy. If you like a thinner shake, use 1½ bananas. *Makes 1 large shake.*

NOTE: From now on, if you like these shakes, keep frozen bananas on hand in freezer.

These shakes are nutritious and an excellent substitute for ice cream shakes or protein drinks. Children *love* this! So do adults.

Fresh Almond Milk:

¼ cup raw almonds
1 cup cold water
2 teaspoons pure maple syrup (optional)

Nut and seed milks were used for centuries in Europe, Asia, and by the American Indians, and they are still used throughout the world as easily digestible substitutes for cow's milk. Those made from almonds or sesame seeds are excellent sources for easily assimilated calcium and they are delicious!

Blanch almonds by adding them to large skillet containing ½ inch boiling water, allowing them to sit in water as it boils for about 30 seconds. The skins will loosen noticeably. Drain and pop skins off. Place blanched almonds in blender with 1 cup cold water. Run blender at high speed for 2–3 minutes until a thick white milk has formed. If you are going to drink almond milk straight, strain it through a fine sieve. If there is a lot of pulp, you have not blended long enough. If you are going to use the milk in a shake, there is no need to strain.

Shakes are an ideal "smoothing out" food after an All-fruit Day. We do not recommend having a shake on any day when you are also having cooked food.

BANANA SHAKE DIVINE

   1 **cup almond milk (see page 438)**
2–2½ **frozen bananas (depending on size and desired thickness of shake)**
   2 **teaspoons maple syrup**
  ⅛ **teaspoon fresh ground nutmeg (optional)**

Place almond milk in the blender. Add frozen bananas in increments with blender running until shake has reached desired thickness. Add maple syrup and nutmeg. Blend briefly. *Yields 1 large or 2 medium shakes.*

CAROB SHAKE

1 **cup almond or sesame milk (see page 438)**
2 **frozen bananas**
2 **teaspoons maple syrup**
1 **tablespoon unsweetened roasted carob powder**

Combine almond milk, frozen bananas, maple syrup, and carob powder in blender. Blend until creamy. *Serves 1 to 2.*

RAINBOW CREAM

This fantastic icy treat requires a Champion juicer for preparation. This alone is worth the investment!

1½ **cups frozen mango or papaya cubes**
 12 **frozen strawberries**
  2 **frozen bananas**

Assemble Champion with the blank. Feed frozen fruit through the feeder tube in the order given. Serve immediately. Can also be used as a topping for your favorite fruit salad. *Serves 3.*

CONCLUSION

HARVEY AND MARILYN:

We all want to have control of our health. No one wants to relinquish control. We want it, but do we have it? Rarely. Most people are overwhelmed and confused about their health as a result of the never-ending onslaught of differing opinions. Not only is it an exercise in frustration to attempt to extract the valuable from the not so valuable, but the situation is compounded by the fact that we are led to believe that we are incapable of determining what is best for ourselves. In fact, we are encouraged *not* to participate in decisions relating to our own health, admonished instead to "check with your doctor" for the slightest abnormality. Then we're expected to follow our doctor's "orders"—blindly, unquestioningly! We're directed to abdicate all responsibility to the "experts," who then can manipulate us in any way they desire. We necessarily pay a dear price for relinquishing this responsibility, both in terms of money and in our health.

It's expensive, isn't it? We Americans pour *over half a trillion dollars a year* into health care—expensive doctors' appointments, expensive hospital stays, and expensive diagnostic tests, resulting in expensive prescriptions and treatments, all topped off with expensive health insurance. We Americans have more doctors, more hospitals, and more costly health plans than any country in the world, and yet we lead the world in occurrences of the degenerative diseases. It certainly appears that being healthy in the United States is an expensive proposition.

But there is a whole world of possibilities open to us. Anyone who studies the vast field of health care knows full well that whatever we know about the subject is but a small fraction of what there is to know. The entire field is still in an embryonic stage. That is why it is so important that there be no attempt by any one group to suppress or reject out of hand the work of another. There must be a free flow of information, ideas, and theories among all those interested in helping others to achieve good health.

No one group has ever been duly elected or appointed to be the final arbiter of truth in health care. There are those who would like to confer upon themselves the all-encompassing and exclusive right to decide what is and what is not "legitimate" information and who is and who is not capable of dispensing it. But the field of health is simply too vast, too fertile, and too unknown for any *self-appointed* group with only *one philosophy* to be in the position of deciding who will and who will not have the right to speak.

Before there were doctors, dietitians, hospitals, million-dollar heart monitoring machines, or prescription pads, there was Mother Nature, waiting patiently in the wings through it all, ready to supply us with *everything* we need, not only to grow and develop but also to maintain our bodies *healthfully!* Mother Nature provides for our health needs every day of our lives. Without her, we can't survive. She offers us *elements of health* to maintain us, prolong our lives, and prevent disease in our bodies—*if we will use them*.

The truth is, **WE KNOW WHAT THE ELEMENTS OF HEALTH ARE BUT WE HAVE *FORGOTTEN* HOW TO USE THEM**. And they are free! They cost nothing! They are part of the deal when we are born into this world, "standard equipment" as it were. You now can see that **THE ELEMENTS OF HEALTH ARE EXTRAORDINARILY EASY TO INCORPORATE INTO YOUR LIFE-STYLE**. By using them, you vastly improve your existence. Without harmful side effects you get results for yourself quickly, effectively, and pleasantly, and *they do not cost you a cent!*

This is not good news for the mammoth machine that depends on your sickness for its profits. In fact, for its very survival, the disease complex requires that you be sick—regularly! For example, the Managing Director of Unichem, a drug wholesaler in Great Britain, once said in a speech, "People are becoming more health conscious. They're eating less, smoking less, and taking more exercise. All that is bad for business."*

*Nutrition Health Review #21, Dec. 1982.

Natural Hygiene is a field that respects the gifts of health provided by Mother Nature. These gifts are simple and obvious and have never been "discovered" by medical "science" because there's no money to be made in discovering them. **NATURAL HYGIENE RECONNECTS US WITH THESE ELEMENTS OF HEALTH**. It shows us as individuals how to use these elements to attain the robust existence that is the natural heritage of the human species.

The words on these pages are intended to help you live your life without the growing fear of falling victim to one of the many diseases we are threatened by, to keep your children out of the leukemia wards and to allow your parents to glide gracefully into their waning years in comfort rather than pain. It is our heartfelt wish that you will see the wisdom of a philosophy toward living that is in harmony with nature, not at odds with it.

There are many chapters of the American Natural Hygiene Society throughout the United States and Canada. To locate the chapter nearest you, contact:

> American Natural Hygiene Society
> P.O. Box 30630
> Tampa, Florida 33630

For information on **Fit for Life** programs and Newsletter write to:

> FIT FOR LIFE
> 2210 Wilshire Blvd.
> Suite #118
> Santa Monica, California 90403

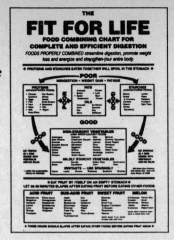

BIBLIOGRAPHY

1. Abdulla, Mohammed, M.D., *et al.* "Nutrient Intake and Health Status of Vegans; Chemical Analyses of Diets Using the Duplicate Portion Sampling Technique." *American Journal of Clinical Nutrition*, Vol. 34, Nov. 1981, p. 2464.
2. Abernathy, R. P., Ph.D., *et al.* "Lack of Response to Amino Acid Supplements by Preadolescent Girls." *American Journal of Clinical Nutrition*, Vol. 25, Oct. 1972, p. 980.
3. Abramowski, O. L. M., M.D. *Fruitarian Diet and Physical Rejuvenation*. Wethersfield, Connecticut: Omangod Press, 1973.
4. —————. *Fruitarian Healing System*. Natal, South Africa: Essence of Health, 1976.
5. Accraido, Marcia M. *Light Eating for Survival*. Wethersfield, Connecticut: Omangod Press, 1978.
6. "Acta." *Medicine Scandinavia*, Vol. 192, Sept. 1972, p. 231.
7. Agranoff, Bernard W., *et al.* "Diet and the Geographical Distribution of Multiple Sclerosis." *Lancet*, Vol. 2, Nov. 2, 1974, p. 1061.
8. Agres, Ted. *Your Food, Your Health*. Chicago: Inter-Direction Press, 1972.
9. Alcott, William A. *Forty Years in the Wilderness of Pills and Powders*. Boston: John P. Jewett & Co., 1859, p. 178.
10. —————. *The Teacher of Health and the Laws of the Human Constitution*. Boston: D. S. King & Co., 1843, pp. 136, 358.

11. Alexandrou, Evangelos. *Yoga and You*. San Jose, California: Christananda Publishing Co., 1975.

12. Allard, Norman, Dr. "Exercise and Its Beneficent Role in Nutrition and Digestion." *Life Science Health System, Lesson #17*. Austin, Texas: Life Science, 1982.

13. Allen, Hannah. "Lesson #33, Why We Should Not Eat Animal Products in Any Form." In: *The Life Science Health System*, by T. C. Fry. Austin, Texas: Life Science, 1984.

14. ——————. *The Happy Truth About Protein*. Austin, Texas: Life Science, 1976.

15. ——————. "Why We Should Not Eat Meat." *Life Science Health System, Lesson #32*. Austin, Texas: Life Science, 1983.

16. ——————. "Why We Should Not Eat Animal Products." *Life Science Health System, Lesson #33*. Austin, Texas: Life Science, 1983.

17. Allen, Lindsay H., Ph.D., *et al*. "Protein-Induced Hypercalcuria: A Long-Term Study." *American Journal of Clinical Nutrition*, Vol. 32, April 1979, p. 741.

18. Aloia, John F., M.D. "Exercise and Skeletal Health." *Journal of the American Geriatric Society*, Vol. 29, 1981, p. 104.

19. Aloia, John F., M.D., *et al*. "Prevention of Involutional Bone Loss by Exercise." *Annals of Internal Medicine*, Vol. 89, Sept. 1978, p. 356.

20. Altchuler, Steven I., Ph.D. "Dietary Protein and Calcium Loss: A Review." *Nutrition Research*, Vol. 2, 1982, p. 193.

21. Alter, Milton, M.D., Ph.D., *et al*. "Multiple Sclerosis and Nutrition." *Archives of Neurology*, Vol. 31, Oct. 1974, p. 267.

22. Altman, Nathaniel. *Eating for Life*. Wheaton, Illinois: Theosophical Publishers, 1974.

23. "Aluminum Exposure & Neurological Abnormalities." *International Clinical Nutrition Review*, Vol. 3, No. 4.

24. American Cancer Society. *Nutrition and Cancer: Cause and Prevention, A Special Report*. Vol. 34, 1984, p. 121.

25. Anand, Chander Rekha, *et al*. "Effect of Protein Intake on Calcium Balance of Young Men Given 500mg Calcium Daily." *Journal of Nutrition*, Vol. 104, Jan./June 1974, p. 695.

26. Anderson, Bonnie M., M.Sc., *et al*. "The Iron and Zinc Status of Long Term Vegetarian Women." *American Journal of Clinical Nutrition*, Vol. 34, June 1981, p. 1042.

27. Anderson, J. "Update of HCF Diet Results." *HCF Newsletter*, Vol. 4, June 1982, Lexington, Kentucky.

28. Anderson, Joseph T., Ph.D., *et al*. "Independence of the Effects of Cholesterol and Degree of Saturation of the Fat in the Diet on Serum Cholesterol in Man." *American Journal of Clinical Nutrition*, Vol. 29, Nov. 1976, p. 1184.

29. Andrews, Arthur D. *Eat Your Way to Glowing Health*. Affton, Missouri: Good Life Publications, 1957.

30. Annand, J. C. "Further Evidence in the Case Against Heated Milk Protein, Atherosclerosis." *Journal of the College of General Practitioners*, Vol. 7, 1964, p. 386.

31. Appleton, Scott B., and Colin T. Campbell. "Inhibition of Aflatoxin Initiated Preneoplasmic Liver Lesions by Low Dietary Protein." *Nutrition and Cancer*, Vol. 3, No. 4, 1982, p. 200.

32. Arroyave, G. "Nutritive Values of Dietary Proteins: For Whom?" *Proceedings 9th International Congress of Nutrition* (Mexico), Vol. 1, 1972, p. 43.

33. Atkinson, Donald T. *Myth, Magic & Medicine*. Cleveland: World Publishing Co., 1956.

34. *Atlanta Journal*, Sept. 24, 1982.

35. Bach, Edward. *Heal Thyself*. London: Daniel, 1946.

36. Bahna, Sami L., M.D. *Allergies to Milk*. New York: Grune & Stratton, 1980.

37. Bahna, Sami L., M.D., *et al*. "Cow's Milk Allergy: Pathogenesis, Manifestations, Diagnoses, and Management." *Advances in Pediatrics*, Vol. 25, 1978, p. 1.

38. Barlow, Wilfred. *The Alexander Technique*. New York: Warner Books, Inc., 1973.

39. Barnard, R. James, *et al*. "Response of Non Insulin Dependent Diabetic Patients to an Intensive Program of Diet and Exercise." *Diabetes Care*, Vol. 5, July/Aug. 1982, p. 370.

40. Baron, Samuel, M.D. *Medical Microbiology*. Menlo Park, California: Addison-Wesley Publishing Co., 1982.

41. Bartlett, R. W. *The Milk Industry*. New York: Ronald Press, 1946.

42. Bauman, Edward, *et al. The Holistic Health Handbook.* Berkeley, California: And/Or Press, 1978.

43. Bealle, Morris A. *The Drug Story.* Spanish Fork, Utah: The Hornet's Nest, 1949.

44. ——————. *The New Drug Story.* Washington, D.C.: Columbia Publishing Co., 1958.

45. Bear, John, Ph.D. *Bear's Guide to Non-Traditional College Degrees*, 9th Edition. Berkeley, California: Ten Speed Press, 1985.

46. Beasley, R. Palmer, *et al.* "Low Prevalence of Rheumatoid Arthritis in Chinese: Prevalence Survey in a Rural Community." *Journal of Rheumatology*, Vol. 10, Nov. 1983, p. 11.

47. Beighton, P. "Rheumatoid Arthritis in a Rural South African Population." *Annals of the Rheumatic Diseases*, Vol. 34, 1975, p. 136.

48. Beiler, Henry G. *Food Is Your Best Medicine.* New York: Random House, 1965.

49. Bell, G. *Textbook of Physiology and Biochemistry*, 4th Ed., p. 167. Baltimore, Ohio: Williams & Wilkins, 1959.

50. Bennett, John G. *Creative Thinking.* Gloucestershire, England: Coombe Springs Press, 1969.

51. ——————. *Sex.* Gloucestershire, England: Coombe Springs Press, 1975.

52. Bennion, Lynn J., M.D., and Scott M. Grundy, M.D., Ph.D. "Risk Factors for the Development of Cholelithiasis in Man." *The New England Journal of Medicine*, Vol. 299, Nov. 1978, p. 1221.

53. Benton, Mike. "Proteins in the Diet." *Life Science Health System, Lesson #8.* Austin, Texas: Life Science, 1982.

54. Bernard, Raymond W. *Eat Your Way to Better Health*, Vol. I & II. Clarksburg, West Virginia: Saucerian, 1974.

55. ——————. *Rejuvenation Through Dietetic Sex Control.* Natal, South Africa: Essence of Health, 1967.

56. *The Best of Food & Wine.* New York: American Express Food & Wine Magazine Corp., 1984.

57. *The Best of Food & Wine 1986 Collection.* New York: American Express Food & Wine Magazine Corp., 1986.

58. Bidwell, Victoria. *The Salt Conspiracy.* Hollister, California: Get Well–Stay Well Publications, 1986.

59. Bien, Edward J., *et al.* "The Relation of Dietary Nitrogen

Consumption to the Rate of Uric Acid Synthesis in Normal and Gouty Men.'' *Journal of Clinical Investigations*, Vol. 32, May 1, 1953, p. 778.

60. Bikle, Daniel D., M.D., Ph.D. "Bone Disease in Alcohol Abuse.'' *Annals of Internal Medicine*, Vol. 103, July 1985, p. 42.

61. Billings, John J., M.D. *The Ovulation Method*. Collegeville, Minnesota: The Liturgical Press, 1972.

62. Bircher-Benner, M. *Eating Your Way to Health*. Baltimore, Maryland: Penguin, 1973.

63. Biser, Samuel. "The Truth About Milk." *The Healthview Newsletter*, Vol. 14, Spring 1978, pp. 1–5.

64. Blume, Elaine. "Protein." *Nutrition Action*, Vol. 14, March 1987, p. 1.

65. Bolourchi, Simin, Ph.D., *et al*. "Wheat Flour as a Source of Protein for Adult Subjects.'' *American Journal of Clinical Nutrition*, Vol. 21, Aug. 1968, p. 827.

66. Bond, Harry C., M.D. *Natural Food Cookbook*. North Hollywood, California: Wilshire Book Co., 1974.

67. *Breads*. Alexandria, Virginia: Time-Life Books, 1981.

68. Bricker, Mildred L., *et al*. "The Protein Requirement of the Adult Rat in Terms of the Protein Contained in Egg, Milk and Soy Flour.'' *Journal of Nutrition*, Vol. 34, July/Dec. 1947, p. 491.

69. Bricklin, Mark. *The Practical Encyclopedia of Natural Healing*. Emmaus, Pennsylvania: Rodale Press, 1976.

70. Briscoe, Anne M., Ph.D., and Charles Ragan, M.D. "Effect of Magnesium on Calcium Metabolism in Man.'' *American Journal of Clinical Nutrition*, Vol. 19, No. 5, Nov. 1966.

71. Broitman, Selwyn A., Ph.D., *et al*. "Polyunsaturated Fat, Cholesterol and Large Bowel Tumorigenesis.'' *Cancer*, Vol. 40, Nov. 1977, p. 2455.

72. Brooks, Karen. *The Complete Vegetarian Cookbook*. New York: Pocket Books, 1976.

73. Buisseret, P. D. "Common Manifestations of Cow's Milk Allergy in Children.'' *Lancet*, Vol. 1, Feb. 11, 1978, p. 304.

74. Burkitt, Denis P., F.R.C.S., F.R.C. "Some Diseases Characteristic of Modern Western Civilization.'' *British Medical Journal*, Vol. 1, Feb. 1973, p. 274.

75. Burstyn, P. G., and D. R. Husbands. "Fat Induced Hyper-

tension in Rabbits, Effect of Dietary Fiber on Blood Pressure and Blood Lipid Concentration." *Cardiovascular Research*, Vol. 14, March 1980, p. 185.

76. Burton, Alec, Ph.D. "Milk." *Hygienic Review*, July 1974.

77. Buscaglia, Leo F., Ph.D. *Bus 9 to Paradise*. New York: Slack Inc., 1986.

78. —————. *Loving Each Other*. New York: Fawcett, 1984.

79. *Cancer Facts and Figures*. American Cancer Society, 1985.

80. Carmichael, Dan. "Milk Surplus Continues to Grow as Price Climbs Even Higher." *St. Petersburg Times*, June 3, 1982.

81. Carque, Otto. *Rational Diet*. Los Angeles: Times Mirror Press, 1923.

82. —————. *Vital Facts About Food*. New Canaan, Connecticut: Keats, 1975.

83. Carrington, Hereward, Ph.D. *The History of Natural Hygiene*. Mokelhumne Hill, California: Health Research, 1964.

84. —————. *The Natural Food of Man*. Mokelhumne Hill, California: Health Research, 1963.

85. —————. *Vitality, Fasting and Nutrition*. New York: Rebman Company, 1908.

86. Carroll, Kenneth K. "Experimental Evidence of Dietary Factors and Hormone Dependent Cancers." *Cancer Research*, Vol. 35, Nov. 1975, p. 3374.

87. Carter, Mary Ellen, and William McGarey. *Edgar Cayce on Healing*. New York: Warner Books, 1972.

88. "The Case Against Meat and Dairy." *Nutrition Health Review*, Vol. 35, July 1985, p. 4.

89. Cheraskin, Emanuel, M.D., W. Ringsdork, M.D., and J. W. Clark. *Diet and Disease*. Emmaus, Pennsylvania: Rodale Press, 1968.

90. Christiansen, Claus, Dr., *et al*. "Prevention of Early Post Menopausal Bone Loss: Controlled 2-Year Study in Normal Females." *European Journal of Clinical Investigation*, Vol. 10, Aug. 1980, p. 273.

91. Claire, Rosine. *French Gourmet Vegetarian Cookbook*. Millbrae, California: Celestial Arts, 1975.

92. Clark, Helen E., Ph.D., *et al*. "Nitrogen Balances of Adult Human Subjects Fed Combinations of Wheat, Beans, Corn, Milk, and Rice." *American Journal of Clinical Nutrition*, Vol. 26, July 1973, p. 702.

93. Clements, John A., *et al*. "Prenatal Origin of the Respiratory Distress Syndrome (ROS) of Premature Infants." *Journal of Applied Physiology*, Vol. 12, March 1958, p. 262.

94. Coe, F. "Eating Too Much Meat Called Major Cause of Renal Stones." *Internal Medical News*, Vol. 12, 1979, p. 1.

95. Colgate, Doris. *The Barefoot Gourmet*. New York: Offshore Sailing School, 1982.

96. Collin, Rodney. *The Mirror of Light*. London: Stuart & Watkins, 1959.

97. Committee on Diet, Nutrition and Cancer: Assembly of Life Sciences National Research Council. *Diet, Nutrition and Cancer*. Washington, D.C.: National Academy Press, 1982.

98. Connor, W. "The Key Role of Nutritional Factors in the Prevention of Coronary Heart Disease." *Preventative Medicine*, Vol. 1, 1979, p. 49.

99. "Consensus Conference: Osteoporosis." *Journal of the American Medical Association*, Vol. 252, 1984, p. 799.

100. Coombs, R. R. A., and P. McLaughlan. "The Enigma of Cot Death: Is the Modified Anaphalaxis Hypothesis an Explanation for Some Cases?" *Lancet*, Vol. 1, June 19, 1982, p. 1388.

101. Cousins, Norman. *Anatomy of an Illness*. New York: Bantam Books, 1979.

102. —————. *The Healing Heart*. New York: Avon, 1984.

103. Crowley, Jerry. *The Fine Art of Garnishing*. Baltimore: Lieba Inc., 1978.

104. Cruse, Peter, *et al*. "Dietary Cholesterol Is Cocarcinogen for Human Colon Cancer." *Lancet*, Vol. 1, April 7, 1979, p. 752.

105. Cummings, J. H., *et al*. "The Effect of Meat Protein and Dietary Fiber on Colonic Function and Metabolism, Changes in Bowel Habit, Bile Acid Excretion, and Calcium Absorption." *American Journal of Clinical Nutrition*, Vol. 32, Oct. 1979, p. 2086.

106. Cunningham, Allan S. "Lymphomas and Animal Protein Consumption." *Lancet*, Vol. 2, Nov. 27, 1976, p. 1184.

107. Cunningham-Rundles, C. "Milk Precipitins, Circulating Immune Complexes and IgA Deficiency." *Proceedings National Academy of Science* (USA), Vol. 75, 1978, p. 3387.

108. Curtis, H. J. *Biological Mechanism of Aging*. Springfield, Illinois: C. C. Thomas, 1966.

109. D'Adamo, Janus, M.D. *One Man's Food*. New York: Richard Marek, 1980.

110. Daniell, Harry W., M.D. "Osteoporosis of the Slender Smoker: Vertebral Compression Fractures and Loss of Metacarpal Cortex in Relation to Post Menopausal Cigarette Smoking and Lack of Obesity." *Archives of Internal Medicine*, Vol. 136, March 1976, p. 298.

111. Dauphin, Lise, N.D. *Recettes Naturiste*. Montreal, Canada: Editions Du Jour, 1969.

112. De Romana, Guillermo Lopez, *et al*. "Fasting and Postprandial Plasma Free Amino Acids of Infants and Children Consuming Exclusive Potato Protein." *Journal of Nutrition*, Vol. 111, July/Dec 1981, p. 1766.

113. Derrick, Fletcher C., Jr., M.D., and William C. Carter, III, M.D. "Kidney Stone Disease: Evaluation and Medical Management." *Postgraduate Medicine*, Vol. 66, Oct. 1979, p. 115.

114. DeVries, Herbert A. *Vigor Regained*. Englewood Cliffs, New Jersey: Prentice-Hall, 1974.

115. Diamond, Marilyn. *The Common Sense Guide to a New Way of Eating*. Santa Monica, California: Golden Glow Publishers, 1979.

116. "Diet and Stress in Vascular Disease." *Journal of the American Medical Association*, Vol. 176, 1961, p. 134.

117. "Diet and Urinary Calculi." *Nutrition Review*, Vol. 38, 1980, p. 74.

118. "Diet for the Prevention and Treatment of Cancer." *The Herald of Health*, Vol. 37, #421, July–Sept. 1914, p. 54.

119. Dole, Vincent P., *et al*. "Dietary Treatment of Hypertension, Clinical and Metabolic Studies of Patients on the Rice-Fruit Diet." *Journal of Clinical Investigation*, Vol. 29, June 12, 1950, p. 1189.

120. Donaldson, Charles, M.D., *et al*. "Effect of Prolonged Bedrest on Bone Mineral." *Metabolism*, Vol. 19, Dec. 1970, p. 1071.

121. Dreyfuss, John. "Majority of the World's Population Suffers Allergic Reactions to Milk." *Los Angeles Times*, Sept. 18, 1984.

122. Dwyer, Johanna T., D.Sc., *et al*. "Nutritional Status of

Vegetarian Children.'' *American Journal of Clinical Nutrition*, Vol. 35, Feb. 1982, p. 204.

123. Dyer, Wayne, Dr. *Gifts from Eykis*. New York: Pocket, 1983.

124. ——————. *What Do You Really Want for Your Children?* New York: William Morrow, 1985.

125. Eastman, Sandy. ''Medications and Bone Loss.'' *Nutrition Health Review*, Vol. 35, June 1985, p. 5.

126. Edwards, Cecile H., Ph.D., *et al*. ''Utilization of Wheat by Adult Man: Nitrogen Metabolism, Plasma, Amino Acids and Lipids.'' *American Journal of Clinical Nutrition*, Vol. 24, Feb. 1978, p. 181.

127. Ehrenreich, Barbara, and Deirdre English. *Witches, Midwives & Nurses*. Old Westbury, New York: The Feminist Press, 1973.

128. Esser, William L. *Dictionary of Man's Foods*. Chicago: Natural Hygiene Press, 1972.

129. Farb, Peter, and George Armelagos. *The Anthropology of Eating*. Boston: Houghton Mifflin Co., 1980.

130. Farnsworth, Steve. ''Plan to Cut Milk Surplus Isn't Working.'' *Los Angeles Times*, March 5, 1984.

131. Fathman, George, and Doris Fathman. *Live Foods*. Beaumont, California: Ehret Literature Publishing, 1973.

132. Feingold, Ben F., M.D. *Why Your Child is Hyper-Active*. New York: Random House, 1974.

133. Ford, Marjorie Winn, Susan Hillyard, and Mary F. Knock. *Deaf Smith Country Cookbook*. New York: Collier Books, 1974.

134. Fraser, David R. ''The Physiological Economy of VD.'' *Lancet*, Vol. 1, April 30, 1983, p. 969.

135. Fredericks, Carlton, Ph.D. *Arthritis: Don't Learn to Live with It*. New York: Grosset & Dunlap, 1981.

136. Fritch, Albert J. *The Household Pollutants Guide*. New York: Anchor Books, Center for Science in the Public Interest, 1978.

137. *Fruits*. Alexandria, Virginia: Time-Life Books, 1983.

138. Fry, T. C. *High Energy Methods, Lessons 1–7*. Austin, Texas: Life Science, 1983.

139. ——————. *Super Food for Super Health*. Austin, Texas: Life Science, 1976.

140. ——————. *Superior Foods, Diet Principles and Prac-*

tices for Perfect Health. Austin, Texas: Life Science, 1974.

141. —————. *The Curse of Cooking*. Austin, Texas: Life Science, 1975.

142. —————. *The Great Water Controversy*. Austin, Texas: Life Science, 1974.

143. —————. *The Life Science Health System, Lessons 1–111*. Austin, Texas: Life Science, 1983.

144. —————. *The Myth of Medicine*. Austin, Texas: Life Science, 1974.

145. —————. *The Revelation of Health*. Austin, Texas: Life Science, 1981.

146. Fuchs, Nan K., Ph.D. *The Nutrition Detective*. Los Angeles: Jeremy P. Tarcher, 1985, p. 140.

147. Gainer, John, Dr. "Protein and Hardening of the Arteries." *Science News*, Aug. 21, 1971.

148. Gale, Bill. *The Wonderful World of Walking*. New York: William Morrow, 1979.

149. Gandhi, Mahatma. *Mohan-Mala*. India: Navajiuan Press, 1949.

150. Garrier, Robert. *Great Salads and Vegetables*. Sydney, Australia: Angus & Robertson, 1965.

151. Garrison, Omar V. *The Dictocrats*. Chicago: Books for Today, 1970.

152. Gaskin, Ina May. *Spiritual Midwifery*. Summertown, Tennessee: The Book Publishing Co., 1980.

153. Gerrard, J. W., D.M., F.R.C.P. "Milk Allergy: Clinical Picture and Familial Incidence." *Canadian Medical Association Journal*, Vol. 97, Sept. 23, 1967, p. 780.

154. Gewanter, Vera. *A Passion for Vegetables*. New York: Viking Press, 1980.

155. Giller, Robert M., M.D. *Medical Makeover*. New York: William Morrow, 1986.

156. Glaser, Ronald. *The Body Is the Hero*. New York: Random House, 1976.

157. Goodhart, Robert S., and Maurice E. Shils. *Modern Nutrition in Health and Disease*, 5th Ed. Philadelphia: Lea & Febiger, 1973.

158. —————. *Modern Nutrition in Health and Disease*. Philadelphia: Lea & Febiger, 1980.

159. Graham, Sylvester, *et al. The Greatest Health Discovery*. Chicago: Natural Hygiene Press, 1972.

160. Gray, Henry, M.D. *Gray's Anatomy*. New York: Bounty Books, 1977.
161. Greenberger, N. "Effect of Vegetable and Animal Protein Diets on Chronic Hepatic Encephalopathy." *Digestive Diseases*, Vol. 22, 1977, p. 945.
162. Gross, Joy. *The Vegetarian Child*. New York: Lyle Stuart, 1983.
163. Guyton, Arthur C., M.D. *Physiology of the Body*. Philadelphia: W. B. Saunders, 1964.
164. ——————. *Guidance Textbook of Medical Physiology*. Philadelphia: Saunders Publishing Co., 1981.
165. ——————. *Physiology of the Human Body*. Philadelphia: Saunders College Publishing, 1984, p. 502.
166. ——————. *Physiology of the Body*. Philadelphia: W. B. Saunders, 1981.
167. Harper, A. E., Ph.D. "Some Implications of Amino Acid Supplementation." *American Journal of Clinical Nutrition*, Vol. 9, Sept./Oct. 1961, p. 553.
168. Hart, P. M., and M. D'Arcy. "The Prevention of Pulmonary Tuberculosis Among Adults in England." *Lancet*, May 8, 1937, p. 1093.
169. Haurylewicz, Ervin J. "Mammary Tumorigenesis by High Dietary Protein in Rats." *Nutrition Reports International*, Vol. 26, Nov. 1982, p. 793.
170. Hazard, Susan, Ph.D. "Rheumatic Diseases." *Life Science Health System, Lesson #72*. Austin, Texas: Life Science, 1982.
171. ——————. "Ulcers." *Life Science Health System, Lesson #76*. Austin, Texas: Life Science, 1983.
172. Heaney, Robert P., *et al*. "Effects of Nitrogen, Phosphorus and Caffeine on Calcium Balance in Women." *Journal of Laboratory and Clinical Medicine*, Vol. 99, 1982, p. 46.
173. ——————. "Calcium Nutrition and Bone Health in the Elderly." *American Journal of Clinical Nutrition*, Vol. 36, Nov. 1982, p. 986.
174. *Heart Facts*. New York: American Heart Association, 1984.
175. Hegsted, D. M. "Minimum Protein Requirements of Adults." *American Journal of Clinical Nutrition*, Vol. 21, May 1968, p. 352.
176. Hegsted, D. M., Ph.D., *et al*. "Lysine and Methionine Supplementation of All-Vegetable Diets for Human Adults."

Journal of Nutrition, Vol. 56, May/Aug. 1955, p. 555.

177. Hegsted, D. M. "Calcium and Osteoporosis." *Journal of Nutrition*, Vol. 116, Nov. 1986, p. 2316.

178. Hegsted, D. M., Ph.D., *et al.* "Protein Requirements of Adults." *Journal of Laboratory and Clinical Medicine*, Vol. 31, March 1946, p. 261.

179. Hegsted, Maren, *et al.* "Urinary Calcium and Calcium Balance in Young Men as Affected by Level of Protein and Phosphorus Intake." *Journal of Nutrition*, Vol. 111, Jan./June 1981, p. 553.

180. Heritage, Ford. *Composition and Facts about Foods*. Mokelhumne Hill, California: Health Research, 1971.

181. Hightower, Jim. *Eat Your Heart Out*. New York: Random House, 1976.

182. Hill, M. "Colon Cancer: A Disease of Fiber Depletion or of Dietary Excess." *Digestion*, Vol. 11, 1974, p. 289.

183. Hill, P., *et al.* "Environmental Factors and Breast and Prostate Cancer." *Cancer Research*, Vol. 41, Sept. 1981, p. 3817.

184. Hill, Peter, Ph.D., *et al.* "Diet and Endocrine Related Cancer." *Cancer*, Vol. 39, April 1977, p. 1820.

185. Hinsworth, H. P. "The Physiological Activation of Insulin." *Clinical Science*, Vol. 1, 1933/1934, p. 1.

186. Hoffman, William S., *et al.* "Nitrogen Requirement of Normal Men on a Diet of Protein Hydrolysate Enriched with the Limiting Essential Amino Acids." *Journal of Nutrition*, Vol. 44, May/Aug. 1951, p. 123.

187. Holt, E. *Protein and Amino Acid Requirements in Early Life*. New York: University Press, 1960, p. 9.

188. *Hors d'Oeuvres*. Alexandria, Virginia: Time-Life Books, 1980.

189. Hotema, Hilton. *Perfect Health*. Natal, South Africa: Essence of Health, no date in book.

190. Hovannessian, A. T. *Raw Eating*. Tehran: Arshavir, 1967.

191. Howe, Jean M., Ph.D., *et al.* "Nitrogen Retention of Adults Fed Six Grams of Nitrogen from Combinations of Rice, Milk, and Wheat." *American Journal of Clinical Nutrition*, Vol. 25, June 1972, p. 559.

192. Howell, W. H., M.D. *The Human Machine*. Ontario, Canada: Provoker Press, 1969.

193. Hunter, Beatrice T. *Consumer Beware: Your Food and What's*

Been Done to It. New York: Simon & Schuster, 1972.

194. Hur, Robin A. *Food Reform—Our Desperate Need.* Herr-Heidelberg, 1975.

195. —————. "Osteoporosis: The Key to Aging." *Life Science Health System, Lesson #32.* Austin, Texas: Life Science, 1983.

196. Hurd, Frank J., D.C., and Rosalie Hurd, B.S. *Ten Talents.* Chisholm, Minnesota: Dr. & Mrs. Frank J. Hurd, 1968.

197. Illich, Ivan. *Medical Nemesis.* New York: Bantam, 1976.

198. Immerman, Alan M., Dr. "Vitamins: The Metabolic Wizards of Life Processes." *Life Science Health System, Lesson #9.* Austin, Texas: Life Science, 1982.

199. Ippoliti, Andrew F., M.D., *et al.* "The Effect of Various Forms of Milk on Gastric-Acid Secretions, Studies in Patients with Duodenal Ulcer and Normal Subjects." *Annals of Internal Medicine,* Vol. 84, March 1976, p. 286.

200. Irwin, M. Isabel, *et al.* "A Conspectus of Research on Protein Requirements of Man." *Journal of Nutrition,* Vol. 101, March 1971, p. 385.

201. Jackson, James C., M.D. *How to Treat the Sick Without Medicine.* Dansville, New York: Austin, Jackson & Co., 1873, p. 307.

202. Jampolsky, Gerald G., M.D. *Love Is Letting Go of Fear.* Berkeley, California: Celestial Arts, 1979.

203. Johnson, Nancy E., *et al.* "Effect of Level of Protein Intake on Urinary and Fecal Calcium and Calcium Retention of Young Adult Males." *Journal of Nutrition,* Vol. 100, July/Dec. 1970, p. 1425.

204. Juan, David, M.D. "The Clinical Importance of Hypomagnesemia." *Surgery,* Vol. 91, No. 5, May 1982.

205. Kalikowski, B., *et al.* "Low Protein and Purine Free Diet in Acute Leukemia in Children." *Polish Medical Journal,* Vol. 5, 1966, p. 558.

206. Kamen, Betty, Ph.D. *Osteoporosis: What It Is, How to Prevent It, How to Stop It.* New York: Pinnacle, 1984.

207. Kempner, Walter, M.D. "Compensation of Renal Metabolic Dysfunction." *North Carolina Medical Journal,* Vol. 6, Feb. 1945, p. 61.

208. Khalsa, Siri V. K. *Conscious Cookery.* Los Angeles: Siri Ved Kaur Khalsa, 1978.

209. Kies, Constance, *et al.* "Determination of First Limiting

Nitrogenous Factor in Corn Protein for Nitrogen Retention in Human Adults.'' *Journal of Nutrition*, Vol. 86, May/Aug. 1965, p. 350.

210. Kime, Zane R., M.D. *Sunlight*. Penryn, California: World Health Publications, 1981.

211. Knapp, John, M.D., *et al*. ''Growth and Nitrogen Balance in Infants Fed Cereal Proteins.'' *American Journal of Clinical Nutrition*, Vol. 26, June 1973, p. 586.

212. Kon, Stanislaw Kazimierz, and Aniela Klein. ''The Value of Whole Potatoes in Human Nutrition.'' *Biochemical Journal*, Vol. 22, 1928, p. 258.

213. Kopple, J. D., *et al*. ''Controlled Comparison of 20g and 40g Protein Diets in the Treatment of Chronic Uremia.'' *American Journal of Clinical Nutrition*, Vol. 21, June 1968, p. 553.

214. Korenblat, Phillip E., M.D. ''Immune Responses of Human Adults After Oral and Parenteral Exposure to Bovine Serum Albumin.'' *Journal of Allergy*, Vol. 41, March 1968, p. 226.

215. Krauss, W. E., *et al*. ''Studies on the Nutritional Value of Milk and the Effects of Pasteurization on Some of the Nutritional Properties of Milk.'' Ohio Agriculture Experiment Station Bulletin #518, Jan. 1933, p. 7.

216. Krok, Morris. *Amazing New Health System*. Natal, South Africa: Essence of Health, 1976.

217. —————. *Formula for Long Life*. Natal, South Africa: Essence of Health, 1977.

218. —————. *Fruit, the Food and Medicine for Man*. Natal, South Africa: Essence of Health, 1967.

219. —————. *Golden Path to Rejuvenation*. Natal, South Africa: Essence of Health, 1974.

220. —————. *Hatha Yoga*. Natal, South Africa: Essence of Health, 1975.

221. —————. *Health, Diet and Living on Air*. Natal, South Africa: Essence of Health, 1964.

222. —————. *Health Truths Eternal*. Natal, South Africa: Essence of Health, 1964.

223. Kulvinskas, Victoras. *Survival into the 21st Century*. Wethersfield, Connecticut: Omangod Press, 1975.

224. Laurel, Alicia B. *Living on the Earth*. New York: Vintage, 1971.

225. Leaf, Alexander, M.D. "Every Day Is a Gift When You Are Over 100." *National Geographic*, Vol. 1, 1973, pp. 93–119.

226. LeBoyer, Frederick. *Birth Without Violence*. New York: Alfred A. Knopf, 1975.

227. —————. *Loving Hands*. New York: Alfred A. Knopf, 1982.

228. Lee, Chung-Ja, Ph.D., *et al*. "Nitrogen Retention of Young Men Fed Rice With or Without Supplementary Chicken." *American Journal of Clinical Nutrition*, Vol. 24, March 1971, p. 318.

229. Lemlin, Jeanne. *Vegetarian Pleasures*. New York: Alfred A. Knopf, 1986.

230. Leonardo, Blanche. *Cancer and Other Diseases from Meat*. Santa Monica, California: Leaves of Healing, 1979.

231. Lewinnek, George E., M.D. "The Significance and a Comparative Analysis of the Epidemiology of Hip Fractures." *Clinical Orthopedics and Related Research*, Vol. 152, Oct. 1980, p. 35.

232. Lindahl, Olov, *et. al*. "A Vegan Regimen with Reduced Medication in the Treatment of Hypertension." *British Journal of Nutrition*, Vol. 52, July 1984, p. 11.

233. Linkswiler, H. "Calcium Retention of Young Adult Males as Affected by Level of Protein and of Calcium Intake." *Transcript New York Academy of Science*, Vol. 36, 1974, p. 333.

234. Linkswiler, Helen M. *Nutrition Review's Present Knowledge in Nutrition*, 4th Ed. The Nutrition Foundation, New York, 1976.

235. Littman, M. L., *et al*. "Effect of Cholesterol-Free, Fat-Free Diet and Hypocholesteremic Agents on Growth of Transplantable Tumors." *Cancer Chemotherapy Report*, Vol. 50, Jan./Feb. 1966, p. 25.

236. Longwood, William. *Poisons in Your Food*. New York: Pyramid, 1969.

237. Lotzof, L. "Dairy Produce and Coronary Artery Disease." *Medical Journal of Australia*, Vol. 1, June 30, 1973, p. 1317.

238. Lucas, Charles P., and Lawrence Power. "Dietary Fat Aggravates Active Rheumatoid Arthritis." *Clinical Research*, Vol. 29, Nov. 5/6/7, 1981, p. 754.

239. MacArthur, John R. *Ancient Greece in Modern America*. Caldwell, Idaho: The Caxton Printers Ltd., 1943.

240. Mallos, Tess. *Complete Middle East Cookbook*. New York: McGraw-Hill, 1982.

241. Margen, S., M.D., *et al.* "Studies in Calcium Metabolism, the Calciuretic Effect of Dietary Protein." *American Journal of Clinical Nutrition*, Vol. 27, June 1974, p. 584.

242. Marks, Geoffrey, and William K. Beatty. *The Precious Metals of Medicine*. New York: Charles Scribner's Sons, 1975.

243. Massey, Linda K., Ph.D., and Kevin J. Wise, B.S. "The Effect of Dietary Caffeine on Urinary Excretion of Calcium, Magnesium, Sodium and Potassium in Healthy Young Females." *Nutrition Research*, Jan./Feb. 1984, p. 43.

244. Mazess, Richard Z., Ph.D., *et al.* "Bone Mineral Content of North Alaskan Eskimos." *American Journal of Clinical Nutrition*, Vol. 27, Sept. 1974, p. 916.

245. McBean, Eleanor. *The Poisoned Needle*. Mokelhumne Hill, California: Health Research, 1974.

246. McCarter, Robert, Ph.D., and Elizabeth McCarter, Ph.D. "A Statement on Vitamins," "Vitamins and Cures," "Other Unnecessary Supplements." *Health Reporter*, Vol. 11, 1984, pp. 10, 24.

247. McClellan, Walter S., *et al.* "Prolonged Meat Diets with a Study of the Metabolism of Nitrogen, Calcium and Phosphorus." *Journal of Biological Chemistry*, Vol. 87, 1930, p. 669.

248. McConnell, R. "Genetic Aspects of Gastrointestinal Cancer." *Clinics in Gastroenterology*, Vol. 5, 1976, p. 483.

249. McDougall, John A., M.D. *McDougall's Medicine*. Piscataway, New Jersey: New Century Publishers, 1985, pp. 231–254.

250. —————. *The McDougall Plan*. Piscataway, New Jersey: New Century Publishers, 1983.

251. McLaren, Donald S. "The Great Protein Fiasco." *Lancet*, Vol. 2, July 13, 1974, p. 93.

252. McNair, James. *Power Food*. San Francisco: Chronicle Books, 1986.

253. —————. *Cold Pasta*. Sydney, Australia: Angus & Robertson, 1986.

254. Medvin, Jeannine O. *Prenatal Yoga and Natural Birth*. Albion, California: Freestone Publishing Co., 1974.

255. Mendelsohn, Robert S., M.D. *Confessions of a Medical Heretic*. New York: Warner Books, 1980.

256. —————. *How to Raise a Healthy Child in Spite of Your Doctor*. Chicago: Contemporary Books, 1984.

257. "Milk Facts." Milk Industry Foundation, New York, 1946–1947.

258. Modesto, Ruby, and Guy Mount. *Not for Innocent Ears*. Arcadia, California: Sweetlight Books, 1980.

259. Montagna, Joseph F. *People's Desk References*, Vol. I & II. Lake Oswego, Oregon: Quest for Truth Publications, 1980.

260. Moore, W. "The Evaluation of Bone Density Findings in Normal Populations and Osteoporosis." *Trans American Clinical Climatological Association*, Vol. 86, 1974, p. 128.

261. Morash, Marian. *The Victory Garden Cookbook*. New York: Alfred A. Knopf, 1982.

262. *Morbidity & Mortality Weekly Report*. Center for Disease Control, Atlanta, Mar. 16, 1979.

263. Muktananda, Swami. *I Welcome You All With Love*. South Fallsburg, New York: Syda Foundation–Om Namah Shivaya, 1978.

264. Murray, A. B. "Infant Feeding and Respiratory Allergy." *Lancet*, Vol. 1, Mar. 6, 1971, p. 497.

265. Nahas, A. M. El, and G. A. Coles. "Dietary Treatment of Chronic Renal Failure." *Lancet*, Vol. 1, March 8, 1986, p. 597.

266. Nasset, E. "Movement of the Small Intestines." *Medical Physiology*, 11th ed. St. Louis: C. V. Mosby, 1961.

267. National Geographic Society. *The Incredible Machine*. Washington, D.C.: National Geographic Society, 1986.

268. Newman, Laura, M.D. *Make Your Juicer Your Drugstore*. Simi Valley, California: Benedict Lust, 1972.

269. Nilas, L., M.D., *et al*. "Calcium Supplementation and Post Menopausal Bone Loss." *British Medical Journal*, Vol. 289, Oct. 27, 1984, p. 1103.

270. Nishizuka, Yasuaki. "Biological Influence of Fat Intake on Mammary Cancer and Mammary Tissue: Experimental Correlates." *Preventative Medicine*, Vol. 7, June 1978, p. 218.

271. Nolfi, Cristine, M.D. *My Experiences with Living Food*. Ontario, Canada: Provoker Press, 1969.

272. "Nutrition and Health." *Nutrition Health Review #37*, Jan. 1986, p. 17.

273. O'Brien, J. R., M.A., D.M., M.R.C.S., L.R.C.P. "Fat Digestion, Blood Coagulation, and Atherosclerosis." *American Journal of Medical Science*, Vol. 234, Oct. 1957, p. 373.

274. Olefsky, Jerrold M., M.D. "Reappraisal of the Role of Insulin in Hypertriglyceridemia." *American Journal of Medicine*, Vol. 57, Oct. 1974, p. 551.

275. Orage, A. R. *On Love*. New York: Samuel Weiser, Inc., 1974.

276. Osborn, Thomas B., *et al.* "Amino Acids in Nutrition and Growth." *Journal of Biological Chemistry*, Vol. 17, 1914, p. 325.

277. Oyster, Nancy, *et al.* "Physical Activity and Osteoporosis in Post Menopausal Women." *Medicine and Science in Sports and Exercise*, Vol. 16, No. 1, 1985.

278. Page, Melvin, and H. L. Abrams. *Your Body Is Your Best Doctor*. New Canaan, Connecticut: Keats, 1972.

279. Parham, Barbara. *What's Wrong with Eating Meat?* Denver, Colorado: Ananda Marga Publications, 1979.

280. Parish, W. E., B.A., B.V.Sc., *et al.* "Hypersensitivity to Milk and Sudden Death in Infancy." *Lancet*, Vol. 2, Nov. 19, 1960, p. 1106.

281. Parke, A. L., M.B., F.R.C.P., and G. R. V. Hughes, M.D., F.R.C.P. "Rheumatoid Arthritis and Food: A Case Study." *British Medical Journal*, Vol. 22, June 20, 1981, p. 2027.

282. Parrette, Owen S., M.D. *Why I Don't Eat Meat*. St. Catherines, Ontario: Provoker Press, 1972.

283. Pasley, Salley. *The Tao of Cooking*. Berkeley, California: Ten Speed Press, 1982.

284. *Pasta*. Alexandria, Virginia: Time-Life Books, 1980.

285. Paterson, C. "Calcium Requirements in Man: A Critical Review." *Postgraduate Medical Journal*, Vol. 54, 1978, p. 244.

286. Patrick, Lee T. "Pets Vulnerable to Human Ailments." *Nutrition Health Review*, Vol. 35, June 1985, p. 8.

287. Paulsen, Jane H. *Working Pregnant*. New York: Fawcett, 1984.

288. Pearce, Joseph Chilton. *Magical Child*. New York: E. P. Dutton, 1977.

289. ——————. *Magical Child Matures*. New York: E. P. Dutton, 1985.

290. Peck, M. Scott, M.D. *The Road Less Traveled*. New York: Simon & Schuster, 1978.

291. Pelletier, Kenneth R. *Healthy People in Unhealthy Places: Stress and Fitness at Work*. New York: Delacorte Press, 1984.

292. Pike, M. C., Ph.D., *et al.* "Age at Onset of Lung Cancer: Significance in Relation to Effect of Smoking." *Lancet*, Mar. 27, 1965.

293. Pinkney, Callan. *Callanetics*. New York: William Morrow, 1984.

294. Pixley, Finoa, *et al.* "Effect of Vegetarianism on Development of Gall Stones in Women." *British Medical Journal*, Vol. 291, July 6, 1985, p. 11.

295. Pottenger, F. M., Jr. "The Effects of Heated, Processed Foods and Vitamin D Milk on the Dental Facial Structure of Experimental Animals." *American Journal of Orthodontics and Oral Surgery*, Aug. 1946.

296. *Poultry.* Alexandria, Virginia: Time-Life Books, 1978.

297. Prosser, C. *Comparative Animal Physiology*, 2nd ed. St. Louis: W. B. Saunders, 1961, p. 61.

298. "Protein and Salt: Calcium Thieves." *Nutrition Health Review*, Vol. 35, June 1985, p. 4.

299. Puska, Pekka, *et al.* "Controlled Randomized Trial of the Effect of Dietary Fat on Blood Pressure." *Lancet*, Vol. 1, Jan 1/8, 1983, p. 2.

300. Ramtha. *Ramtha.* Eastsound, Washington: Sovereignty Inc., 1986.

301. Randolph, Theron G., M.D., and Ralph W. Moss, Ph.D. *An Alternative Approach to Allergies*. New York: Lippincott/ Crowell, 1979.

302. Reddy, Bandaru S., Ph.D., *et al.* "Metabolic Epidemiology of Large Bowel Cancer." *Cancer*, Vol. 42, Dec. 1978, p. 2832.

303. Reddy, Vinodini, M.D., D.C.H. "Lysine Supplementation of Wheat and Nitrogen Retention in Children." *American Journal of Clinical Nutrition*, Vol. 24, Oct. 1971, p. 1246.

304. Rensberger, Boyce. "Research Yields Surprises About Early Human Diets." *The New York Times*, May 15, 1979.

305. Reuben, David, M.D. *Everything You Always Wanted to Know About Nutrition*. New York: Avon, 1979.

306. Richards, Valerie. "The Dietary Dilemma." *Nutrition Health Review*, Vol. 29, Jan. 1984.

307. Richter, Vera. *Cook-Less Book*. Ontario, Canada: Provoker Press, 1971.

308. Rüs, Bente, M.D., *et al*. "Does Calcium Supplementation Prevent Post Menopausal Bone Loss?" *The New England Journal of Medicine*, Vol. 316, Jan. 22, 1987, p. 173.

309. Roberts, H. "Potential Toxicity Due to Dolomite and Bonemeal." *Southern Medical Journal*, Vol. 76, 1983, p. 556.

310. Robertson, W. "The Role of Affluence and Diet in the Genesis of Calcium-Containing Stones." *Forteschritte der Urologie and Nephrologie*, Vol. 11, 1979, p. 5.

311. Robinson, Victor. *The Story of Medicine*. New York: The New Home Library, 1943.

312. Rombauer, Irma S., and Marion R. Becker. *Joy of Cooking*. New York: Signet, 1973.

313. Rose, William C., *et al*. "The Amino Acid Requirements of Adult Man—The Role of the Nitrogen Intake." *Journal of Biological Chemistry*, Vol. 217, Nov./Dec. 1955, p. 997.

314. Rosenblum, Art. *The Natural Birth Control Book*. Philadelphia: Aquarian Research Foundation, 1982.

315. Rothschild, Bruce M., and Alfonse T. Masi. "Pathogenesis of Rheumatoid Arthritis: A Vascular Hypothesis." *Seminar Arthritis Rheumatoid*, Vol. 12, Aug. 1982, p. 11.

316. Rouse, Ian L., *et al*. "Blood Pressure Lowering Effect of a Vegetarian Diet: Controlled Trial in Normotensive Subjects." *Lancet*, Vol. 1, Jan. 1/8, 1983, p. 5.

317. Sacca, Joseph D., M.D., F.A.C.A. "Acute Ischemic Colitis Due to Milk Allergy." *Annals of Allergy*, Vol. 29, May 1971, p. 268.

318. Sahni, Julie. *Classic Indian Cooking*. New York: William Morrow, 1980.

319. *Salads*. Alexandria, Virginia: Time-Life Books, 1980.

320. Sandler, Sandra and Bruce. *Home Bakebook of Natural Breads and Cookies*. Harrisburg, Pennsylvania: Stackpole, 1972.

321. Sandoz, Mari. *These Were the Sioux*. New York: Dell, 1961.

322. Scharffenberg, John A., M.D. *Problems with Meat*. Santa Barbara, California: Woodridge Press, 1979.

323. Schell, Orville. *Modern Meat*. New York: Random House, 1984.

324. Schuette, Sally A., *et al*. "Studies on the Mechanism of Protein-Induced Hypercalciuria in Older Men and Women." *Journal of Nutrition*, Vol. 110, Jan./June 1980, p. 305.

325. Schuller, Robert. *The Be Happy Attitudes*. Waco, Texas: Word Books, 1985.

326. Schuman, L. M., and J. S. Mandel. "Epidemiology of Prostate Cancer in Blacks." *Preventative Medicine*, Vol. 9, Sept. 1980, p. 630.

327. Select Committee on Nutrition and Human Needs, U.S. Senate. *Dietary Goals for the United States*. Washington, D.C.: U.S. Government Printing Office, 1977.

328. Shah, P. J. R., and Rosemary Farren. "Dietary Calcium and Idiopathic Hypercalciuria." *Lancet*, Vol. 1, April 4, 1981, p. 786.

329. Shapiro, Jay R., M.D. "Osteoporosis: Evaluation of Diagnosis and Therapy." *Archives of Internal Medicine*, Vol. 135, April 1975, p. 563.

330. Shelton, Herbert M., Ph.D. "Are Humans Meat Eaters?" *The Life Science Health System, Lesson #88*. Austin, Texas: Life Science, 1983.

331. —————. *Exercise*. Chicago: Natural Hygiene Press, 1971.

332. —————. "The Digestion of Milk." *Hygienic Review*, Aug. 1969.

333. —————. *Human Beauty, Its Culture and Hygiene*. San Antonio, Texas: Dr. Shelton's Health School, 1968.

334. —————. *Human Life, Its Philosophy and Laws*. Mokelhumne Hill, California: Health Research, 1979.

335. —————. *The Hygienic Care of Children*. Bridgeport, Connecticut: Natural Hygiene Press, 1981.

336. —————. *The Hygienic System*, Vol. I, II, & III. San Antonio, Texas: Dr. Shelton's Health School, 1934.

337. —————. *The Natural Cure of Cancer*. San Antonio, Texas: Dr. Shelton's Health School, 1935.

338. —————. *Natural Hygiene, Man's Pristine Way of Life*. San Antonio, Texas: Dr. Shelton's Health School, 1968.

339. —————. *Principles of Natural Hygiene*. San Antonio, Texas: Dr. Shelton's Health School, 1964.

340. —————. *Rubies in the Sand*. San Antonio, Texas: Dr. Shelton's Health School, 1961.

341. —————. *Superior Nutrition*. San Antonio, Texas: Dr. Shelton's Health School, 1951.

342. Sherman, Henry C., M.D. *Essentials of Nutrition*, 4th ed. New York: Macmillan, 1957.

343. Shettles, Landrum B., M.D., and David M. Rorvik. *How to Choose the Sex of Your Baby*. Garden City, New York: Doubleday, 1984.

344. Shillam, K. W., *et al*. "The Effect of Heat Treatment on the Nutritive Value of Milk for the Young Calf: The Effect of Ultra-High Temperature Treatment and of Pasteurization." *British Medical Journal*, Vol. 14, Nov. 10, 1960, p. 403.

345. Shippen, Katherine B. *Men of Medicine*. New York: New Viking, 1957.

346. Simmons, Richard. *Reach for Fitness*. New York: Warner Books, 1986.

347. Singer, Peter, and Jim Mason. *Animal Factories*. Bridgeport, Connecticut: Natural Hygiene Press, 1980.

348. Singh, Charan. *The Master Answers*. New Delhi, India: R. S. Satsang Beas, 1966.

349. Singh, Inder, and M. B. Rangoon, F.R.F.P.S., M.R.C.P.E. "Low-Fat Diet and Therapeutic Doses of Insulin in Diabetes Mellitus." *Lancet*, Vol. 1, Feb. 26, 1955, p. 422.

350. Sirtori, C. R., *et al*. "Soybean Protein Diet in the Treatment of Type II Hyperdipoproteinemia." *Lancet*, Vol. 1, Feb. 5, 1977, p. 275.

351. Sivamanda, Swami. *Bhagavad Gita*. Bombay, India: Divine Life Society, 1983.

352. Smith, Everett L., Jr. "Physical Activity and Calcium Modalities for Bone Mineral Increase in Aged Women." *Medical Science of Sports and Exercise*, Vol. 13, 1981, p. 60.

353. Smith, Jeff. *The Frugal Gourmet*. New York: William Morrow, 1984.

354. "Smoking, Alcohol and Bone Degeneration." *Nutrition Health Review*, Vol. 35, June 1985, p. 4.

355. *Snacks & Sandwiches*. Alexandria, Virginia: Time-Life Books, 1980.

356. Solomon, L., M.D., F.R.C.S., *et al*. "Rheumatic Disorders

in the South African Negro, Rheumatoid Arthritis and Ankylosing Spondylitis.'' *South African Medical Journal*, Vol. 49, July 26, 1975, p. 1292.

357. Solomon, L. "Osteoporosis and Fracture of the Femoral Neck in the South African Bantu." *Journal of Bone and Joint Surgery*, Vol. 50B, Feb. 1968, p. 2.

358. *Soups.* Alexandria, Virginia: Time-Life Books, 1979.

359. *Southern California Dental Association Journal*, Vol. 31, No. 9, Sept. 1963.

360. Spencer, R. P. *The Intestinal Tract*. Springfield, Illinois: Charles Thomas Publishers, 1960.

361. Spenser, James T., Jr., M.D. "Hyperlipoproteinemias in the Etiology of Inner Ear Disease." *Laryngoscope*, Vol. 85, Jan. 11, 1973, p. 639.

362. Stevenson, J. C., and M. I. Whitehead. "Post Menopausal Osteoporosis Regular Review." *British Medical Journal*, Vol. 285, Aug. 28/Sept. 4, 1982, p. 585.

363. Stroud, R. M., *et al*. "Comprehensive Environmental Control and Its Effect on Rheumatoid Arthritis." *Clinical Research*, Vol. 28, Nov. 6/7/8, 1980, p. 791.

364. Studervant, Richard A. L., M.D., M.P.U. "Increased Prevalence of Choletithiasis in Men Ingesting a Serum Cholesterol Lowering Diet." *The New England Journal of Medicine*, Vol. 288, Jan. 4, 1973, p. 24.

365. Su-Huei, Huang. *Chinese Appetizers and Garnishes*. Taipei, Taiwan: Huang Su-Huei, 1983.

366. Sunset International. *Vegetarian Cookbook*. Menlo Park, California: Lane Publishing, 1983.

367. Swank, Roy L., M.D., Ph.D. "Multiple Sclerosis: Twenty Years on Low Fat Diet." *Archives of Neurology*, Vol. 23, Nov. 1970, p. 460.

368. Sweeny, Shirley J., M.D. "Dietary Factors That Influence the Dextrose Tolerance Test." *Archives of Internal Medicine*, Vol. 40, 1927, p. 818.

369. "Symposium on Human Calcium Requirements: Council on Foods and Nutrition." *Journal of the American Medical Association*, Vol. 185, 1963, p. 588.

370. Talamini, R., *et al*. "Obesity, Milk and Cancer in Italy." *British Journal of Cancer*, Vol. 53, 1986, p. 817.

371. Tannahill, Reay. *Food in History*. New York: Stein & Day, 1981.

372. Thomas, Anna. *The Vegetarian Epicure*, Books I & II. New York: Alfred A. Knopf, 1972.

373. Tilden, John H., M.D. *Toxemia Explained*. Denver, Colorado: Health Research, 1926.

374. —————. *Food: Its Composition, Preparation, Combination* . . . Denver: J. H. Tilden, 1916, p. 211.

375. —————. "Cancer." *A Stuffed Club*, Vol. 1, 1900–1901, p. 28. Also references in Vols. 3, 10, 12–15. *A Stuffed Club* becomes *Philosophy of Health* in Vol. 16. *Philosophy of Health* Vols. 18, 19, 21 also contain references to cancer.

376. Tobe, John H. *Hunza: Adventures in a Land of Paradise*. Ontario, Canada: Provoker Press, 1971.

377. Tommori, J., and Pal Osvath, Hajnalka Marton, and Helga Lehotzky. "Study of the Frequency of Cow's Milk Sensitivity in the Families of Milk-Allergic and Asthmatic Children." *Acta Allergol*, Vol. 28, July 1973, p. 107.

378. Trall, Russell T., M.D. *The Hygienic System*. Battle Creek, Michigan: The Office of the Health Reformer, 1872.

379. —————. *The Hydropathic Encyclopedia*. New York: Fowlers & Wells, 1854, p. 347.

380. Trop, Jack D. *Please Don't Smoke in Our House*. Chicago: Natural Hygiene Press, 1976.

381. —————. *You Don't Have to Be Sick*. New York: Julian Press, 1961.

382. Truelove, S. C., M.D., M.R.C.P. "Ulcerative Colitis Provoked by Milk." *British Medical Journal*, Vol. 1, 1961, p. 154.

383. Truswell, A. Stewart, M.D., *et al.* "The Nutritive Value of Maize Protein for Man." *American Journal of Clinical Nutrition*, Vol. 10, Feb. 1962, p. 142.

384. Tzu, Lao. *Tao Teh King*. New York: Frederick Ungar Publishing Co., 1972.

385. United Nations Food and Agriculture Organization. *FAO Production Yearbook*, Vol. 37, 1984, p. 263.

386. —————. *Food Balance Sheets: 1979–1981 Average*. Rome, 1984.

387. United States Senate Report: *Dietary Goals for the U.S.* Washington, D.C.: Government Printing Office, 1977.

388. Upton, Arthur C., M.D., Director National Cancer Institute. Statement on the Status of the Diet, Nutrition and Cancer Program Before the Subcommittee on Nutrition. Senate

Committee on Agriculture, Nutrition and Forestry, Oct. 2, 1972.

389. "Urinary Calcium and Dietary Protein." *Nutrition Review*, Vol. 38, 1980, p. 9.

390. Vanecek, Karel, and Alois Zapletal. "Sensibilization of Guinea Pigs with Cow's Milk as a Model of Sudden Death in Infants and Children." *Acta University Carolina Medica*, Vol. 13, 1967, p. 207.

391. *Vegetables*. Alexandria, Virginia: Time-Life Books, 1979.

392. Verrett, Jacqueline, and Jean Carper. *Eating May Be Hazardous to Your Health*. New York: Simon & Schuster, 1974.

393. Wachman, Ammon, M.D., and Daniel B. Bernstein, M.D. "Diet and Osteoporosis." *Lancet*, Vol. #1, May 4, 1968, p. 958.

394. Walker, Alan, Dr. "Research Yields Surprises About Early Human Diets." *New York Times*, May 15, 1979.

395. Walker, Alexander R. P., D.Sc. "Colon Cancer and Diet with Special Reference to Intakes of Fat and Fiber." *American Journal of Clinical Nutrition*, Vol. 29, Dec. 1976, p. 1417.

396. —————. "The Human Requirement of Calcium: Should Low Intakes Be Supplemented?" *American Journal of Clinical Nutrition*, Vol. 25, May 1972, p. 518.

397. —————. "Osteoporosis and Calcium Deficiency." *American Journal of Clinical Nutrition*, Vol. 16, Mar. 1965, p. 327.

398. Walker, A. R. P., *et al*. "The Influence of Numerous Pregnancies and Lactations on Bone Dimensions in South African Bantu and Caucasian Mothers." *Clinical Science*, Vol. 42, Feb. 1972, p. 189.

399. Walker, N. W., D.Sc. *Become Younger*. Phoenix, Arizona: Norwalk Press, 1949.

400. —————. *Diet and Salad Suggestions*. Phoenix, Arizona: Norwalk Press, 1971.

401. —————. *Fresh Vegetables and Fruit Juices*. Phoenix, Arizona: Norwalk Press, 1978.

402. —————. *Natural Weight Control*. Phoenix, Arizona: O'Sullivan Woodside & Co., 1981.

403. —————. *Vibrant Health*. Phoenix, Arizona: O'Sullivan Woodside & Co., 1972.

404. —————. *Water Can Undermine Your Health*. Phoe-

nix, Arizona: O'Sullivan Woodside & Co., 1974.

405. Walker, Ruth M., *et al*. "Calcium Retention in the Adult Human Male as Affected by Protein Intake." *Journal of Nutrition*, Vol. 102, July/Dec. 1972, p. 1297.

406. Walser, Mackinzie, M.D. "Does Dietary Therapy Have a Role in the Predialysis Patient?" *American Journal of Clinical Nutrition*, Vol. 33, July 1980, p. 1629.

407. Weisburger, John H., Ph.D., B.S., *et al*. "Nutrition and Cancer—On the Mechanisms Bearing on Causes of Cancer of the Colon, Breast, Prostate and Stomach." *Bulletin New York Academy of Medicine*, Vol. 56, Oct. 1980, p. 673.

408. Welch, Raquel. *Raquel*. New York: Fawcett, 1984.

409. Whitaker, Julian M., M.D. *Reversing Heart Disease*. New York: Warner Books, 1985.

410. White, Ellen G. *Counsels on Health*. Mountain View, California: Pacific Press Publishing Association, 1923.

411. "Whole Milk Linked with Cancer." *Nutrition Health Review*, Spring 1983.

412. Wigmore, Ann. *Be Your Own Doctor*. Boston: Hippocrates Health Institute, 1973.

413. ——————. *Recipes for Longer Life*. Wayne, New Jersey: Avery Publishing Group, 1978.

414. Wilder, Alexander. *History of Medicine*. New Sharon, Maine: New England Eclectic Publishers, 1901.

415. Williamson, Francis. "Exercise and Activity for Bone Health." *Nutrition Health Review*, Vol. 35, June 1985, p. 3.

416. ——————. "Osteoporosis: The Silent Thief of Body and Bone." *Nutrition Health Review*, Vol. 35, June 1985, p. 2.

417. Winter, Ruth. *Beware of the Food You Eat*. New York: Signet, 1971.

418. Woolsey, Raymond H. *Meat on the Menu, Who Needs It?* Washington, D.C.: Review & Herald Publishing, 1974.

419. Wright, Ralph, M.D., D.Phil., M.R.C.P., *et al*. "A Controlled Therapeutic Trial of Various Diets in Ulcerative Colitis." *British Medical Journal*, Vol. 2, July 17, 1965, p. 138.

420. Wynder, E. "The Dietary Environment and Cancer." *Journal of American Dietetic Association*, Vol. 71, 1977, p. 385.

421. Yerushamy, J., Ph.D., and Herman E. Hilleboe, M.D. "Fat

in the Diet and Mortality from Heart Disease.'' *New York State Journal of Medicine*, Vol. 57, July 15, 1957, p. 2343.

422. Yudkin, John, M.D. *Sweet and Dangerous*. New York: Bantam, 1972.

423. Zollner, N. "Diet and Gout." *Proceedings of the 9th International Congress of Nutrition* (Mexico), Vol. 1, 1972, p. 267.

INDEX

abdominal breathing, 67–73
  exercises for, 71–73, 344
"Abuses of Bathing, The," 214
Acciardo, Marcia, 347
accreditation, 15–16, 17–19
acetaldehyde, 77
acetonitrile, 78
acid-alkaline balance, 86–88, 258
acid foods, 87
acrolein, 76
Action on Smoking and Health
  (ASH), 80
advertising:
  of processed food, 113–15,
    274–76, 279
  of smoking, 78, 82
aerobic exercise, 142–63, 356
  "Perfect Workout" for,
    147–63, 184
  rebounding, 145–60
Afghanistan, 283
Agriculture Department, U.S.,
  79, 273, 287
AIDS, 108
air, 62–91
  deep breathing and, 66–74
  detoxification and, 310
  exercise and, 65–66, 71–73,
    139
  fresh, prejudices against, 62
  good, 64–65
  night, 62
  polluted, 63

sleeping and, 74, 139, 343
smoking and, 74–91, 218
air fresheners, 217–18
alcohol, 75, 208, 211, 289
  calcium absorption and, 258
alkaline foods, 87
Allen, George, 271
Allen, Woody, 88
allergies, 243
almonaise, Diamond's, 388–89
almond milk, 293, 438
  pulp of, 216
almond surprise, 370
alternate nostril breathing, 72–73,
  344
alternative health care:
  resurgence of, 15–17
  suppression of, 15–17
  see also Natural Hygiene
aluminum chloride, 215
aluminum filings, 103–04
Alzheimer's disease, 76, 104,
  215
American Association for the Advancement of Science, 119
American Cancer Society, 236
  dietary recommendations from,
    288–89
American College of Health Science, 15, 17, 19, 334
American Dietetic Association
  (ADA), 18, 21
American Heart Association, 22

472